BIOLOGICS, A HISTORY OF AGENTS MADE FROM LIVING ORGANISMS IN THE TWENTIETH CENTURY

STUDIES FOR THE SOCIETY FOR THE SOCIAL HISTORY OF MEDICINE

Series Editors: David Cantor
Keir Waddington

TITLES IN THIS SERIES

1 Meat, Medicine and Human Health in the Twentieth Century
David Cantor, Christian Bonah and Matthias Dörries (eds)

2 Locating Health: Historical and Anthropological Investigations of
Place and Health
Erika Dyck and Christopher Fletcher (eds)

3 Medicine in the Remote and Rural North, 1800–2000
J. T. H. Connor and Stephan Curtis (eds)

4 A Modern History of the Stomach: Gastric Illness, Medicine and
British Society, 1800–1950
Ian Miller

5 War and the Militarization of British Army Medicine, 1793–1830
Catherine Kelly

6 Nervous Disease in Late Eighteenth-Century Britain:
The Reality of a Fashionable Disorder
Heather R. Beatty

7 Desperate Housewives, Neuroses and the Domestic Environment,
1945–1970
Ali Haggett

8 Disabled Children: Contested Caring, 1850–1979
Anne Borsay and Pamela Dale (eds)

9 Toxicants, Health and Regulation since 1945
Soraya Boudia and Nathalie Jas (eds)

10 A Medical History of Skin: Scratching the Surface
Jonathan Reinarz and Kevin Siena (eds)

11 The Care of Older People: England and Japan, A Comparative Study
Mayumi Hayashi

FORTHCOMING TITLES

BIOLOGICS, A HISTORY OF AGENTS MADE FROM LIVING ORGANISMS IN THE TWENTIETH CENTURY

EDITED BY

Alexander von Schwerin, Heiko Stoff and Bettina Wahrig

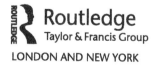

Routledge
Taylor & Francis Group

LONDON AND NEW YORK

First published 2013 by Pickering & Chatto (Publishers) Limited

Published 2016 by Routledge
2 Park Square, Milton Park, Abingdon, Oxfordshire OX14 4RN
711 Third Avenue, New York, NY 10017, USA

First issued in paperback 2015

Routledge is an imprint of the Taylor & Francis Group, an informa business

BRITISH LIBRARY CATALOGUING IN PUBLICATION DATA

Biologics : a history of agents made from living organisms in the twentieth century. – (Studies for the Society for the Social History of Medicine)
1. Biologicals – Europe – History – 20th century.
I. Series II. Schwerin, Alexander von editor of compilation. III. Stoff, Heiko editor of compilation. IV. Wahrig, Bettina editor of compilation.
615.3'6'094'0904-dc23

ISBN-13: 978-1-138-66297-1 (pbk)
ISBN-13: 978-1-8489-3430-6 (hbk)

Typeset by Pickering & Chatto (Publishers) Limited

CONTENTS

ACKNOWLEDGEMENTS

The original workshop on which this book is based was sponsored by the European Science Foundation (ESF) Research Networking Programme 'Standard Drugs – Drug Standards. A Comparative Historical Study of Pharmaceuticals in the Twentieth Century' (DRUGS) and the Technical University Braunschweig in Germany. We wish to thank the other members of the 'Biological drugs' team of DRUGS who met in Paris and encouraged us to conduct the workshop on 'Drugs, Living Things and the Problems of Standardization' at the Technical University Braunschweig in March 2010.

With one exception, the essays in this volume were originally presented at the Braunschweig workshop and have been substantially revised in light of the conference discussion. We owe an anonymous reviewer a debt of gratitude for his/her comprehensive and helpful comments. The editors would also like to thank the steering committee of ESF DRUGS for supporting the publication of this volume. Finally, we thank Eileen Kwiecinski and Julia Saatz for editing the manuscript.

LIST OF CONTRIBUTORS

Klaus Angerer studied Cultural Studies and Spanish at the Humboldt-University in Berlin. Currently he is working on his PhD thesis on the investigation, the uses and the transformations of collected biological materials in intermediary institutions in Europe, with fieldwork undertaken especially in a natural-product company, university departments and a botanical garden. Recent publications are 'Frog Tales – On Poison Dart Frogs, Epibatidine, and the Sharing of Biodiversity', *Innovation. The European Journal of Social Science Research*, 24:3 (2011), pp. 353–69; 'Die Natur der Bioprospektion: Die Welt als biochemisches Labor', *Zeitschrift für Kulturwissenschaften*, 2 (2009), pp. 91–102.

Beat Bächi is a Research Associate at the Archives of Rural History in Bern, Switzerland, where he works in a project funded by the Swiss National Science Foundation on the scientization and industrialization of agriculture, especially on the history of cattle breeding since the mid-nineteenth century. He has published in the history of technology, the history of medicine and the history of knowledge. Among his publications are *Vitamin C für alle! Pharmazeutische Produktion, Vermarktung und Gesundheitspolitik, 1933–1953* (Zurich: Chronos, 2009); 'Zur Krise der westdeutschen Grenzwertpolitik in den 1970er Jahren. Die Verwandlung des Berufskrebses von einem toxikologischen in ein sozioökonomisches Problem', *Berichte zur Wissenschaftsgeschichte*, 33 (2010), pp. 419–35 and 'Chemopolitik und Reproduktionstechnologien: Hormone, Vitamine und Tranquilizer in der Rindviehzucht (1920–1985)', *Blätter für Technikgeschichte*, 74 (2012), pp. 93–113.

Sven Bergmann is a Post-Doctoral Researcher currently working at the Institute for the History of Medicine, Charité Berlin, in a research group about 'cultures of madness'. He holds a PhD in European Ethnology and has worked on medical mobilities, kinship and reproductive technologies. Recent publications include: 'Resemblance that Matters: On Transnational Anonymized Egg Donation in Two European IVF Clinics', in M. Knecht, M. Klotz and S. Beck (eds), *Reproductive Technologies as Global Form: Ethnographies of Knowledge, Practices, and Transnational Encounters* (Frankfurt and New York: Campus,

2012), pp. 331–55; 'Fertility Tourism: Circumventive Routes that Enable Access to Reproductive Technologies and Substances', *Signs*, 36:2 (2011), pp. 280–9; 'Reproductive Agency and Projects: Germans Searching for Egg Donation in Spain and the Czech Republic', *Reproductive BioMedicine Online*, 23:5 (2011), pp. 600–8.

Sophie Chauveau is Professor for the History of Sciences and Technology at the Technological University of Belfort-Montbeliard. She has worked on the history of the relationships between the French state and pharmaceutical firms in the twentieth century. Her most recent works include research on blood transfusion organizations in France and sanitary scandals and studies of the medical uses of human body parts. Recent publications include: *L'affaire du sang contaminé (1983–2003)* (Paris: Les Belles Lettres, 2011); 'Organ and Blood Donations', in D. Southerton (ed.), *Encyclopedia of Consumer Culture* (London: CQ Press/ Sage Publications, 2011), pp. 1065–7; 'Le corps comme ressource. Éthique de la greffe', in Collège des enseignants de sciences humaines et sociales en médecine et santé (ed.), *Médecine, santé et sciences humaines. Manuel* (Paris: Les Belles Lettres, 2011), pp. 637–48; 'L'Etat et l'innovation thérapeutique: la transfusion sanguine en France depuis les années 1960', in P. Fridenson and P. Griset (eds), *Entreprises de haute technologie, État et souveraineté depuis 1945* (Paris: Comite pour l'histoire économique et financière de la France, 2013), pp. 195–212.

Jean-Paul Gaudillière is Senior Researcher at the *Institut National de la Santé et de la Recherche Médicale* and director of the Center for Research on Science, Medicine, Health and Society (CERMES3) in Paris. His work has addressed many aspects of the history and sociology of the biomedical sciences during the twentieth century, looking in particular at the dynamics of research in the life sciences and its relations to technological developments. His present research focuses on the changing relations between biology and the drug industry, the various ways of regulating drugs and the post-war globalization of pharmacy. Among other publications, he has edited 'How Pharmaceuticals Became Patentable in the Twentieth Century', a special issue of *History and Technology*, 24:2 (2008) and co-edited, with Volker Hess, *Ways of Regulating Drugs in the 19th and 20th centuries* (Basingstoke: Palgrave Macmillan, 2012).

Christoph Gradmann is Professor in the History of Medicine at the University of Oslo. He has published widely on a variety of fields, his main focus being the history of infectious disease and experimental medicine in the nineteenth to twentieth century, the history of standardization in modern medicine and historical biographies. Some recent publications include 'Magic Bullets and Moving Targets: Antibiotic Resistance and Experimental Chemotherapy 1900–1940', *Dynamis*, 31 (2011), pp. 29–45; with J. Simon (eds), *Evaluating and*

Standardizing Therapeutic Agents 1890–1950 (Houndsmills Basingstoke: Palgrave Macmillan, 2010); *Laboratory Disease: Robert Koch's Medical Bacteriology* (Baltimore, MD: The Johns Hopkins University Press, 2009); 'Locating Therapeutic Vaccines in Nineteenth-Century History', *Science in Context*, 21 (2008), pp. 145–60; 'Alles eine Frage der Methode. Zur Historizität der Kochschen Postulate 1840–2000', *Medizinhistorisches Journal*, 43 (2008), pp. 121–48.

Lea Haller holds a Post-Doctoral position at ETH Zurich. Her research interests cover the history of science and technology, the history of medicine and body politics, and economic history. She completed her PhD in 2011 with a dissertation on the history of cortisone, focusing on the correlation between hormone theory, pharmaceutical standardization and changing conceptions of health and disease: *Cortison. Geschichte eines Hormons, 1900–1955* (Zurich: Chronos, 2012). Her current project is a history of global commodity trade in the twentieth century that focuses on Swiss trading companies (funded by a Branco Weiss Fellowship). During the academic year 2012/13 Lea Haller was a visiting scholar at Sciences Po, Paris. In 2013/14 she will be a fellow at the Center for European Studies at Harvard University.

Pim Huijnen is a Post-Doctoral Researcher at the University of Utrecht where he studies the uses of digital methods to analyse transfers of knowledge. His research focuses on the cultural history of genetics and eugenics in the Netherlands and Germany and on the impact of Americanization on Dutch culture. He did his PhD research on the history of vitamin research in the Netherlands and the relations between academic science and applied research before the Second World War, resulting in *De belofte van vitamines. Voedingsonderzoek tussen universiteit, industrie en overheid 1918–1945* (Hilversum: Verloren, 2011). In 2011 he was a visiting research fellow at the Max Planck Institute for the History of Science in Berlin.

Jonathan Simon is *maître de conférences* at Université Lyon 1 where he teaches history and philosophy of science. He has worked on the history of chemistry and pharmacy and is a member of the research team S2HEP (EA 4148). His publications include (with B. Bensaude-Vincent) *Chemistry: the Impure Science* (London: Imperial College Press, 2nd edn, 2012) and *Chemistry, Pharmacy and Revolution* (Aldershot: Ashgate, 2005). His 2007 article 'Emil Behring's Medical Culture: From Disinfection to Serotherapy' received the 2008 Estes Award from the American Association for the History of Medicine.

Heiko Stoff is Guest Professor for the History of Science and Technology at the Technical University of Braunschweig. His research focuses on the history of things, body history, gender studies and theories of history. Recent publications explore the history of biologically active substances and food additives. Stoff has also worked on the cultural and science history of rejuvenation, aging and beauty. He is the author of *Ewige Jugend. Konzepte der Verjüngung vom späten 19. Jahrhundert bis ins Dritte Reich* (Cologne and Weimar: Böhlau, 2004) and *Wirkstoffe. Eine Wissenschaftsgeschichte der Hormone, Vitamine und Enzyme, 1920–1970* (Stuttgart: Steiner, 2012).

Ulrike Thoms is a Researcher at the Institute for the History of Medicine, Berlin. Her publications examine the history of consumption and its linkages with the history of medicine and science, such as food history and the history of the body. Her current research is on the history of pharmaceutical marketing and the role of drugs in agribusiness. Apart from numerous articles, she has published *Ansaltskost im Rationalisierungsprozess. Die Ernährung in Krankenhäusern und Gefängnissen im 18. und 19. Jahrhundert* (Stuttgart: Steiner, 2005) and edited (with E. Engstrom and V. Hess) *Figurationen des Experten. Ambivalenzen der wissenschaftlichen Expertise im ausgehenden 18. und beginnenden 19. Jahrhundert* (Frankfurt a.M: Lit Verlag, 2005) and (with M. Middell and F. Uekötter) *Verräumlichung, Vergleich, Generationalität. Dimensionen der Wissenschaftsgeschichte* (Leipzig: Universitäts-Verlag, 2004). She is currently writing a book on the history of the pharmaceutical representative and preparing an edited volume on the history of pharmaceutical marketing: *Drugs and the Birth of Scientific Marketing.*

Alexander von Schwerin is Research Scholar at the Department for the History of Pharmacy and Science at the Technical University Braunschweig. His research focuses on the history of genetics and biomedicine, historical and political epistemology, the history of things and regulation. His publications include studies on animal models, eugenics and molecular biology: *Experimentalisierung des Menschen. Der Genetiker Hans Nachtsheim und die vergleichende Erbpathologie*, 1920–1945 (Göttingen: Wallstein, 2004); 'From Agriculture to Genomics: The Animal Side of Human Genetics and the Organization of Model Organisms in the Longue Durée', in B. Gausemeier, S. Müller-Wille and E. Ramsden (eds), *Human Heredity in the Twentieth Century* (London: Pickering & Chatto, 2013). His most recent research on radiation biology in Germany will be published in 2014 as *Strahlen. Biologie und Politik staatswichtiger Substanzen. Die Deutsche Forschungsgemeinschaft und Strahlenforschung, 1920–1970* (Stuttgart: Franz Steiner Verlag).

Bettina Wahrig is Professor of History of Science and Pharmacy at the Technical University Braunschweig. She has worked on the experimental history of nineteenth-century physiology, on metaphors of organism and the state in the seventeenth century, on the history of pharmaceutical and medical professions, on questions of gender and science, and on the history of precarious substances, especially of poisons. Her publications include: B. Wahrig, V. Balz, A. Schwerin and H. Stoff (eds), *Precarious Matters/Prekäre Stoffe. The History of Dangerous and Endangered Substances in the Nineteenth and Twentieth Centuries*, Preprint series 356 (Berlin: Max-Planck-Institut für Wissenschaftsgeschichte, 2008); '"Fabelhafte Dinge": Arzneimittelnarrative zu Coca und Cocain im 19. Jahrhundert', *Berichte zur Wissenschaftsgeschichte*, 32 (2009), pp. 345–64; 'Systeme in pragmatischer Hinsicht: Lehrbücher der Toxikologie in Deutschland, England und Frankreich 1785–1929', in C. Friedrich and W-D. Müller-Jahnke (eds), *Gifte und Gegengifte in Vergangenheit und Gegenwart* (Stuttgart: Wissenschaftliche Verlagsgesellschaft, 2012), pp. 99–133.

LIST OF FIGURES

BIOLOGICS: AN INTRODUCTION

Alexander von Schwerin, Heiko Stoff and Bettina Wahrig

Over the past century, our bodies have increasingly become exposed to the pharmaceutical action of incorporated biological substances. Some of these have become so ubiquitous that we have even stopped thinking about them as 'biologics'. We swallow our daily vitamin pills; we rely on vaccines and antibiotics when microbes proliferate; we account for the adverse effects of cortisone; we live a more-or-less normal life thanks to regular injections of insulin or an organ transplant; and we place our faith in monoclonal antibodies when a tumour has been diagnosed. One recent textbook definition of biologics provides us with still more examples:

> By definition biologics are proteins and/or derivatives thereof that modulate the immune system, downregulate the inflammatory response or support tumor specific defence. Biologics – also known as 'biologicals' or 'recombinant therapeutics' – do not represent one homogeneous group of drugs. Monoclonal antibodies, fusion proteins (along with other proteins, toxins and radionucleotides) and recombinant proteins, growth factors, anti- and pro-angiogenic factors, and expression vectors generating proteins in situ may all be included as members of this class of pharmaceuticals.[1]

This recent definition does not include vitamins, hormones, antibiotics or vaccines, although they have been and sometimes still are categorized as 'biologics' or 'biologicals'.

The term 'biologics' first emerged in connection with national health-care legislation and the control of vaccine production in the US more than a hundred years ago. For a long time, there existed no equivalent expression in Europe, where terms like *Naturstoffe, Wirkstoffe (biologische Arzneimittel)* or *médicaments biologiques* were common. These terms encompassed a broader range of substances like hormones, vitamins, enzymes, as well as plant extracts, especially if they worked in ways comparable to animal enzymes. Thus, all of these terms had different meanings and connotations, while sharing a common reference to 'natural products' in one way or another. Their introduction into pharmaceutical terminology opened up a semantic field that proliferated wildly and exuberantly both in the US and in Europe throughout the twentieth century. In the first half of that century, the adjective 'biological' was often used to indicate a 'life reformist' or 'naturalist' understanding of the human body. 'Biological' agents, which in spite of their small quantity had such intense effects, became prototypes for ideas of naturalness and purity. This characterization of biological enzymes, toxins, antitoxins, etc. resonated with broader efforts and rhetorical strategies to redefine the boundaries between nature and technology: in chemistry for example, the new technique of catalysis was ennobled by the fact that nature seemed to have invented it. However, this beneficial nature turned into a threat when catalysis involved microbial contaminants.

The aim of this volume is not to provide another definition of biologics, but to introduce the concept of biologics as a fruitful perspective for the history of pharmaceuticals, medicine and science. The fact that in many Western countries a great number of very heterogeneous substances were subsumed under a small number of terms, all of which captured their biological origins, demonstrates the importance of industrially produced 'biological' scientific objects and pharmaceuticals in the twentieth century. Hence, the notion of biologics 'is less a problem of natural versus artificial ontology, than of socio-technical order'.[2] Biologics have posed specific scientific, industrial, medical and legal problems and are hence of particular interest to any deeper understanding of the so-called therapeutic revolution, its scientific bases and its relationship to the standardization of medicinal drugs, the dynamics of regulation and risk-management policies, the industrialization of precarious substances, the economics and politics of 'natural' things and the development of biotechnology since the late nineteenth century.[3]

Since biologics are both of natural origin and produced using advanced industrial methods, the historical study of biologics provides a useful research perspective, enabling new insights into the genealogy of industrial and consumer medicine and of the life sciences. It also contributes to the historicization of the production of naturalness, alongside the corresponding processes of representation and intervention.[4] The very practical context, in which terms like 'biologics' emerge, already indicates that biologics transgress the conceptual (and material) boundaries between the inanimate and the living, between the organism as a whole and its organic and inorganic contents, as well as between nature and its technical modification. Accordingly, this volume highlights different, but interdependent aspects of biologics: the production and regulation of substances made from living organisms and the signification of biological remedies as both powerful drugs and agents of naturalness. In light of the today's rapid development of new biological entities such as recombinant DNA-derived products, biomolecules and biosimilars, this book offers historical perspectives that stretch far back from our age of biotechnologically processed substances and that illuminate the changing relations between laboratories, clinical services, industrial settings and regulatory bodies.

In this introduction, we will provide an outline of the historical study of biologics. A suitable approach to the topic is to examine the emergence and evolution of the terms 'biologics' and 'biologicals' and so the first three sections will concentrate on the fate of these and related concepts in both the US and Europe. Historical examination of discourses on biologics reveals this group of substances to be a distinct historical object that becomes tangible as a result of different contingent processes in the medical, technological, economic and social history of the twentieth century.

In the last three sections of this introduction we will further explain this perspective by introducing the main categories used to characterize biologics as historical subjects. Those categories reflect the larger subdivisions of the present volume and outline a comprehensive historiographical perspective on biologics. While there have been many studies on blood, vaccines, hormones, vitamins or flavonoids, our aim is to relate these substances to discourses and practices such as standardization, naturalization, politicization, industrialization and regulation. It is therefore necessary to begin with an outline of the regulatory and cultural concept of biologics and to use this term as an analytical tool for acquiring new perspectives on the history of pharmacology, health-care legislation and biomedicine.

The authors of this volume deal with the production, regulation and control of biologics and include gendered, colonial and consumer perspectives. The contributions originated from a workshop held at the Technical University Braunschweig in Germany during the foggy days of March 2010. The workshop was one of a series funded by the European Science Foundation's network DRUGS.[5] It represented the first attempt to bring together the histories of different substances and materials, such as vaccines and sera, plant extracts, genetically engineered proteins, cells, tissues and organs. Given the complexity of these substances, we hope that the contributions to this volume will encourage readers to take a comparative perspective on the history of biologics in the twentieth century.

Standardizing Biologics in the US in the First Half of the Twentieth Century

The term 'biologics' first emerged in the United States in the early twentieth century. It was inextricably connected with governmental efforts to standardize and control therapeutic, prophylactic and diagnostic agents like sera, viruses, vaccines and antitoxins. Although it is difficult to establish exactly when these terms were introduced, it is clear that federal statutes and regulations played a crucial role in bringing a range of different substances together within the conceptual framework of 'biologics' and 'biological products'.[6]

In some respects, the history of biologics begins with the diphtheria anti-toxin. By 1895, laws regulating biological products had been enacted by the governments of France, Germany, Italy and Russia. In the United States, many people were concerned about the safety of vaccines, given that they were injected and could have rapid and adverse effects if contaminated. Nevertheless, these products were initially rushed to market and their use proceeded without regulatory safeguards.[7] But the reluctance to regulate these new substances changed in 1901, when thirteen children died after being treated with a diphtheria anti-toxin made from the blood of a tetanus-infected milk-wagon horse named Jim.[8] Soon thereafter, a similar tragedy in Camden, New Jersey resulted in deaths and injuries that were attributed to a tainted biological product. In 1902, the executive body of the National Convention for Revising the Pharmacopoeia decided to include *Serum Antidiphtherium*, the most important serum product of the time, in the Pharmacopoeia of the United States because of the increasing use of it and other serum products.[9]

That same year, discussions about the risks of vaccination also resulted in more stringent government regulations. Under an Act of Congress in 1902, all viruses, sera and toxins sold in the United States were required to conform to established standards. This law marked the beginning of a 'regime for licensing of biologics and vaccines' that, according to Carpenter, ultimately evolved into the Food and Drug Administration (FDA), which today is responsible for the control of biologics in the US.[10] Indeed, when the FDA celebrated the seventy-fifth anniversary of the Food and Drugs Act of 1920, it also celebrated the 'Biologics Control Act' of 1902, thus implicitly suggesting a continuity in the regulation of biological products.[11] However, in the original law of 1 July 1902 there was no mention of 'biologics', 'biologicals' or 'biological products'.[12] Instead, it was officially designated as 'An Act to Regulate the Sale of Viruses, Serums, Toxins and Analogous Products in the District of Columbia, to Regulate Interstate Traffic in Said Articles, and for Other Purposes'.[13] The law's scope was defined to include 'any virus, therapeutic serum, toxin, antitoxin, or analogous product applicable to the prevention and cure of diseases of man'.[14] Obviously, the advent of biologics as a new category of therapeutic substances was steeped in the history and science of immunization.[15] The law's main targets were vaccines, but its reference to 'analogous products' began paving the way to include other biological products.[16]

With this new legislative framework in place, subsequent years witnessed the emergence of various labels to describe these products. The first documented use of 'biologics' occurred in 1912 when the pharmacological editor of the *California State Journal of Medicine*, Fred Lackenbach, used the term in an overview to describe a variety of different substances. Unlike other contemporary drugs, the use of these substances would demand 'accurate clinical and bacteriological diagnosis' and a thorough knowledge of the indication, dosage and mode of administration.[17] To the benefit of pharmacists and physicians, this implied that 'biologics' were products ill-suited to the huge market for self-medication being served by department stores and mail-order houses.

Lackenbach considered the year 1902 to have been crucial in the formation of this new class of pharmaceutical products. For that year saw not only the 'Act to Regulate the Sale of Viruses, Serums, Toxins', but also a second, related act approved on 1 July that sought to reorganize the US Public Health and Marine Hospital Service (later designated simply as the Public Health Service or PHS) and entrusted its Hygienic Laboratory with the task of performing all necessary tests and inspections.[18] Together, both acts established the legal framework for federal regulation of biological products designed for human use and 'established the authority of federal institutions to regulate biological products and ensure their safety for the American public'.[19] Subsequently, the PHS went about establishing a regime of vaccine control and it was in this context that several new generic terms emerged. The *Annual Report of the Surgeon General of the PHS* in 1908 harked back to the tragedy of 1901 in explaining that 'all possible care should be taken for the exclusion of the tetanus bacillus from all biologic products'.[20] Other authors referred to 'biological products' or substances of a 'biologic nature', but all of these terms were used only sporadically.[21]

It seems that the catchy term 'biologics' emerged only when economic and business interests were at stake. In his overview, Lackenbach used the term 'biologics' in addressing the commercial pharmacist (i.e. 'the man who handles these products for revenue').[22] Similarly, the Commercial Interests Section of the *Journal of the American Pharmaceutical Association* published a summary entitled 'the sale of biologicals' in which the terms 'biologicals' and 'biologics' were used synonymously.[23] In 1917, the Biological Department of Eli Lilly and Company published a small treatise on 'Elements of Biologics' designed to provide the company's representatives with standard knowledge about antitoxins and vaccines. The definition used for biologics read: 'A line of products, including serums, smallpox and rabies vaccine viruses, bacterial vaccines, antigens, and extracts, toxins, etc., the manufacture of which depends upon the use of bacteria and bacterial products'.[24] Lilly's instructions suggest that the market for antitoxins and vaccines was expanding. And indeed, by 1921, some 41 establishments were licensed to sell no less than 102 different sera, toxins and analogous products, posing considerable challenges to federal regulators.[25]

The use of generic terms became more and more common as federal authorities invented new structures to cope with the regulatory challenges in the 1920s. In 1923, *Public Health Reports* compiled a list of national agencies and organizations associated with the regulation of 'biologics'.[26] Around the same time, the Revision Committee of the US Pharmacopoeia established the 'Sub-Committee on Biologics'.[27] The most important federal agency was the Hygienic Laboratory of the PHS, given its responsibility for testing biological products and licensing manufacturers (see Figure I.1).

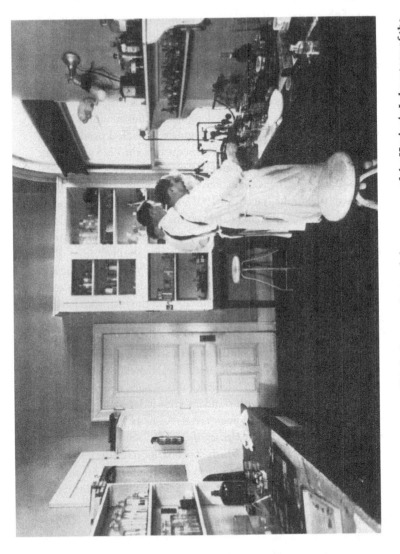

Figure I.1: The regulation of biologics severely taxed the resources of the Hygienic Laboratory of the Public Health Service at Bethesda, Maryland, US. Source: Bethesda: National Institutes of Health, 1930. Reproduced courtesy of the National Library of Medicine.

Under the 1902 Act, all Diphtheria Antitoxins sold in the United States were required to conform to the standard established by the PHS. This standard was based on the Ehrlich Immunity Unit preserved at the Royal Institute for Experimental Therapy in Germany – the first biological standard in the world, prepared by Paul Ehrlich himself in 1897.[28] During the First World War, this no longer seemed acceptable and the Hygienic Laboratory began developing its own biological standards.[29] 'Activities in viruses, serums, toxins, and analogous products' were conducted under the supervision of the laboratory's director and using personnel drawn from its four divisions: pathology and bacteriology, zoology, pharmacology and chemistry. The laboratory was increasingly responsible for enforcing the law, regulating the sale and routine inspection of businesses, as well as conducting research (see Figure I.2).[30] Ensuring the purity and efficacy of sera and other agents was the specific task of the Division of Pathology and Bacteriology. In 1920, these responsibilities were classed under the heading 'Biologics (routine examination)'.[31] And in 1923, all of these activities were brought together in a fifth division responsible for the 'Control of Biologic Products'.[32] In 1930, the Hygienic Laboratory was re-named as the National Institute of Health (NIH).[33] Finally, in 1937, work on biologics control was granted its own division within the NIH, the Division of Biologics Control.[34]

Institutionalizing the control of biologics involved expanding existing regulations on vaccines, sera and antitoxins to include arsenical drugs, blood and blood products. The scope of the Hygienic Laboratory's activities increased accordingly, especially after 1917 when the United States entered the First World War.[35] Before the war, the US had depended on Germany for its supply of salvarsan and neosalvarsan, arsenical drugs used in the treatment of syphilis. With the entry of the United States into the war, the Federal Trade Commission abrogated German patent rights and licensed American manufacturers to produce their own arsenical drugs: 'It seemed a logical step to bring the testing and control of arsenicals under the same system as biologics, and so the Hygienic Laboratory was given this responsibility'.[36] In 1920, the Surgeon General complained that routine controls of biologic products had come to dominate the work of the Division of Pathology and Bacteriology – with 3,525 'biologic products' examined in that fiscal year – and that as a result other research problems were being neglected.[37] Furthermore, blood products became a main focus of the Laboratory's research activities. In 1934, the NIH issued the first licenses to manufacturers for the production of a human blood product, a preparation of protein from human placental extract that was designed to immunize against measles.[38]

After the entry of the United States into the Second World War, many of the scientific advances were driven by the need to provide US military personnel with the best medical care possible, including ready access to safe blood products and protection against diseases. Throughout this time, the Division of Biolog-

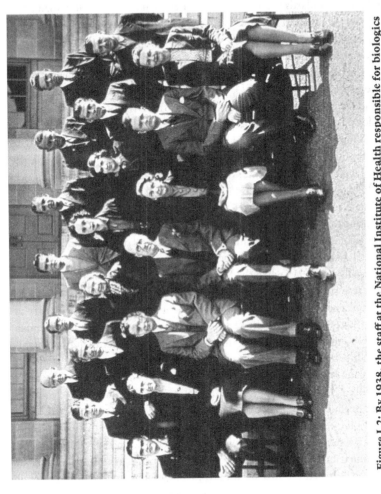

Figure I.2: By 1938, the staff at the National Institute of Health responsible for biologics control had increased markedly. Source: Bethesda: National Institutes of Health, 1938. Reproduced courtesy of the National Library of Medicine.

ics Control established standards for a number of blood products.[39] Korwek suggests that the 'whole blood or plasma language' was added as a result of the use of blood transfusions during the Second World War.[40] Obviously, the constant redefinition of terms was necessitated by developments that modified the practice and regulatory scope of biologics control. But a number of scandalous incidents also contributed to the flux of terminologies. In the 1930s, over a hundred people, among them many children, died after consuming an improperly prepared sulfanilamide medicine, 'Elixier Sulfanilamide'.[41] The manufacturer Massengill & Company had used diethylene glycol as a solvent, resulting in mass poisoning in 1937 and a huge public outcry. To strengthen consumer protection in the emerging national food marketing system, the Pure Food and Drugs Act of 1906 was replaced in 1938 by the Federal Food, Drug and Cosmetic (FD&C) Act, which now defined biological products as drugs. From then on, both the 1902 'Biologics Control Act' and the FD&C Act comprised a 'dual legal system' responsible for the regulation of biologics.[42] Subsequently, when the Public Health Service Act was re-codified in 1944, the dual status of biological products turned out to be the main issue of concern to legislators. According to Section 351 of the PHS Act – which at the time was often confusingly referred to as the Biologics Act –, the term 'biologics' now included any

> virus, therapeutic serum, toxin, antitoxin, vaccine, blood, blood component or derivative, allergenic product, or analogous product, or arsphenamine or its derivatives (or any other trivalent organic arsenic compound), applicable to the prevention, treatment, or cure of diseases or injuries of man.[43]

Standardizing Substances made from Living Organisms in Europe

The example of the United States illustrates the emergence of biologics at the intersection of government regulation and the economy. 'Biologics' was a regulative term introduced to enable state-controlled production of these substances and it played a major role in the institutionalization of drug control in the US. However, there existed no equivalent term in Europe, although the standardization and regulation of substances made from living organisms was common in most European states from the late nineteenth century onward. Instead, other generic terms emerged from different contexts, first and foremost the term '*biologische Wirkstoffe*' (biologically active substances). As the European case shows, rather than confining historical analysis solely to the topic of standardization, one must instead consider the institutionalization, regulation, activation and casual use of these agents, as well as their hybrid status, their semantic fields, their political meanings and socialized actions.

In the nineteenth century, state vaccination policies – be they based on consent or compulsory – were common in many European countries, such as England, France, Prussia, Germany, Italy and Russia.[44] Laws fostering and regulating vaccination had already been enacted by the 1860s and 1870s. In England, it was the responsibility of the General Board of Health in conjunction with the Epidemiological Society to supervise vaccinations mandated by the Vaccination Acts from 1867, 1871 and 1874. In Germany, the smallpox epidemic of 1871 had prompted the *Reichs-Impfgesetz* (Imperial Vaccination Law) of 1874 which, after 1876, was implemented by the Imperial Health Office (*Reichsgesundheitsamt*). The law introduced compulsory vaccination as part of the state welfare system.[45] The introduction of sera therapy highlights some of the problems characteristic of biological substances, the most urgent one being the difficulties of ensuring their efficacy, i.e. defining their effective dose. There was no stable relationship between the absolute quantity of any kind of serum and its effectiveness against a specific disease such as diphtheria. Ever since the tuberculin affair of 1891, when Robert Koch's cure for tuberculosis spectacularly failed, serum and antitoxin therapy in Germany had been viewed with suspicion. Regardless of their therapeutic and economic viability, sera were considered to be precarious substances in need of state control and evaluation (*Wertbestimmung*). The new imperial law of 1895 regulated the production and distribution of sera, restricting their sale to pharmacies and declaring them prescription drugs. In addition, only state-certified serum was allowed on the market.[46]

The situation was different in France, where the Pasteur Institute had been granted a monopoly on the rabies vaccine and was also exempt from regulations concerning diphtheria serum. Under the heading 'prophylactic and therapeutic agents for use against contagious diseases', the French law of 25 April 1895 grouped together attenuated viruses, therapeutic sera, modified toxins and analogous products.[47] The fabrication of these biological products required governmental permission and only authorized institutes could produce and distribute serum in France. Pasteurism resulted in the Public Health Law of 1902.[48] Unlike Germany, where the safety of the new substances was broadly monitored, the French government's main goal was to exclude ineffective serum. And so French legislation was limited to defining approved producers and leaving quality control in their hands.[49]

According to Canguilhem, the bacteriological age, notably the development of sera and vaccines, was characterized by a semantic shift from health to prevention to protection. In response to this shift, medicine had to assume the appearance of a 'biological technology'.[50] Canguilhem concluded that if medicine ever attained the status of a science, it did so in the era of bacteriology. The research and development of remedies such as Emil Behring's diphtheria serum, which involved large-scale sera production and regulation by government agencies, was all based upon the use of bacteriology and hygiene as political tools of social regulation.[51] Hence, vaccines, sera and antitoxins in nineteenth-century Europe can be interpreted as boundary objects that not only exemplify the co-productivity of the state, industry and science, but that also (as argued below) link physiology, the new field of organic chemistry and alternative medicine movements.[52]

Standardization and regulation were important characteristics of these new substances and the main focus of American biologics' legislation. Although European 'biologics' were also discussed and regulated along similar lines, focusing only on them is insufficient. While the history of vaccination and serotherapy in Europe has been explored at length in recent years, the conceptualization of biological substances is historically more complex and convoluted. One must therefore trace a different path back to the long tradition of medicinal substances prepared from living organisms and compiled in the different pharmacopoeias. Medicinal substances prepared from plants constituted an important part in the *materia medica* literature. Although preparations from animal bodies were also integrated into the *materia medica*, their status was very different. Often, traditional drugs were products that used animal parts, like dried viper flesh, to prevent or counteract poisoning. Concrements from goats' stomachs – also thought to be effective against poisoning – were not comprised of organic matter in the modern sense, since they contained mostly minerals. The same holds for rasped or calcinated deer horns or corals. All these preparations entered into the traditional tripartite classification of drugs as mineral, animal and vegetable substances.[53] Preparations based on entire organs (livers, spinal cords, placentas) and body fluids (animal blood) were also part of most pharmacopoeias.[54] In the nineteenth century, authors like early pharmacologist Heinrich Böhnke-Reich tried to integrate regional German pharmacopoeias, thereby systematizing 'animal and vegetable-based drugs' ('*Arzneistoffe aus dem Thier- und Pflanzenreich*') according to pharmacognostic and chemical criteria. The list ranged from lard and staghorn to musk and cod liver oil and also included leeches.[55] Böhnke-Reich was one of several authors who compiled items from different German pharmacopoeias in order to create a unified and modern body of pharmaceutical knowledge. He retained the conventional, tripartite categories and included traditional remedies from the vegetable and animal realms. The entries reflected both traditional *materia medica* and new knowledge based on chemical and physical methods. Many of these remedies, including a number of chemical compounds and new drugs, were listed in the first *Pharmacopoeia Germanica* (1872), the most important reference work of pharmacists in the German Reich. The *Pharmacopoeia Germanica*, however, circumvented the problem of systematization by simply listing the substances in alphabetical order.

But classifications had already started to change with the development of organic chemistry, which made it possible to produce organic substances out of inorganic ones. The famous first case was the synthesis of uric acid by German chemist Friedrich Wöhler in 1822. In the second half of the nineteenth century, when cyclic compounds had come to be understood and later produced in the laboratory, organic chemistry began to branch off from inorganic chemistry, serving as a catalyst for changes in the systematization of the pharmaceutical *materia medica*. The new chemistry helped to blur the distinction between the animal and mineral realms by drawing on notions like '*Tierchemie*', the precursor to 'biochemistry', which was introduced by the German chemist Justus Liebig, and also by successfully synthesizing organic substances that could be used in medicine, such as chloroform or acetyl-salicyclic acid.[56] Proteins, amongst them the enzyme pepsin, were marketed as substances to aid digestion.[57] Unlike the 'chemical saga' recounting the rise of the pharmaceutical industry, *material medica* was primarily composed of biologics and not chemicals.[58] By the turn of the century, 'the vast majority of drugs used by doctors were prepared from plants, with little insight into their molecular structure or into the chemical properties of active principles'.[59] This gradually changed with the emergence of biologically active substances and new ideas of organic regulation. In this regard, it's worth reassessing the concept of biology itself. As Foucault famously remarked, the concept of biology relied on an idea of life itself, on a 'functional homogeneity' as its hidden foundation.[60] The new discipline of biology or life science (*Lebenslehre*) that was institutionalized in the 1850s was always more than just a counterpart to physics as a science of the inorganic world. More so than elsewhere, biology in Germany was shaped decisively by romantic and holistic world views.[61] From the 1890s onward and on the basis of organological semantics, the adjective 'biological' strongly connoted natural health, alternative medicine and the new life-reform movement. Biological medicine (*Biologische Medizin*) was both Hippocratic rhetoric and body politics. In 1908, a medicinal-biological society (*Medizinisch-biologische Gesellschaft*) was founded, bringing together naturopaths, homeopaths, writers and artists, all of whom were critical of scientific medicine and advocates of holism. The adjective 'biological' signified not only the knowledge production of an institutionalized scientific discipline, but also an organological narrative that led to early twentieth-century biopolitics positioning life as the basis of politics.[62]

Biological medicine was not just a reaction to the so-called crisis of medicine in Germany, but also combined hereditary thinking with the utopian politics of human enhancement. In this regard, biological remedies were defined as those natural agents that protected bodies from deficiencies and so-called diseases of civilization and that simultaneously enabled utopian visions of human enhancement.[63] Notably, the physicians Erwin Liek and Karl Kötschau propagated a holistic, precautionary lifestyle that favoured preventive care (*Vorsorge*) instead of welfare (*Fürsorge*). Biological medicine combined prevention, eugenics and holism and translated a biological discourse into politics.[64] In 1929, Heinrich Meng, a Viennese psychoanalyst and subsequent founder of psycho-hygiene in Basel, compiled all the practices of biological medicine in his medical almanac (*Ärztliches Volksbuch*). Nine years later, the physician and entrepreneur Gerhard Madaus (1890–1942) published a famous three-volume textbook of biological remedies (*Lehrbuch der biologischen Heilmittel*); and in 1939, a research institute for biological remedies (*Forschungs- und Prüfungsinstitut für biologische Heilmittel*) was founded at the Paracelsus-Institute.[65] Madaus' products ranged from homeopathic preparations of metals to hormones, enzymes or combinations of bacterial antigens, but most of all plant derivatives. Such combinations of therapeutic agents, analysed according to their physiological effects, dosage, thresholds and sensibility, were also found in France in the 1930s, but there, restrained by the *visas des spécialités pharmaceutiques* of 1941, herbalists lost their official status and control of medicinal plants passed completely to pharmacists.[66]

Biologically active substances like organ extracts, hormones, vitamins and enzymes played a crucial role in life-reformist discourse. In 1889, the physiologist Charles-Édouard Brown-Séquard tested Claude Bernard's assumptions about internal secretion in a spectacular self-experiment, convincing him that the use of efficient substances produced by glands held out the promise of physical rejuvenation. Brown-Séquard's so-called 'organotherapy' was validated by the British physiologist George R. Murray's successful therapeutic treatment of myxoedema with an active substance from the thyroid gland of sheep in 1891. The substitution, grafting or re-implantation of glands substantiated the curative efficacy of certain internally secreted, but unknown substances.[67] Around 1900, many 'organotherapeutics' were in use and there was a common understanding of their efficacy: extracts from endocrine organs were thought to replace a patient's failing bodily functions. When the British physiologist Ernest Starling coined the expression 'hormone' in 1905, he had in mind very specific substances that acted as chemical messengers 'speeding from cell to cell along the blood stream' and coordinating the activities and growth of different parts of the body.[68] Likewise, the concept of vitamins as 'accessory food factors' followed the logic of internal secretions and of efficient agents that could cure deficiency states. Hormones and vitamins were both drug-like and communicative substances; they could be industrially produced while they defined and explained the modern body.[69] This new physiology, based on problematizations of gender, sex, reproduction, nutrition and degeneration and situated in military and colonial medicine, created a new concept of a homeostatic body regulated by chemical substances.[70] To describe this class of substances, the German-speaking research community invented a term that fascinated not only researchers but also the general public in the 1920s: the afore-mentioned *biologische Wirkstoffe* (biologically active substances).

This newly invented term was specifically used to describe powerful, physiological substances such as hormones, vitamins and enzymes. In this context, chemistry and biology merged into a chemistry of natural substances (*Naturstoff-chemie*) that brought chemical skills, biological knowledge and life-reformist beliefs together with the interests of the pharmaceutical industry. The production of biologically active substances was a pharmaceutical procedure, i.e. a chemical process based on biological assays. During the first third of the twentieth century, research on biologically active substances and the mass production of biological compounds depended on the action of raw materials – urine, testicles, adrenal glands, fruits and vegetables – and the development of biological assays stabilize effectiveness and activate efficient agents. The isolation of natural substances from animal organisms and the synthesis of bioactive molecules became the main purpose of the highly productive cooperation between life scientists and the pharmaceutical industry – a cooperation that resulted in new molecules, patents, and a new physiology that seemed to hold great potential for enhancing the efficiency of the human body. The successful cooperation led to mass production of hormones and vitamins in Germany, Switzerland, England, the Netherlands and the US.[71] In a brief period from 1921 to 1934, biological substances like insulin (1921), vitamin D (1927), estron (1929), androsteron (1931), ascorbic acid (1932) and progesterone (1934) were isolated and synthesized. Moreover, in the first half of the 1930s, the list of biologically active substances and isolated natural substances was expanded by 'unnatural' synthetic derivatives.

Vitamania and the rejuvenation craze were worldwide phenomena in the 1920s. But in German-speaking countries they took on special meaning because of their association with the life-reformist concept of 'nature'. Organs and the various substances they secreted, as well as accessory food factors, soon became the prime movers of biological medicine and public health policies involving prophylactic practices.[72] In Germany, research and development on biologically active substances was part of the biomedical and political discourse. While the new concept of a biological body, clearly defined by natural laws, was the basis for Nazi Germany's biopolitics, *Wirkstoffe* as drugs with a seemingly vital ability to strengthen human efficiency came to play a central role in National Socialist war policies.[73] Biological medicine, organized in Nazi Germany as a New German Therapy *(Neue deutsche Heilkunde)*, deeply influenced German concepts of health for over half a century and well into the post-war years.[74] Biological remedies, biologically active substances (*Wirkstoffe*) and vital substances (*Vitalstoffe*) all held out the promise of sound health, an organological and natural way of living and a biological identity.

The Widening of the Concept of Biologics: The Biotechnological Transition until Today

The decades after the Second World War, especially from the 1950s to the 1980s, were dynamic years for biologics, as the number and variety of biologics – as well as the challenges facing regulators – continued to grow. Especially when recombinant drugs emerged on the market, scientists, regulators and the public tended to treat them as new kinds of substances that became denoted as 'biologicals'. However, this transition, which was often labelled as a 'biotechnological revolution', needn't be viewed as something entirely new, but rather as a recent variation in the episteme, technology and economy of biologics. The 'colossal change in our abilities to use and appropriate living organisms', as Gaudillière claims, started much earlier than common narratives of the so-called biotechnological revolution proclaim.[75]

After the spectacular introduction of penicillin in the 1940s, the biotechnological exploitation of fungal metabolisms invigorated the search for magic bullets.[76] Likewise, the amazing effects of the hormone cortisone raised expectations and drove pharmaceutical industries in their search for initial extracts from exotic plants.[77] Another advance in post-war research that significantly influenced the development of biologics was made in 1949 at Boston Children's Hospital, where scientists successfully grew a human virus, the Lansing Type II polio virus, in a human tissue cell culture.[78] The ability to grow human viruses easily and safely outside of a living host wasn't just a breakthrough that led to an explosion of research in vaccinology, but also a 'precondition for discoveries and changes relevant to biologics in the second half of the twentieth century'.[79] From the 1950s onward, vaccine research flourished. In the mid-1960's, pioneering work resulted in the first experimental live virus vaccine against German measles (rubella). 'Test inoculations conducted in West Africa led to a combined measles-smallpox product, the first commercial combined live virus vaccine'.[80] The growth of industrial biochemistry also established important prerequisites for the biotechnological transitions. The late 1960s and 1970s brought about a revival of interest in enzymes and their applications. Enzymatic reactions had been in use for some time, but now they began to play a central role in certain branches of production and triggered new developments. Increasingly, biological agents became recognized as an important field of future research.[81]

The new technologies were also subject to regulation, especially inasmuch as biologics were employed in food production or conservation. The food industry made increasing use of enzymes and enzymatic systems that were biotechnologically produced from non-toxic micro-organisms. The Joint FAO/WHO Food Standards Programme therefore included enzymatic preparations in its comprehensive efforts to develop food standards and codes of practice.[82] But the use of biologics for food preservation also raised concerns. Pharmaceutical firms began to massively promote the use of antibiotics as preservatives in fresh food.[83] Although attitudes towards this practice differed from country to country, West German regulations completely banned the use of antibiotics as food preservatives in 1958.

These developments not only changed the meaning of biologics, but also the ways of handling them. The fate of the Division of Biologics Standards, which stood at the centre of the re-organization of the NIH in the US, is a case in point. In 1955, after the so-called 'Cutter incident' involving the deaths of eleven people due to an impure polio vaccine sold by Cutter Laboratories, the status of biological control within the NIH was improved: to strengthen and expand its operations, the Division became an independent entity within the NIH.[84] Around 1970, the Division's review activities were criticized for not being 'as well institutionalized and not as clear and effective as the equivalent work being performed for the control of medicinal drugs'.[85] And in July 1972, both the authority to administer the drug provisions of the FD&C Act for all biological products and the responsibility for implementing the Biologics Act was delegated to the FDA.[86] The Division of Biologics Standards was transferred from the NIH to the FDA and renamed the Bureau of Biologics (BoB). In one sense, the merger with the FDA was a foregone conclusion because a 'biological product' as defined by the 1944 PHS Act also fell within the jurisdiction of the earlier 1938 FD&C Act. Thus, the jurisdictional and regulatory provisions of the 1902 Biologics Act and the FD&C Act were combined under *one* authority. When the BoB was merged with the FDA Bureau of Drugs in 1982, the evaluation of 'drugs' and 'biologics' was bundled into one institution, the National Center for Drugs and Biologics (NCDB). The FDA journal, *FDA Consumer*, sought to justify this merger as early as 1977: 'Vaccines are just one of a group of drug products that are called "Biologics" because they are made from or with the aid of living organisms that are produced in man or animals'.[87]

These changes in institutional organization reflected major scientific changes related to the beginnings of the biotechnological transition in the 1970s. In short, the distinction drawn between a drug and a biologic, or a device and a biologic, became ever more blurred.[88] Contemporary definitions of biotechnology focused attention on the biotechnological processing of 'biological agents' in general, even though they were initially intended for industrially useful enzymes.[89] Hence, biotechnology was already attracting increased attention when the next step in its development occurred, i.e. when recombinant DNA technology appeared on the scene in the 1970s.

With the advent of genetic engineering, the modification of micro-organisms opened up new possibilities in industrial processing, agriculture and biomedicine. The biotechnological production of clinically relevant molecules became the main challenge faced by early biotech companies in the 1970s and

1980s. Geneticists such as Joshua Lederberg time and again emphasized the potential benefits of genetic engineering.[90] Some of the further steps in the development of genetic engineering have been well researched.[91] Insulin was one of the proteins that embodied the aspirations of the New Biology and its promise of new products. A team at the University of California, San Francisco, associated with Herbert Boyer, who in April 1976 founded the small company Genentech (Genetic Engineering Technology), used the bacterium *Escherichia coli* to produce insulin and claimed success in September 1978. The FDA finally approved the drug in 1982. Despite the claims that molecular biology would revolutionize the whole industry, the main focus of attention after insulin turned to other potential money-spinners: human growth hormone and interferon, a protein that the body itself produces to fight viruses and that thus promised to be a miraculous cure for viral diseases. By 1980, Biogen was producing interferon through recombinant DNA after human DNA was transferred to bacterial DNA.[92] In the case of interferon, the promised magic bullet in the fight against viral infections never materialized and several companies shifted their attention elsewhere. A new, *immunological* approach emerged, based on interleukin-2, which was hailed as the new 'natural' weapon against cancer.[93] As Pieters summarizes, such substances represented a process of molecularizing medicine that originated in the engineering, preparation and purification of so-called recombinant protein drugs.[94]

Retrospectively, the transgenic transformation of biotechnology from the 1980s onward has been interpreted as a major break, either in terms of politics, technology and research practices, or in terms of the mode of knowledge production.[95] This rupture found expression in the proliferation of a term used to denote the recombinant DNA products: biologicals. The WHO began to use the term 'biologicals' exclusively after its department of 'biological standardization' was renamed 'biologicals' in the mid-1970s and from the 1980s onwards the term was used only in connection with advances in biotechnology and 'new biological products prepared using recombinant DNA techniques'.[96] Generally, the common term 'biologicals' came to be associated with the biotechnological age of recombinant DNA technology, while the term 'biologics' was more closely affiliated with the regulatory context of traditional biological substances such as vaccines. In his history of the FDA, Carpenter points to the simultaneous and sometimes confusing use of both terms ever since that period:

> Molecular entities are usually distinguished from 'biologics'. The world of biologics is often wrongly conflated with the world of 'biotech', when in fact most biotechnology drugs are not vaccines or otherwise bioactive. A more pervasive difference is between 'small' and 'large' molecules, such that the larger molecules represent proteins and antibodies that are 'biologically active' whereas the smaller molecules stand in for more traditional drugs.[97]

However, this distinction represents only a snapshot in the history of biologics and their definitions. As in the story of interferon, there was no clear-cut break between conventionally produced substances and the substances of the biotech transition since both originated in the preparation and purification of biological material.[98] Likewise, since the 1980s, the terms and classifications have again become contested, reflecting the challenges of regulation and developments in the biotech industry. By 1988, five proteins from genetically engineered cells had been approved as drugs by the FDA: insulin, human growth hormone, hepatitis B vaccine, alpha-interferon and tissue plasminogen activator (tPA) for lysis of blood clots.[99] In a reaction to this slow progress, research policies in the US and in Europe began developing new strategies.[100] This shift was described in a 1990 report of Britain's science advisory committee ACOST: 'Whereas efforts so far have been concentrated on the generation of biologically important molecules, the next phase is likely to lead to the engineering of higher levels of biological organization: the engineering of pathways and cells'.[101] This new situation has contributed to ongoing negotiations about the very definition of biologics, which in turn has been reflected in the steady reorganization of regulatory bodies. In 1988, the FDA again split biologics from the more general drug review process.[102] Since then, the FDA has been busy distributing and redistributing the responsibility for an ever-growing number of biological products. The FDA Center for Biologics Evaluation and Research (CBER) became responsible for some therapeutic proteins, such as monoclonal antibodies, but control of these was later transferred to the Center for Drug Evaluation and Research (CDER).[103] Some other drugs, such as certain anticoagulants and plasma volume expanders, have remained under the control of CBER. Meanwhile, the list of biologics continues to grow, including not only new substances but also cell products and organs such as human cell tissues, xenotransplantation, gene therapy and human cloning.[104] Similar ongoing redefinitions and regulatory reorganizations occurred in Europe as well. The first European pharmaceutical directive of January 1965, Directive 65/65/EEC 1965, provided only a rough sketch of efforts to harmonize European drug regulation and listed a range of substances, including a variety of biological products derived from human, animal, vegetable and chemical sources.[105] This list was updated some thirty years later when the London based European Agency for the Evaluation of Medicinal Products (EMEA) – set up 1995 and later renamed as the European Medicines Agency, EMA – established a Biologics Working Party (BWP) to provide recommendations to the EMA scientific committees 'on all matters relating to quality and safety aspects relating to *biological and biotechnological medicinal products*'.[106] In 2001, the European Union updated the 1965 directive to include a rearranged list of biologics that reflected the new system of drug approval. The 'Community code relating to medicinal products for human use' differentiates four approval procedures. Notably, the various biological products were not grouped into one category, but distributed across all four categories depending on the specific characteristics of the medicinal approval process.[107] However, one has to be careful with all these definitions since the terms and uses depend on the legislative and the administrative context. For instance, while the EMA differentiates 'biologics' and 'biologicals' ('biotechnological medicinal products'), the Directive 2001/83/EC does not refer to 'biologics' at all; instead, it uses the somewhat analogous terms 'biological medicinal products' and 'biological medicines' respectively.[108] Even more confusingly, additional terms such as 'biomedicines' have come into use with the proliferation of biologics, agencies, markets and with practices related to biological products.[109]

The realm of biologics has evolved throughout the twentieth century and the metamorphosis of objects and concepts remains unfinished. In the future, we will see more substances and new classes of substances enter the stage and change our understanding, classification and regulation of biologics. One very recent example is the advent of biosimilars, i.e. the analogues of generics in the field of biotechnologically produced medicines. Future work may reveal more details of the semantic field of biologics and dig deeper into linguistic and conceptual layers and transitions such as the biotech transition. But for the moment, what can we learn from this overview?

Biologics in the History of Medicine, Pharmacy and Science

There is no easy, apodictic way to determine the object of biologics studies. The previous sections have examined biologics as a semantic field containing different denotations, such as natural substances, *Naturarzneien*, organotherapeutic substances, *Wirkstoffe*, biological products, biologics, biologicals, *médicaments biologiques*, biopharmaceuticals and biological medicinal products. Such diverse nomenclature reveals that the history of biologics is truly multifaceted and difficult to grasp. Generic terms such as 'biologics' and 'biologicals' played an important role in the US, whereas European scientists and regulators were reluctant to adopt them. In Germany, the term *biologische Wirkstoffe* was introduced in the context of hormone and vitamin research, but it signified something quite different compared to the regulatory environment in the US, where the terms 'biologics' or 'biological products' included allergens and immune-based products, but not hormones.[110] And so, as the semantic overview suggests, attributions have been made according to actual and practical needs, forcing historians of medicine and pharmacy to account not just for the common features of biologics, but also for their specific historical development. For instance, the concepts of mid-twentieth century pharmacy cannot adequately explain why arsphenamine – a class of arsphenical substances – was subjected to the Biologics Control Act 1944. Most probably this was due to the fact that it posed regulatory problems analogous to sera and vaccines and was equally important, since it was administered in the fight against syphilis.[111]

But how can we define biologics when the categories in the semantic field have been blurred throughout history? Biologics have been defined in terms of sources, chemical properties, immunogenicity, macromolecular size or structure, or function. They have been characterized as complex macromolecules, as proteins, as derived from living organisms, natural sources and so on. In his splendid analysis of the 'language of biologics', Korwek stepped into deeper waters in analysing categories such as 'use', 'mechanism' and 'origin' as the shifting points of reference for regulatory definitions over time. For instance, 'use' was an important aspect of original statutory language that focused on disease prevention. The 'prevention and cure of diseases' language of the 1902 human biologics statute was revised in 1944 to include the 'prevention, treatment, or cure of diseases or *injuries* of man' since 'injuries' had become the main rationale for blood transfusions during the Second World War.[112] Korwek's analysis of the language of biologics once again emphasizes the significance of the practical historical context for the definition of biological products. What people denoted as 'biological products', 'biologics', or 'biologicals' was embedded in the context of regulation and legislation.

The language of biologics reveals these substances as cultural, political, economic and socio-technical entities. Biologics are at the same time natural resources, experimental representations, technical devices, visions, products, medical and clinical measures, cultural practices and legal entities. In fact, some of the historical approaches we considered in the previous section already suggest as much. Take for example an amendment to the directive of 2001, in which the EU Commission eventually tried to define biological products. Notably, this definition did not explain what biological products are as a group of substances, but instead described a feature that they share: what biologics have in common is the fact that they are *made* out of 'any substance of biological origin'.[113] For instance, biologics such as vaccines are substances produced in highly elaborated procedures of maceration, filtration, digestion, distillation, evaporation, sterilization, desiccation, levigation, dialysis, precipitation and physiological assay of living organisms. By adopting a pragmatic approach towards the history of biologics, the authors of this volume avoid ontological presuppositions about the nature of biologics, focusing instead on the technical context of biologics and the way they are produced. Synthetic drugs consist of pure chemical substances and their structures are known. 'Biologics, however, are complex mixtures that are not easily identified or characterized'.[114]

These conceptual insights can be incorporated into a characterization of biologics as substances that (1) are specific kinds of drugs, (2) have a 'biological origin', (3) are processed and (4) are more complex than drugs in general.[115] For the purposes of historical analysis, it is important to emphasize that this is not a characterization that relies on any putative 'nature' of biologics, but instead simply a helpful heuristic tool for use within an ever-changing common field of historical objects. Hence, none of these four traits are timeless and there are substances that do not satisfy these criteria. The following examples illustrate some pitfalls: first-generation antibiotics were described as any substance produced by a micro-organism that is antagonistic to the growth of other micro-organisms. With advances in medicinal chemistry, most of today's antibacterials are semisynthetic modifications of various natural compounds. There are different classification systems in use for antibacterial compounds, based either on their origin, their mechanism of action, their chemical structure or their biological activity. Again, we are confronted with the question of what 'biological origin' means. The case of the synthetic drug DES (Diethylstilbestrol) also belies easy definition. In the 1950s, DES was used in farming in spite of debates about the health risks it posed.[116] The pharmaceutical industry invented DES as a medical treatment for certain conditions, including breast and prostate cancers. It was not until the 1970s that DES was found to be an 'endocrine disruptor', i.e. a chemical that interferes with the hormone system in animals and humans.[117] These and many other examples illustrate that origins alone do not suffice in transforming substances into biologics.[118] They show that the field of biologics is historically determined and actualized by experimental configurations and trajectories, discourses, marketing strategies, regulatory practices and legal definitions.

Biologics studies will contribute to the history of pharmaceuticals and medicine in as much as they illustrate the epistemes, cultures, policies and economies of connections and demarcations that constituted biologics as specific kinds of drugs and, hence, as historiographic objects in their own right. These studies will draw on the histories of individual substances to teach us more about the specific relationship between biologics and politics, science, industry and culture. Although this introduction focuses mainly on regulation and legislation, the history of biologics is not limited to these contexts. An impressive number of excellent case studies have already been published that examine biological substances as objects of scientific inquiry, the pharmaceutical industry, public health policy and reform movements. We therefore advocate a comprehensive perspective that will stimulate future work and that will incorporate a panoply of connections to the stories we tell about the development of single substances such as diphtheria serum, vitamin D, estrogen, or interferon and their characterization as biologics.

The essays published in this volume suggest three main domains that contributed to the shaping of biologics as economic, political, social and cultural objects and that are best suited to grasping the historical contingencies of these heterogeneous substances and materials.

These domains, which constitute the organizational structure of this book, are (1) the production of nature, (2) the body politics of biologics and (3) the making of contested biologics.

The Production of Nature

The first part of the book focuses on one of the basic problems of drug production and on a fundamental technique of the modern industrialized world: standardization. Standardization became a key part of the research, production and regulation of pharmaceutical chemicals and was therefore an important concern in the nascent market for modern drugs from the nineteenth century onwards.[119] In the history of biological products, the standardization and regulation of vaccines, sera and antitoxins have garnered the most scholarly attention.[120]

Standardization was usually equated with the development of reliable biological assays. Up to the present day, these assays have been major targets of industrial as well as administrative forms of regulation. Both the variability of the biological raw material and the uncertainties regarding the composition of extracts made standardization essential, but difficult. It is no coincidence that the early strategies of *Wertbestimmung* combined statistical procedures with easily observable phenomena (e.g. the percentage of deaths prevented by a certain quantity of serum in a given animal population). Experiences with biological products have repeatedly resulted in their impure origin 'from nature' being problematized. To name just one early, prominent case: in the 1850s, the French physiologist Claude Bernard tested extracts made from strychnea by different Parisian pharmacies and came to the conclusion that they differed by a factor of six.[121] Successfully isolating a hormone or vitamin, enabling an adequate chemical method for its measurement and synthetically producing the pure principle all involved the use of biological tests and, hence, standardization. As British pharmacologist Henry Dale proclaimed, the only property by which an active principle can be recognized and measured is its action on the living animal or isolated organ, which must somehow be made the basis of what is called a 'biological standardization' or 'biological assay'.[122] Questionable 'purity' and the equivocal results of clinical observation are often two sides of the same coin. The story of anti-diabetic agents derived from plants leads directly to the problematic qualities that, time and again, are ascribed to biologics. And it illustrates how the model of biological effects served as a bridge linking pharmacognostical and biochemical plant research with animal and clinical studies. In general, the pharmacological effects of biological preparations lacked reliability.[123]

The point here is that the problems posed by biologics were associated with particular forms of production that included not just standardization (the bioassays), but also 'characteristic routes of production (extraction, fermentation, or enzymatic synthesis), and a special legal status'.[124] The specificities of biologic production shaped science, industry and regulation. In most European countries, therapeutic agents were not patentable. When the German pharmacopoeia was enacted in 1872, the normal objects of drug regulation were still considered to be pharmaceutical substances produced according to the rules of the pharmacopoeia. But a number of new substances were already being manufactured outside the pharmacies, which merely inspected and tested them, and so their synthesis was not described by the pharmacopoeia. Patented medicines with secret ingredients were also marketed. Most biologics were not included in the traditional pharmacopoeias because there were no generally accepted verification procedures and pharmacies were often unable to conduct appropriate testing. The realm of pharmaceutical biological drugs witnessed the introduction and tentative implementation of several forms of patenting and intellectual property rights protection.

In his essay on the introduction and production of diphtheria serum in France, **Jonathan Simon** argues that what set sera apart from patent medicines was their intimate connection with the promise of innovative scientific research, notably in microbiology. The special status of biologics was based on the precarious qualities generally assigned to them. Contamination was the first difficulty ascribed to the production of biological products. As they were derived from living organisms, this procedure brought with it the potential for the transmission of infectious diseases. In 1927, the US office of biologics control concluded:

> The products covered by the law and regulations – viruses, serums, toxins, antitoxin and analogous products applicable to the prevention or cure of diseases of man – are collectively referred to as biologic products and by their very nature are particularly prone to become contaminated, or, in some instances, rapidly to lose their curative properties. It was *because of these peculiar properties of this class of products* that the necessity for some method of accurate control of their manufacture and sale was early recognized.[125]

The need for purity in research, production and control evoked an apparatus of practices and facilities that facilitated standardization. Purity was a time-consuming and expensive necessity in the production of biologics. Producing isolated or synthesized substances on a large scale became a question of techniques, patents and costs. Last but not least, this transformation into a remedy was determined by economic and material constraints.

Research as well as commercial production of biologics depended on the use of natural resources, frequently in very large quantities. An often-cited example is the production of extracts and hormones out of tons of animal organs acquired from slaughterhouses. In most cases, however, the trajectories of biologics were interconnected with colonial history: the exploitation of resources, the appropriation of indigenous knowledge and the transformation of both into an industrial context.[126] As described in **Jean-Paul Gaudillière**'s contribution, the invention of drugs from extracts of kola nuts grown in sub-Saharan, tropical West Africa depended on colonial economies and politics. He concludes from his case study that kola extracts became drugs – elaborate, albeit impure compositions – only once a series of practical and social arrangements had been performed: Biologics were not just remedies 'made' out of biological things. 'They were technical objects, at once socially and culturally associated with nature and at the same time elaborated through industrial mass-preparation.'[127]

Another obstacle that has often been highlighted as a common feature of biological products is their complexity. Biological products are more difficult to identify and characterize than chemical products, and accordingly it is more difficult to ensure that their identity remains unaltered under different manufacturing conditions. The FDA has therefore customarily required clinical testing of any product manufactured *at a new site* before it will license production there.[128] A recent definition of biologics makes reference to these problems: 'In contrast to most drugs that are chemically synthesized and their structure is known, most biologics are complex mixtures that are not easily identified or characterized.'[129] Today, more and more modern biological products can be standardized using chemical analysis and there are numerous attempts being undertaken to produce biologics in the same way that other pharmaceuticals are made. Therefore, some proponents argue that biologics should no longer be generally considered as complex mixtures.[130] Nevertheless, complexity has shaped the production of biologics, from research on the mysterious effects of extracts and the industrialization of these substances to the regulatory mechanisms governing them.

Standardization and problems arising out of the production of biologics became keystones of specific social, legal and commercial configurations. Some sera – like antidiphtheric serum – were standardized in Germany, but they were not subject to drug legislation around 1900 because they were not marketed through pharmacies. Instead, special laws regulated them. As mentioned above, the production procedures of some standard, industrially produced chemical preparations were for the first time no longer defined in the pharmacopoeia. Thus, the advent of biologics coincided with a major shift in medicinal culture. The question of who controls and markets which substance has continued to be a bone of contention up to the present day, and it always hinges on legal and scientific categories. From the outset, regulatory bodies such as the US Public Health Service's Hygienic Laboratory focused on 'biological standardization'.[131] Furthermore, the unfolding of standardization strategies should be analysed as social and economic processes that influenced both the substances and the protagonists involved, thereby also affecting research and the drug development process, as well as the wider social context.

For instance, shortly after its establishment in 1921 and under the presidency of Thorvald Madsen, Director of the State Serum Institute in Copenhagen, the

League of Nations' Health Organization declared that establishing standards for biologicals was one of its most urgent tasks.[132] In 1921, it initiated a meeting of international experts that finally agreed on Ehrlich's unit for diphtheria antitoxin and arranged for the production of an international standard preparation to be deposited in Copenhagen.[133] This conference was followed by further meetings in 1923 and 1925 to discuss digitalis, pituitary posterior lobe extract and insulin, in 1931 to find stable standards and define units for vitamins and in 1932 and 1935 to specify biological tests, names and units for sex hormones.[134] International standard preparations for oestrus-producing hormones, androsterone and progesterone were kept at the National Institute for Medical Research in Mill Hill on the outskirts of London. It can be argued that these activities, based as they were on the generic problems of biologics, influenced the health-care policies of the League of Nations in general and that the League's 'Standardisation Commission' became an important means by which the League advanced its agenda of peace through international cooperation.[135]

Later on, biological standardization certainly became one of the main concerns of the WHO: to date, the WHO Expert Committee on Biological Standardization has published 59 reports. And it has cooperated with national agencies like the Division of Biological Standards of the National Institute of Medical Research in London in its work on interferon.[136] The history of interferon is an example that illustrates how, in spite of improvements in both the production and regulation of biologics, the problem of standardization remained rampant, because, as in the case of many other biologics, purifying the substance and establishing its biological definition proved especially challenging.

The process of standardization was not just a scientific and technical procedure, but also deeply entangled with social and economic factors and interests. Standardized products shaped and were shaped by this heterogeneous cluster of scientific practices, social actors, material structures, administrative routines and the industrial logic of valorization.[137] As mentioned above, historical studies on biologics have to take into account the institutionalization, regulation, activation and casual use of these agents. From this perspective, their standardization has been multifaceted, involving different kinds of laboratory, economic and regulatory standards. Absolute control was more of an ideal than a reality and some of the contributions to this volume focus on experimental systems and the difficulties encountered while attempting to stabilize biological material. As **Lea Haller** shows in the case of cortisone, the procedures for standardizing and purifying biologics would sometimes destabilize the entire experimental system and thereby effect a change in therapeutic rationale.[138] The process of stabilization, activation and processing of biologics modified experimental systems as well as the social and economic conditions of their use.

The Body Politics of Biologics

The second part of this volume considers the use of biologics in various forms of intervention in the human body, as well as their impact on the creation of bodily concepts. Biological substances enabled new ways of intervening in fundamental bodily processes and provided new options for bodily perfection and human enhancement. We assume that the ambiguous character of biologics – viewed both as chemical agents, technical objects and matters of natural origin – had a major impact on their production and commercialization. The transformation of natural substances into pharmaceuticals, which was the subject of public debate and was shaped by the influence of several interest groups, was a major task in the early twentieth century. Standardization, regulation and activation of biologics should therefore be analysed as scientific and political discourses and practices that connect molecules and organisms in a historically specific regime of knowledge and power.

In illustrating this point, vaccines, sera and antitoxins are again a good place to start. The initial successes of bacteriology in the 1890s called into serious question the fundamental paradigms of medicine. Bacteriological knowledge became a new framework in which to conceptualize not only the causes of diseases, but also the relationship between the human body and its environment. Bacteriological knowledge was a battlefield of contagion and the body's own defences.[139] The body was an 'irritable machine', both physiologically and mechanically, from which hygienic knowledge and strategies could be derived.[140] Hygienic strategies targeted both the environment and individual behaviour (washing one's hands, using a handkerchief). 'The individual that preferred health as an aim in life and therefore submitted to medical-scientific principles – the "homo hygieni-cus" – was a scientific construct of bacteriology'.[141] This body politics of self-care was enacted through governmental surveillance and health-care policies, most prominently in the form of vaccination programmes that aimed at the body's physiological defences. Substances derived from biological material sometimes played a decisive role when new representations of the body intermingled with body politics, as in the case of Sigmund Freud's coca studies. Freud used the famous dynamometer to transform the 'Indian' habit of chewing coca leaves into a measurable effect of cocaine on the modern, working body. As **Beat Bächi** argues, Freud thereby linked the consumption of cocaine to emerging modern concepts of fatigue and to norms of the productive body. The power of biological substances to activate the exhausted body further elucidates the relationship between the production and commercialization of biologics on the one hand, and body concepts on the other. From this perspective, the emergence of different types of biologics around 1900 triggered a commercial success story, linking the fates of new biological molecules like cocaine and cortisone with the promises of organotherapy.

From the 1920s onward, concepts of biological regulation acquired more and more chemical connotations. The complex interplay of antagonistic and synergistic chemical reactions and chemical metabolism justified hormone or vitamin therapies. Up until the mid-1930s, the isolation of natural substances from animal organisms and the synthesis of bioactive molecules provided the raison d'etre for a highly productive collaboration between life scientists and the pharmaceutical industry that produced numerous molecules, patents and a new physiology that seemed to hold great potential for enhancing the efficiency of the human body. The aim of reshaping or even rejuvenating the body was based on the experimental physiological use of organs or nutrients to compensate for deficiencies.[142] But only biologically active substances (*biologische Wirkstoffe*) that could be extracted and chemically synthesized (such as hormones and vitamins) were able to transform this area of research into an industrial and commercial project. **Heiko Stoff**'s overview of this field of research and its histories shows that the isolation of biologically active substances combined knowledge production about the body with the activation of natural products and their transformation into pharmaceuticals. In pledging to produce efficient bodies and to protect consumers' rights to fitness, health and youthfulness, hormones and vitamins were decidedly modern and – in some respects – even a catalyst of modernity. In this regard biologics not only merged laboratory research and industrial production, but also linked practices of representation and intervention. However, research and development on biologically active substances came along with a new 'biological body', clearly defined by natural laws. In Germany, this concept became the basis for Nazi Germany's biopolitics. *Wirkstoffe* as drugs with a seemingly vital ability to strengthen human efficiency played a central role in National Socialist war policies.[143]

The 'natural option' became a central theme of body politics that targeted the exhausted and deficient body. That body can be described as being both industrial and non-industrial because one has to differentiate between the cultural reservoir of 'meanings' associated with biologics as opposed to industrial strategies and calculations. The marketing of biologics as therapeutics or prophylactics and the new physiology of an organism regulated by chemical agents share the same origins. Even though biologics have long been artificially and/or industrially produced, they have retained their image of being 'more natural' than drugs synthesized from inorganic substances.[144] The twentieth century witnessed the creation of new consumers of biologics and brought forth markets that were grounded in a discourse about naturalness, life and vitality.

This understanding of biologics as 'natural substances' continued into the late twentieth century, when a new wave of biologics arose that relied upon biotechnologically produced materials. For instance, although company officials of Wellcome, Roche and Schering-Pough had difficulty defending the costly interferon research and development, they were ultimately successful in depicting interferon as an opportunity: unlike most chemical drugs, these genetically engineered biologics could be viewed in their 'natural' (physiological) role as regulators or modifiers of a variety of pharmacologically interesting *biological* mechanisms.[145] Biomedical technologies not only evolved new options in the realm of molecular biology, but also in the handling, treatment, storage and application of bodily organs, tissues and cells. Like the technical transformation of cell mechanisms into engineering tools, these new biologic regimes turned the human body into a resource of biological treatment.

In his ethnographic study of the procedures of assisted reproduction, **Sven Bergmann** follows the transformation of body parts and the making of reproductive substances using procedures like purification, preparation and classification. At the same time, these objects are loaded and attached with meaning and allusions that remind us that living material has a separate social life. **Sophie Chauveau** tackles the process that transforms human body parts into organ and tissue transplants. Her analysis is linked to themes from the first part of this volume and presents an analysis of standardization as a process of change: human body parts are transformed into products, like drugs or surgical equipment, and then into commodities. But there are differences, because like tissue or entire organs, human body parts are more akin to 'living things' than biologics in the narrower sense. This conclusion may point to essential problems that accompany organ transplantation, since this medical practice depends on a radical shift in our understanding of what a living body is and what 'living' means in this context, as illustrated in debates about the brain-death criterion. Hence, organ transplantation is a contentious political issue that brings us to the next part of this book.

The Making of Contested Biologics

This final section addresses another basic aspect of biologics: their precarious qualities. Modern pharmaceuticals are well known to have potentially deleterious effects. Indeed, most of the substances discussed in this volume have their own ambiguities in so far as their effects can oscillate between desirable and harmful outcomes. A common way of referring to these problems is to speak of 'side effects'. However, this term disguises the fact that harmful effects are not an accidental quality, but rather a basic feature of modern pharmaceutical research.[146] This holds for drugs in general, but it is especially pronounced in the case of biologics since these problems seem to be specifically connected to their historical characterization. We have already argued that the basic qualities continually being ascribed to biologics tend to evoke specific problems: it is difficult to appropriate them within laboratory regimes, to stabilize their effects and to standardize their production. As Pieters concludes in his story of interferon: 'As far as the pharmaceutical industry was concerned most biologicals had a problematic developmental track record. They were tricky to produce – requiring elaborate and expensive production, safety testing and standardization procedures – and difficult to quantify and store'.[147]

Rheinberger has pointed to this intrinsic ambivalence of standardization as an emblematic process within modern societies. There is always a flip-side to processes of normalization, standardization and stabilization. 'We could possibly even go so far as to claim that the desire for standardization is the expression of that flip-side. And sure enough, standardization never results in complete control'.[148] Precariousness is a concept that has been used to describe this intrinsic relationship and that is especially pronounced in the case of biological substances.[149] The precariousness of biologics results from their historical constitution as both natural and artificial objects. Their 'naturalness' guaranteed their special effectiveness, but this 'natural promise' made their control even harder. Their autonomy was not obliterated after being disciplined in the laboratory and standardized in industrial production, but was in fact expanded. Since enhancing and improving their benefits was (and is) a redundant feature of the processing of biological substances, their risks are likewise amplified.[150] In this respect, the molecularization and chemical definition of biologically active substances not only dissolved the boundaries between natural and artificial substances, but also created a tension between the chemical identity of therapeutic substances and the cultural merits of naturalness. **Ulrike Thoms** compares the practices of regulation in Canada and Germany and the respective instabilities arising from the development of standards designed to reduce the precariousness of insulin. Here again, the obstacles posed by standardization, purification and calibration are a useful starting point. In the early 1920s, the German Insulin Committee recognized the risks of insulin preparations, but at this point its members left developments to market forces that they believed would limit the dangerous effects. 'The entire biotechnological task of standardising insulin as a substance was left to industry, while physicians were responsible only for a final quality check'.[151] The instabilities of biologics resulted in ongoing negotiations and changes in the practices and relationships between the actors involved.

Biologics also highlight the role of industry in coping with these ambiguities. The perception of biologicals 'as profitable but troublesome and high-risk commodities' played an important role in preventing drug companies from diving into research on biological substances such as interferon.[152] **Pim Huijnen** uncovers unprecedented consequences in his study of the introduction of vitamin preparations in the Netherlands, where from the outset science-based quality control, standardization processes and marketing were heavily entangled. In the Netherlands, the ambiguities and the lack of uncontested standards were not necessarily problems that had to be overcome, but rather assets that helped sell vitamins. Increasingly over the course of the twentieth century, regulation was publicly debated and negotiated, not least because it involved consumer interests as well as life-reform discourses. In this vein, studying risk management brings together the history of consumer culture, public problematizations of natural substances and scientific definitions of risks. Biologics might have been risky and in need of trials to ensure their efficacy and safety, but they could also function as a surrogate for nature gone missing. In so far as biologics differed from chemical compounds due to their epistemological status as natural substances, they transported discourses of purity, naturalness and vitality. The juxtaposition of natural and artificial substances not only informed public discourse on 'healthy' biologics such as plant products, organotherapeuticals or vitamins versus 'risky' synthetic pharmaceuticals, but also influenced scientific debate and practice itself. As we have argued in this introduction, the shifts and conflicts within the discourse on 'natural' substances or on their 'naturalness' have persisted to this day, since those substances have always been both biological and chemical, both natural and synthetic.

One of the early examples of this can be seen in the history of the public's concerns about vaccination. The animal origins of the inoculating agents was one of several facts that evoked public concern. Ideally, smallpox vaccination was derived from well-tested calf lymphs. This seemed to juxtapose animal substances and human lives, and the image of organic substances from different species being mixed with the human body elicited deep anxieties. But because calf lymphs were scarce and difficult to store, vaccination was also performed from arm to arm.[153] Yet, the transfer from human to human raised apprehensions as well, since numerous cases of infection – most prominently with syphilis – were known to have occurred. In both Germany and England, vaccination programmes provoked vehement protests on religious, political, scientific and moral grounds. Should healthy people, notably children, be put in jeopardy of contracting an infectious disease or suffering harmful side effects? After several epidemics in the early 1870s, statistics provided evidence for both proponents and adversaries of compulsory vaccination. The death toll seemed to be as high in populations that had been almost completely vaccinated as in those that had not been. German legislators reacted by making not only vaccination, but also revaccination after ten years compulsory, whereas in England the ongoing debate about compulsory vaccination resulted in the 1898 act allowing a large percentage of the population to opt out of vaccination. Here, a policy that relied more on local public health administration than on vaccination, won the upper hand.[154] This was in line with the strong European hygiene movement that demanded epidemiological studies and strategies that focused on the environment rather than the body. Long before the famous Lübeck scandal of 1930, when over seventy babies died from a tuberculosis vaccine that had been contaminated with virulent bacteria, vaccination had become a bone of contention.[155]

The invention of biologics brought with it scepticism, protest and fear. While vaccines and sera were *too* biological and raised doubts and anxieties about purity and contamination, synthesized hormones and vitamins were *too* chemical and elicited concerns about toxicity and alienation.[156] However, biologics also became contested as 'natural resources' originating from countries with long colonial and imperial histories. Colonial and imperial possessions were used as sources of natural products that could be developed into biologics, such as the *Strophantus* species from West Africa, sisal from East Africa and yam (*Dioscorea*) from Mexico that were used in cortisone production.[157] There is an enormous literature on these kinds of material relations that, in fact, brings together topics of imperial exploitation of the natural world and the history of biologics.[158] That literature demonstrates that access to certain substances has been a key factor in the relationship between botany, commercial activities and politics, something that hasn't changed to this day.[159] Between 1991 and 2003, pharmaceutical companies annually imported 467,000 tons of medical plants from twelve 'developing' countries for use in the production of plant medicines.[160] With the rise of the New Social Movements and the internationalization of nature conservation, these companies have become embroiled in the politics of colonial and imperial power relations. The last contribution to this volume offers an example of the politicization of assembling practices. **Klaus Angerer** focuses on the trajectory of epibatidine, an alkaloid isolated from poison frog skins that had been collected during several field trips to Ecuador during the 1970s and 1980s. But the acquisition practices used by researchers to obtain the frog skins were called into doubt by the regulation of the trade in specimens of wild animals and plants in 1987 ('Washington Convention') and by the emerging fight against 'biopiracy' and subsequent negotiations that led to the Convention on Biological Diversity (CBD) in 1992. Thus, the case of epibatidine illustrates the politicization of biologics production and the social conflicts of a globalized economy. Furthermore, epibatidine can serve as a reminder of additional issues not dealt with in this volume, such as biologics produced from recombinant DNA. The history of genetically modified crops, of transgenic animals and of biotechnologically produced biologicals such as monoclonal antibodies will have to take into account the social protests, political conflicts and popular scepticism that accompanied the invasion of these kinds of synthetic biologics. This may be one of the lessons to be drawn from a comparative history of biologics.

1 STANDARDIZATION AND CLINICAL USE: THE INTRODUCTION OF THE ANTI-DIPHTHERIA SERUM IN LYON[1]

Jonathan Simon

The use of serum to treat diphtheria, a deadly childhood disease, was a ground-breaking therapy in many respects. Its production involved inducing immunity to a specific pathogen in horses (they initially used a culture of the bacteria responsible for diphtheria to induce this immunity, and later replaced this culture with the purified toxin produced by the bacteria) and using the serum separated from the animal's blood to treat human victims of the disease. While it can be viewed as an extension of the techniques used for vaccination – the manipulation of a living organism (specifically its immune system) to produce a medicament for use in another species – its status as a treatment for a widespread and deadly disease put it in a class of its own.[2] Furthermore, serum production, starting in 1894, required microbiological techniques and savoir-faire that were beyond the reach of the majority of pharmacists and medical doctors at that time. This is a key reason why, unlike the majority of medicines that were still prepared in the pharmacist's laboratory according to directions provided by the pharmacopoeia, the serum was produced in relatively large quantities at a small number of specialized facilities.

One particularly challenging element in the serum production process was the evaluation of its therapeutic or immunization potential. The active principle of the serum (if, indeed, there was such a thing as an active principle) did not correspond to any known single component, making it different from a chemical medicine, the potency (and, in principle at least, efficacy) of which could be evaluated by simply weighing the physiologically active compounds. Determining the serum's efficacy therefore involved the use of a number of experimental animals and a series of protocols that governed the serum being tested, a sample of standardized diphtheria toxin, and often a standard serum as well.[3]

The particular problems posed by the production and assessment of the therapeutic virtue of this serum opened up a new area of pharmaceutical standardization, which will be the subject of the first part of this essay. I use the term

industrial standardization to characterize this process, an approach to the evaluation of the serum that relied on clearly defined and monitored protocols. These
were aimed at limiting variability in the production process, so that the units of
production and the personnel could be replaced without interrupting or redefining the activity. In a second section, I want to consider the introduction of
this medicine into the clinic, using the example of the diphtheria ward at the
Charité hospital in Lyon. In this part, after surveying views about diphtheria and
its treatment before the introduction of serotherapy, we will see how serum was
used in a hospital ward. Behind the apparently haphazard nature of the serum's
clinical use, I want to argue the case for what I term *clinical standardization*. This
alternative form of standardization, while it is predicated on an increasingly consensual vision of what constitutes appropriate treatment, affirms the autonomy
of the individual clinician in implementing the accepted therapy, leading to a
large diversity in the application of emerging norms.

Anti-Diphtheria Serum, the First *Biological*?

One reason that this anti-diphtheria serum is of interest, is that in an uncritical
history of therapeutics it would, alongside earlier vaccines, qualify as one of the
first biological medicines. Looking at present-day European legislation we find
the following definition of biologics:

> A biological medicinal product is a product, the active substance of which is a biolog-
> ical substance. A biological substance is a substance that is produced by or extracted
> from a biological source and for which a combination of physico-chemical-biological
> testing and the production process and its control is needed for its characterisation
> and the determination of its quality.[4]

It is easy to detect the influence of the history of sera in this definition, in particular with the emphasis placed on product testing. The second part of the
definition orients us towards the issue of forms of quality control that rely on
test organisms. This approach to quality control, termed *Wertbestimmung* in
German, has grown out of the evaluation of the therapeutic sera that appeared
at the end of the nineteenth century, first the serum used to treat diphtheria and
then the serum to treat tetanus.[5] The fact that the sera have influenced this modern definition of biologics makes it logical, if not tautological, to consider them
among the first biological medicines. Nevertheless, as Jean-Paul Gaudillière
argues elsewhere in this volume, why should we not consider all the products
derived from natural sources that are not prepared as pure synthetic molecules
to be biologics? Interpreting the term this widely would open up the category
considerably, and the sera would lose any claim to pioneer status, with homoeopathic remedies having a claim to be considered biological medicines, to take an
extreme example. Nevertheless, it seems to me that counting homoeopathic rem-

edies (as well as other traditional vegetable extracts) as biologics would involve a deliberate misinterpretation of the intention of those who drafted the text cited above. The target of the definition is clearly sera (more particularly monoclonal antibodies), hormones, blood products, and other medicines or vaccines of this type. Even this brief reflection on the question shows how indefinite the term 'biological medicines' is in principle, however well circumscribed its application might be in practice.

The modern definition of biological medicines serves to recall two important aspects of the history of the serum: its production and its evaluation, two processes that provide an entry-point into the issue of standardization. Indeed, the innovations that sera represented in these areas were tightly bound to the establishment of production, managerial and metrological standards.

Something that all products of biological origin (vaccines, sera and, later, hormones) had in common was the impossibility of defining and isolating an active ingredient uniquely responsible for their therapeutic or prophylactic effects. This would not necessarily have posed a problem had these effects been completely invariant (meaning in the case of diphtheria treatment, the same effect for the same volume of blood serum prepared under similar conditions), but the variability inherent in living beings and their natural products meant that the serum manufacturer could not be sure that a new batch would have a level of efficacy similar to that of an old one. This was the case even when the serum came from the same horse, let alone when it came from a different one. Of course with regard to pharmaceuticals, there are two aspects to this problem of variability: that of the product itself and that of the person receiving the treatment. Although we should bear this in mind when we consider the use of the serum in the clinic, we will leave the second aspect to one side for the moment and concentrate our attention on the first one, the variability of the product. The systems that were developed around the serum in order to master this variability conformed to the logic of what I term industrial standardization.

Diphtheria Serum, Evaluation and Industrial Standardization

In Germany, Paul Ehrlich took the lead in successively developing more sophisticated evaluation procedures that came to depend on a standard dose of toxin. The lethal dose – the volume of toxin (per weight) capable of killing guinea pigs within a fixed amount of time – became the touchstone within a system populated by fluctuating products and animals. Thus, Ehrlich based his comparison of different sera on the lethal dose of toxin, and he increasingly used dried standards to compensate for the variability of these products over time.[6] In France, where the production and evaluation processes were not subject to the same pressures for innovation as in Germany, Emile Roux and his successor in charge of serum production, Louis Martin, stuck with an early version for evaluating the potency of the serum, using a technique initially developed by Behring himself. This procedure involved injecting guinea pigs with a proportion of their weight of the serum under test (one 1/50,000 of its weight the other 1/100,000) followed by a lethal dose of toxin. If only the first guinea pig survived, the serum was classed as 150 units, and if they both survived this rose to 200.[7]

While the details of the evaluation method differed between the producers in France and Germany, what I want to emphasize for the sake of comparison are the features of 'industrial standardization' that were common to both. The idea is to draw out the most significant elements of this type of standardization in order to compare it with the 'clinical standardization' that was developed in Lyon (and elsewhere) after the serum became available starting in 1894. In their book on standardization in evidence-based medicine, Timmermans and Berg present four types of standards: design, terminological, performance and procedural.[8] Although these categories (especially performance and procedural) can account for much of the standardization in this context, I believe it is more useful to think of the industrial standardization of the production of serum in more global terms. Thus, this kind of industrial standardization relies on centralized production with a system of sampling and testing that evaluates the products in terms of both their quality and their efficacy. This system of control is tied to bureaucratic procedures that accompany the process, duplicating it on paper and thereby providing a form of traceability and administrative proof that the production process was carried out according to the established norms and that the finished product conformed to the testing standards.[9] This documentation also gives unity to a process that can be broken up through the division of labour at various stages of production. Protocols specifying the materials to be used and procedures to be followed allow different specialists to execute the same steps in the production process. The personnel (like the producing units – in this case the horses) can thus be replaced by others, although this does not mean that we can neglect the importance (and variability) of the specialized skills possessed by each individual technician.

These features mark the difference compared with artisanal production, where the individual manufacturer brings his or her skills to bear in the fabrication of each product. While the products of such an industrial system may be no more uniform than those of the artisan, they are nevertheless subject to a different regime of control, where well-defined procedures and systematic checks form the core of what we are calling 'industrial standardization'. This term, therefore, covers the norms of production, their application and their enforcement, as well as the corollary of the interchangeability of personnel. While it might seem that industrial standardization would require a certain minimum scale of production, this is not a fundamental factor in the present case. For example, the scale of serum production in Lyon was very modest compared to the output of the Pasteur Institute in Paris (two horses versus over one hundred and thirty), and yet the details of production were just as clearly defined.

The Epidemic in Oullins – The Triumph of the Infectious 'Germ'

Having outlined this industrial culture of serum manufacture and the standardization that it implied, I now want to turn to the question of the clinical use of the serum. How was the serum employed once it had been distributed and was no longer under the control of the manufacturers? This section explores the use of the serum in Lyon starting in late 1894, but I also want to expand the perspective to include the place of diphtheria in this city prior to the introduction of serotherapy. This provides relevant context for what I have to say about the issue of standardization in the use of the serum for the treatment of diphtheria in Lyon. Furthermore, I will consider the discussions about serotherapy that took place in medical circles in 1894–5. Nevertheless, in reviewing these debates over the serum that appeared in the medical press, I have found nothing suggesting that the fact that serum was a product taken directly from an animal was of pressing concern for either the patients or the administering doctors. While it might appear surprising from the perspective of the standards embodied in today's health-care regulations that so little attention was paid to a biological product intended to be injected in large doses into young children, it did not seem to shock the doctors or patients at the end of the nineteenth century.

In Lyon, as we shall see, the debate was displaced onto other issues (in particular, onto debates that pre-dated the introduction of serotherapy and would continue for decades afterwards). As we have argued elsewhere, the justification for the widespread use of this relatively untested product was the gravity of the disease itself.[10] The fact that the disease was so lethal, particularly among children, justified a treatment that could well have been rejected in less drastic circumstances. The important place that the serum occupied relatively quickly, particularly in hospitals, did not, however, prevent criticisms of its use and investigations into its potential dangers for the patients. Thus, Saturnin Arloing, a professor of both veterinary and human medicine in Lyon who oversaw local serum production for the region, conducted a number of tests on animals in order to clarify these risks, in spite of the fact that he was producing the serum. We will return to consider Arloing's studies and their motivation at the end of this chapter.

To introduce the historical analysis, I want to consider an epidemic of diphtheria that dates from before the introduction of serotherapy in Lyon. This has the advantage of illustrating not only how the medical community viewed diphtheria and its outbreaks, but also the range of treatments that were available in the second half of the nineteenth century. Thus, I will be looking at a description of an outbreak of the disease in the Lyon area in 1888, i.e. shortly before the introduction of the serum and at a time when the microbial nature of the disease was already well established in the medical community – at least among those doctors who kept themselves informed about these developments. Furthermore, doctors, particularly hospital doctors, were increasingly availing themselves of the possibility of detecting the presence of the 'germ' responsible for diphtheria by means of the microscopic analysis of throat cultures. Thus, while there was no general agreement concerning any 'standard' treatment – a point we will return to later – the means for diagnosing and more generally 'understanding' the disease was becoming more consensual.

In September 1888, the first cases of diphtheria appeared in Oullins, an industrial community on the outskirts of Lyon (population *c.* 8,000). Louis Bard, a young local doctor, gave a full account of the resulting epidemic in the *Lyon Médical* for 1889.[11] This account was presented in the form of an investigation aimed at identifying the cause of the epidemic.[12] Indeed, for all practical purposes, Louis Bard effectively replaced the official *inspecteur des épidémies de Lyon*, Professor Peroud, investigating the outbreak and conducting a case-by-case analysis in order to shed some light on its origins. He divided the epidemic up into different periods, but was mainly interested in the moment when the first cases appeared, hoping it would provide the answers he sought. In this initial period from September to November 1888, there were twenty-nine cases among children brought to the attention of the doctors in the area, with sixteen deaths, a typically high mortality rate for this disease. As I said, Bard offers us a case-by-case analysis of the spread of the disease, but I shall leave these individual accounts aside to consider what we can learn from his investigation about a certain 'enlightened' or elite medical community's perception of the disease and its outbreaks.

One important element that emerges from Bard's account of the spread of diphtheria in Oullins concerns the issue of therapeutic intervention, or rather the lack of it. It seems that doctors felt they could do little when called to homes stricken by the disease. The most active measure involved the hospitalization of the afflicted children (or adults), especially on the diphtheria ward of the *Charité* hospital in Lyon. This ward was under the charge of François Rabot, an important figure in the local history of diphtheria, and we will return later to his handling of the disease before and especially after the introduction of serotherapy. It is perhaps surprising that doctors didn't intervene more directly and radically when called to examine children in their homes, but experience had no doubt taught them that there was little they could do. The relationship with the hospital is interesting, as it suggests that for diseases like diphtheria it had already become an important therapeutic alternative – especially when the prognosis was poor – even before the introduction of serotherapy. While this remains a difficult point to prove, the orientation towards specialized services suggests that the generally acknowledged rise in credibility of hospitals depended on more than a series of technological advances.[13]

Epidemics, Hygiene and the Multiplicity of Therapeutic Techniques before Serotherapy

The analysis of the diphtheria outbreak in Oullins offered by Bard is in line with Bruno Latour's argument concerning the 'pasteurization' of France. In his *War and Peace of the Microbes*, Latour argues that it was Pasteur's mobilization, or annexation, of the existing networks of doctors working more traditionally on questions of hygiene that permitted him and his successors to establish their germ theory so widely and so rapidly in France.[14] Indeed, Bard's hunt for the cause of the diphtheria outbreak nicely illustrates the alliance between microbiology and hygiene. He points to poor hygiene as the most likely background cause of the epidemic, notably the presence of fowl and goats in the vicinity of the school, as well as the recent surfacing of the roads in the neighbourhood using ballast drawn from the polluted Rhône river.[15] Another prime *hygienic* suspect was the Yzeron, a stream carrying local sewage that flowed into the Rhône at Oullins. While Bard found the roadworks to be a particularly interesting potential cause of the contagion, he eventually settled for something else, something more in line with the microbial age in which he was living, as the driving force behind the epidemic. In the end, his main positive argument was that the patients themselves had served as vectors for the germ responsible for the disease – leaving the origin of the epidemic unexplained. Paradoxically, he attributed the cause of the public health problem to those who had survived the disease, since they remained contagious for around a month, while those who died took their infectious material with them to the grave. Bard's attention was attracted to the school as a particularly 'promiscuous' environment, although he concluded that it was not the classroom itself that was the culprit because the 'lateral juxtaposition' of the children did not favour contagion. For him, the privileged sites for propagation were the playground and the school entrance where children circulated freely, providing propitious conditions for contamination.[16]

As I have already mentioned, a number of the children who contracted diphtheria during the epidemic at Oullins were sent to the *Charité* hospital in Lyon for treatment. Thus, it's worth considering the contemporary practices in such hospitals, in Paris as well as in the provinces. Looking at reports from hospitals, we see a much more interventionist approach than was the case at Oullins, although different places favoured different regimes, depending on the preferences of the doctor in charge of the diphtheria ward. Tracheotomy, following its promotion by Bretonneau, had become widespread, notably to prevent suffocation by the membrane that formed in the throat, a characteristic of diphtheria as

a clinical condition. In the 1880s, tracheotomy was replaced or at least comple-
mented by 'intubation' using a whole range of specialized surgical equipment.
The O'Dwyer tube enjoyed particular success, and was used early on in Lyon.
Nevertheless, it seems that by the 1890s, Rabot, in his diphtheria ward at the
Hospices civils, was trying to limit the use of intubation as much as possible due
to infections associated with its use. Thus, he preferred to use opium and topical
disinfection applied directly to the membrane in the hope that young patients
would recover before any more radical (surgical) intervention was needed. In a
medical thesis defended in Paris in 1893 (again, just before the introduction of
the serotherapy), Eugène Aschkinazi presented a survey of current treatments of
diphtheria. In essence, his presentation involved variations on the same theme,
namely the topical disinfection of the membrane (with adjuvant use of surgery),
and he took the opportunity of reviewing the disinfectants to promote his own
preferred product, 'stérésol'.[17]

Thus, we can observe a variety of non-standardized therapeutic practices used
to treat diphtheria, each heavily dependent on the doctor in charge. This being
said, a large number seemed to have involved using a favoured topical disinfect-
ant combined with tracheotomy or intubation in cases of imminent suffocation.
The hospital treatment of diphtheria would change relatively rapidly following
the introduction of serotherapy, although it did not represent as radical a break
with past practices as one might imagine.

The Serum Arrives in Lyon and the Practice of Serotherapy on the Hospital Ward

Emile Roux's presentation of the success he had enjoyed in Paris using the serum
to treat diphtheria at the *Hôpital des enfants malades* was quickly transmitted
around France, including Lyon.[18] While from the outset the newspaper *Le Figaro*
enjoyed a privileged relationship to the French diphtheria serum, other newspapers were quick to reprint its stories. Indeed, *Le Figaro*'s front-page story of
Roux's announcement at the international hygiene conference held in Budapest
was reprinted and commented upon in Lyon's *Le Salut Public* on 7 September
1894. The optimistic picture of the treatment already offered by Roux and *Le
Figaro* was reproduced in the *Salut Public*:

> As for its use, nothing could be simpler, with a single injection almost always being
> sufficient. M. Roux has never given more than two injections to any child with diph-
> theria. He injects 20 cubic centimetres in one shot under the skin at the side (of the
> abdomen); straight away the temperature drops and the false membranes that suf-
> focate the patient stop growing within twenty-four hours, and detach after thirty-six,
> and the bacillus disappears from the throat.[19]

Bearing in mind the high rate of mortality (particularly among young children) of a typical epidemic like the one at Oullins, this treatment must have seemed like a miraculous breakthrough. Nevertheless, more than a month passed before the first doctor used the serum to treat diphtheria in Lyon. This doctor was François Rabot, the head of the diphtheria ward at the *Charité* hospital, part of Lyon's *Hospices civils*. In December 1894, he reported his experience with the serum to Lyon's Medical Society. Like the wider public, he had been alerted to the existence of the serum by the news reports of Roux's presentation in Budapest, and had initially tried to obtain the treatment directly from the Pasteur Institute in Paris. But like many of his colleagues, his request was also denied. Coupled with the inflated promotion of the serum, this rejection spawned a certain bitterness that was probably widespread among specialists outside Paris. This is what Rabot had to say about the experience:

> I cannot say anything about the serum from the Pasteur Institute because I have never had any. I cannot, however, remain silent concerning the curious situation in which provincial doctors find themselves. There is now an infallible remedy for diphtheria, but this remedy can only be used in Paris.[20]

Thus, it wasn't until 15 October 1894 that Rabot was able to use the serum on the diphtheria ward of the *Charité* to treat his first patient, the two-year-old Jacques Cohen, whom he injected with Behring's serum manufactured by Meister, Lucius and Brüning in Hoechst.[21] Closer to Geneva than to Paris, Lyon had received its first batches of serum via Switzerland. But Rabot was able to obtain only limited quantities, and he complained that he could not apply the treatment regime he would have liked before the end of the year due to the scarcity and cost of the serum. From his report, we know that he was already able to perform microbiological diagnoses on site. A sister on the ward – the hospital was, like most, operated by a religious order – was apparently particularly good at taking samples of the membrane; and Brother Seyve served as the head of Rabot's makeshift laboratory, where he cultured and then examined the specimens under the microscope. Based on the results of such diagnoses – often made only after the administration of the serum – Rabot stressed the importance of associated microbes (staphylococcus in particular) in the prognosis. He also pointed out the presence of the *corynebacterium* in the ganglions of those who had died from diphtheria, arguing against a theory of the localization of the *germ* in the false membrane.

In 1894 François Rabot published the first results of the use of the Behring serum in the *Salle Sainte Jeanne* of the *Charité* in Lyon. Between 15 October and 3 December 1894, he had treated seventeen cases of sore throat (he uses the general term '*angine*' as opposed to '*croup*') and eight of them died.[22] Nevertheless, delving into the details of the cases, Rabot concluded that using the serum had resulted in a mortality rate of only 34 per cent, which compared favourably with his estimation of a prior rate of around 50 per cent. While not effusive (perhaps because of his initial assessment of the serum as an *'infallible cure'*), Rabot still considered this change to be a dramatic improvement. In his conclusion, he emphasized the shortage of serum that limited the treatment he could offer.[23] Indeed, he seems to have only treated the most serious cases at first, and could not always give the patients as much serum as he would have liked.

Thanks to a medical thesis from 1895, we have a more complete picture of the treatment at this time. Its author, Pierre Patet, offers a certain amount of information on every case of suspected diphtheria treated by serotherapy at the *Charité* in Lyon between October 1894 and March 1895.[24] I now want to turn to the data on the first hundred cases to see what it can tell us about the early use of the serum in Lyon.

During this initial period, Rabot used serum from three different sources: the Behring serum from Hoechst (in versions of 600 or 1,000 units), the Roux serum from Paris and the Arloing serum produced in Lyon. The introduction of these different sera corresponds with their availability in Lyon, with the Paris serum being used for the first time at the end of December 1894, and the Lyon serum in early February 1895. Nevertheless, while these dates mark the beginning of the use of the new product, they do not signal the end of the use of the others. Rabot remained particularly faithful to the Behring serum, which he continued to use regularly throughout this period.

Looking at the reports of the cases, we see that the Behring No 1 serum (600 immunization units) was used in quantities varying from ten to sixty cubic centimetres (hereafter cc), without any evident criteria for this modulation. The only indications that emerge from the brief case reports are that smaller quantities were reserved for very young babies and that the administration of serum was repeated when the circumstances were judged to be particularly serious. There were similar variations in the quantities of the Parisian serum (from ten to forty cc), with larger amounts usually given over two days. The choice between the Roux or the Behring (or the Arloing) serum does not appear to have been based on any strategy, although the use of the different strengths of serum (Berhing no 1 versus Behring no. 2 – 1,000 immunization units) was once again a decision that depended upon the perceived clinical severity of the disease at the time the treatment was started.

In his own report of 1894, Rabot also recounts the prophylactic use of one cc doses of serum amongst the families of diphtheria victims. Overall, then, we can conclude that there was no fixed protocol for the use of serum at the *Charité* in Lyon, and that the quantities of serum administered varied significantly as a function of each individual case. Indeed, the use of the serum was, I would suggest, determined by the twin factors of clinical judgement and clinical experimentation. While the clinicians now had at their disposal a rudimentary microbiological laboratory attached to the ward, the length of time required to make the microbial cultures meant that the choice to use serum preceded the results of any such tests. Thus, while serotherapy was promoted based on its specific effectiveness against a well-identified '*diphtheria microbe*', it was difficult to integrate the new laboratory technique with the treatment and so treatment went ahead independently of the results of the analyses.

Thus we can observe an increasingly standard therapeutic approach to diphtheria (the use of serum), albeit varying considerably with respect to the details of its application. Although I do not have the complete statistics, it appears that the use of serum was becoming the standard treatment for suspected cases of diphtheria from the time serum became readily available at the beginning of 1895. Initially however, serotherapy did not simply replace other treatments, but instead supplemented pre-existing regimes, with '*tubage*' or '*intubation*' continuing to be used regularly even after the adoption of serum.

When we look in detail at how the serum was administered, we see that the practice of serotherapy was far from uniform, notably in terms of the quantity of serum administered. Nor was this variety in the use of the serum restricted to Lyon. The situation as reported in Le Mans, for example, looks very similar, with doses of the Paris serum varying between ten and sixty cc for each patient during a similar period. This approach is an example of what I would term 'clinical standardization', i.e. a consensus around the general approach to treatment – in this case serotherapy – combined with a certain variety in its application. The form that this approach assumed is largely due to the primacy of clinical judgement in determining the details of an appropriate treatment. While the explicit justification might involve differences between individual patients (their susceptibility to diphtheria as well as to the treatment), the underlying reason was a belief in the reliability of the clinician's judgement born of his specialist experience with the disease in question.

While one might object that what I am describing as clinical standardization was no standardization at all, I believe that this question can be usefully turned around. What can we learn about standardization from this type of approach? Standardization always leaves a place for variability even when the intention behind the procedures is to establish unbending uniformity. A more flexible notion of standardization that accounts for variety from the outset is perhaps closer to the reality in most contexts where some kind of standardization is sought, particularly in the domain of living organisms. While there is a general tendency to impose industrial models on any discussion of what counts as standardization, it might be useful to broaden the sense of standardization and in turn rethink the nature and goals of industrial standardization itself.

While, as I have suggested, the variation of serum use resulted from the clinical assessment of the patient and the disease, there also seems to have been a certain amount of more or less deliberate experimentation. Thus, for example, in Le Mans, when an intern mistakenly injected twenty cc instead of ten cc of serum into a baby, the positive result was reported with some interest. Rather than a source of embarrassment, this mistake was instead presented as a source of useful information about the serum's application. At the beginning of this 'heroic' period of serotherapy, the lack of serum could also lead to extremely experimental forms of treatment by default. When Dr Bonafoux contracted diphtheria in the course of his medical practice in Montpellier, he was injected with the blood of a child recovering from the disease before finally being able to receive treatment with the Behring serum from Hoechst.[25]

The Acceptability and Criticism of the Serum in the Lyon Medical Community

We have already seen how quick the Lyon medical press was to publish the results of the serotherapy. They also kept the public informed about Lyon's efforts to produce its own serum. This project was undertaken by the above-mentioned Saturnin Arloing, a professor at both the Faculty of Medicine and the Faculty of Pharmacy in Lyon, who had been introduced to the practice of microbiology through Emile Roux's courses in Paris. Indeed, it was the *Société des Sciences médicales de Lyon* (Lyon Medical Sciences Society) that, on 12 November 1894, initiated the subscription to pay for Lyon's own serum production. The initiative was also supported by city authorities, with Gabriel Roux, the doctor in charge of public health services in Lyon, recommending local production in a report of 6 November. In this report, Roux reassured the mayor, who was himself a prominent doctor, that the serum posed no risk.[26] He reasoned that the risk associated with vaccines based on attenuated bacteria came from the living pathogen itself, but that the serum contained no such pathogens. The fact that a toxin rather than any bacteria (living, attenuated or killed) was used to induce immunity meant that the serum derived from the immunized horse was safe. As so often in these debates, the example used to illustrate potential dangers was Koch's tuberculine. The failure of this treatment for tuberculosis and the possibility that it might have aggravated the condition or even killed some of the patients who received it cast a pall of suspicion over any similar microbiological products.[27]

Reviewing the local medical journal *Lyon Médical* for 1895, we can identify two distinct phases of the reaction to serotherapy. The initial publications simply informed readers (mostly doctors) about who was producing the serum and where the doctors could obtain it. During this early period, the journal also published upbeat reports from the diphtheria ward at the *Charité*, first by François Rabot and then by one of his interns on the ward, who was even more positive in his assessment of the therapy. But in May 1895 the journal published a long three-part article by a certain Dr Zolot-Nisky entitled the *Revers de la médaille* (the other side of the coin).[28] Zolot-Nisky argued not that the serum was ineffective or particularly dangerous, but rather that it had been overestimated and had benefited from a biased interpretation of the clinical evidence. He stressed the reports of accidents thought to have been provoked by the serum, and pointed out all the various reasons for thinking that the drop in mortality rates proclaimed throughout Europe and the United States might be as much the product of the new bacteriological diagnosis and the interest around the serum as of any therapeutic action of the serum itself. The apparent motivation for this publication was a traditional conception of medicine and the expertise of the doctor. Zolot-Nisky was concerned about what he saw as a therapy imposed by public enthusiasm rather than by the force of clinical judgement. Furthermore, the use of the serum was for him another example of the modern tendency to treat the disease rather than the patient – a play on the words *maladie* and *malade* that does not translate into English.[29] Thus we see the same logic of the independence of clinical judgement that we have just been discussing emerge in a different form. Rather than insisting on the modulation of the treatment in light of clinical judgement, Zolot-Nisky suggests that serotherapy be dropped altogether.

It is interesting that the Lyon Society of Medicine publicized such scepticism at the very moment the city began its own serum production. Indeed, Saturnin Arloing started immunizing four horses at the end of 1894, and by February 1895 two were producing anti-diphtheria serum. In February 1895, the serum was available for sale at the pharmacy of the *Hôtel-Dieu* hospital at the price of five francs per phial. But Zolot-Nisky was not the only doctor to raise doubts about the serum. Arloing himself published an article in 1895 which suggested that the treatment might represent a risk to patients. Informed by his experience of immunizing horses in order to produce the serum in Lyon, Arloing published his observations concerning this process.[30] Here, he assessed the paralysis of horses and the property of the diphtheria culture, like tuberculine, to reveal the presence of earlier infections. While it is a little surprising to see the producer of the Lyon serum raise doubts about the safety of his own product, the critical articles of Arloing and Zolot-Nisky do not seem to have dampened medical enthusiasm for this new therapy.

Conclusion

The serum to treat diphtheria represents a landmark in microbiology-based therapeutics. In terms of the theory and technology of production, it comprises a double intervention, requiring first the immunization of an animal against a specific disease and the subsequent extraction of its blood as altered by the first intervention (which sets it apart from *classic* opotherapy, a therapeutic approach based on the extraction and preparation of *unaltered* animal organs). The absence of a clear chemical basis for the serum's therapeutic action meant that no '*active ingredient*' could be isolated and weighed and so the expected therapeutic effect was determined using a guinea-pig/toxin system.[31] It is easy to be seduced by the sophistication of this system that enabled the serum producers to put precise numerical values – the 'immunization power' – on their phials of serum and to see it as a precursor of modern treatment protocols based on standardized pharmaceutical products. Nevertheless, when we look at the clinical use of the serum, we see that the culture of standardization that developed alongside serum production – what I have termed industrial standardization – was not mirrored in the hospital wards. The attending physicians adjusted treatment in accordance with their clinical judgement of the particular case at hand, using different quantities and different strengths of serum as they saw fit. The operators were not interchangeable, as clinical judgement was essentially personal and not shared. While this judgement could be learned, it could not be imposed; and this clinical logic resisted rationalization, let alone standardization. Thus, a physician who replaced another on a children's ward was unlikely to make the same decisions concerning the use and quantity of serum as his predecessor, even when confronted with very similar cases.

Nevertheless, we can observe an increasing standardization in the global therapeutic approach to diphtheria that placed the serum in the first line of treatment. This rapid integration of the serum as the treatment of choice is easy to see in the hospital records, and it is mirrored by the proliferation of microbiological investigations aimed at identifying the germ responsible for the disease. Thus, we see the biological (as opposed to clinical) aspect of the diagnosis reinforced by the biological medicine that was being used. While the particular form of the serum's uptake in the hospital probably owed something to the innovative nature of the treatment, the most radical effects of its biological origins were to be found in the production process. Nevertheless, while our attention as historians is more readily drawn to the functioning and effects of industrial standardization, the phenomenon that I have termed clinical standardization is an important element in the constitution of modern medicine.

2 BIOLOGICS IN THE COLONIES: EMILE PERROT, KOLA NUTS AND THE INDUSTRIAL REORDERING OF PHARMACY[1]

Jean-Paul Gaudillière

The historiography of twentieth-century pharmaceuticals has, for a long time, shown a strong bias in favour of narratives that focus on the alliance between chemistry and industry, on the generalization of molecular screening and on the trajectories of synthetic drugs. Nonetheless, recent work in the field reminds us that therapeutic preparations based on biological entities, i.e. animals' bodies and plants, dominated the world of pharmacy until the Second World War, that is to say, long after industrial specialties had begun to flood the drug market.[2] Assumptions that equate the rise of chemicals with the industrialization of therapeutic agents are therefore of little use if one seeks to understand the dynamics of drug innovation and standardization that characterized the first half of the twentieth century.

The period was indeed a time of major transformation in pharmacy. This reordering involved the gradual marginalization of the professional regime of drug invention, production and use – a regime associated with the figure of the pharmacist as an expert in *materia medica*, i.e. in all the substances and remedies deemed professionally legitimate and included in the national pharmacopoeia, and which the pharmacist knew how to prepare. As the number of ready-made specialties grew, this pharmacist was slowly replaced by two figures: that of the apothecary turned retailer, and that of the (much more prestigious) industrial entrepreneur, who owned factories that, increasingly, were coupled with in-house laboratories. The rise of biologics, meaning the growing emphasis placed on animal or plant preparations as a source of specific, highly potent, physio-logically tested 'natural' entities, was a means of adjusting this transformation process, a way of preserving and modernizing *materia medica* using practices of mechanization and standardization. Although less visible than hormones or vitamins, medicinal plants, or better put their extracts, were major mid-century biologics. They had become raw materials in the production of scientific pills within the larger group of natural therapeutic agents, including hormones, vita-mins, sera and vaccines.

This process elicited more than a little opposition, resistance and open conflict. These tensions focused not only on the economic rewards of local pharmacists whose competencies and revenues were reduced. They also revolved around the very definition of pharmaceutical science, around questions of what comprised good remedies, how drugs should be sought, characterized, produced and marketed. Considering this profound reorganization, the perspective adopted in the following chapter is that biologics surfaced as a major category and peculiar way of inventing, producing, selling and regulating drugs during the first half of the twentieth century; they were signposts and consequences of pharmacy's industrial reordering. Biologics were not just therapeutics 'made' out of biological things. They were technical objects, at once socially and culturally associated with nature and at the same time elaborated through industrial mass-preparation. Their importance before the 1960s (thus before the advent of biotechnological and biochemical biologicals) is certainly rooted in the relations that sera, hormones or enzymes – these 'new' products of nature bearing the aura of frontier science – maintained with physiology and the experimental life sciences (hence the strong consensus regarding their therapeutic potency). But the visibility of biologics – and this is the hypothesis being defended in this chapter – also derived from the fact that the category included old and new plant extracts, thus creating a porous boundary between the passing professional order of pharmacy, with its emphasis on local preparations, and the industrial order centred on standardized specialties.

To illustrate this double status of biologics, the chapter follows the trajectory of kola extracts in France in order to address and discuss the advent of biologics and this industrial reordering. Long before they became the sort of food supplements we all know from of their use in Coca-Cola, kola extracts surfaced in most European pharmacopeia as plant-based preparations, as sources of alkaloids, as anti-fatigue medications, as stimulants containing caffeine and, more than anything else, as valuable products of the French colonies.

Kola, *Materia Medica* and Industrial Mixtures

Kola extracts entered the French Codex when it was revised in 1908. Unlike the hormones or vitamins of the interwar period, they were not made of simple and purified entities. Like most plant derivatives of *materia medica*, they were complex mixtures. Turning kola into a drug was less of an ontological problem than a question of the practical and social arrangements involved in inventing, producing, using and selling the extracts. In France, kola preparations – like hundreds of herbal compositions – were embedded in a professional world that included the Codex, *materia medica* laboratories in the faculties of pharmacy, multiple techniques for manipulating plants and composing formulations and, last but not least, a legal framework that excluded the possibility of patenting pharmaceuticals.

Considering the trajectories of hormones or vitamins, one might think that the industrialization of kola extracts that occurred alongside their adoption into the Codex was predicated upon the mobilization of chemical knowledge. Chemistry was actually mobilized in two different ways: first, as a global analysis of composition that focused on general categories of plant chemistry (for instance oils or alkaloids); and second, as a list of 'active ingredients', i.e. isolated combinations whose potency had been tested in animals or humans. However, the case of Madaus – the most important German firm producing medicinal plant extracts in the 1920s and 1930s – illustrates that industrializing *materia medica* did not necessarily imply the disappearance of preparations and mixtures or the abandonment of the search for pure – if not synthesized – chemicals.[3] Madaus's most widely advertised product was 'Teep', a plant powder mixed with sugar and used to make pills in an entirely mechanized process. In the eyes of the firm's owners and scientists, its value resided precisely in the fact that it preserved most, if not all of the plants' native components.[4]

How were the tensions between isolation and combination, specificity and multiple effects, preparation and mass-production managed in the case of kola extracts? The French literature on kola nuts and their physiological properties expanded from the 1880s onward. One early promoter of their use was the navy pharmacist Edouard Heckel, professor of botany at the Faculty of Sciences in Marseille and director of the local Colonial Institute and Colonial Museum.[5] Heckel's first paper on kola was published in 1883 in the *Journal de Pharmacie*.[6] It was predicated – as were subsequent publications – upon the supply of commercial nuts obtained from merchants associated with the Marseille Chamber of Commerce, which was the main sponsor of his Museum and Institute.[7]

Heckel's studies linked the kola nuts with what was then a major focus of physiological research: the question of fatigue. Building on the multiple testimonies of *voyageurs*, who argued that people in sub-Saharan Africa used to chew kola nuts as stimulants that facilitated long marches and physical work, he advocated the value of kola preparations as energy savers, as a means to avoid both fatigue and nervous exhaustion. These remarkable properties were traced back to the composition of the nuts, i.e. to their richness in alkaloids, especially caffeine. In Heckel's eyes, extracts of the kola nuts could prove to be useful in the treatment of a wide range of conditions, including chronic diseases, convalescence, neurasthenia and other psychic disturbances, as well as intellectual burnout. But the most important application remained physical fatigue. In order to investigate the effects of kola, Heckel relied on good relations with the military, as Marey had done before him while working on the physiology and visualization of movement.

Accordingly, Heckel's main essay on the drug, published in 1893, reported dozens of experiments conducted with the kola biscuits he had invented and supplied to French soldiers.[8] His evidence rested on the testimonies of officers participating in experiments. The experiments consisted of little more than feeding the troops with the biscuits, observing their physical performances and tacitly comparing them with routine situations and normal nutrition.[9] For instance, a certain captain Rodel explained with a clear note of enthusiasm that:

> A few officers and myself tested the biscuit. I took one biscuit at 11 am without any previous food. I rode my horse, participated in the unit's maneuvers, wrote, etc. ... without any sign of fatigue, any sensation of hunger and any uneasiness. Far from that, I felt a sort of general and constant well-being. I am convinced that this food can provide many benefits to the troops as well as to the officers if it is adopted and if soldiers are permitted to eat it while waiting for more substantial nourishment. It would be desirable – of course with proper financial compensation – for Dr. Heckel to provide us with larger quantities of the biscuits in order to conduct assays with the whole regiment during our garrison maneuvers. Signed J. Rodel and Tanchot.[10]

The question of purification and composition was an essential dimension of this early work. One typical controversy brought Heckel into conflict with the German pharmacist E. Knebel.[11] Looking at the two main alkaloids of the nuts, caffeine and kola red, they adopted divergent interpretations. Knebel argued in his doctoral thesis (1892) that kola red is inactive and that all the effects of the drug were attributable to caffeine. For his part, Heckel explained that the nuts contained at least two active substances, kola red and caffeine, and that their combination was an important dimension of the global and specific effects of the nuts.

In his responses to Knebel, Heckel also emphasized laboratory experiments. These experiments mobilized Marey's graphic method in order to objectify and visualize the temporal dynamics of muscular activity and the gradual appearance of fatigue.[12] Heckel liked to cite a series of experiments conducted by a certain Dr Marie, another fellow of the Marseille Faculty of Science, who contrasted the curves of the muscular activity of volunteers lifting weights after ingesting caffeine with those obtained after ingesting kola powder or isolated kola red. The former revealed an initial increase of work followed by rapid decline due to fatigue, while the latter showed both an increase of work and a slower decline, thus suggesting a much broader enhancement of performance.

Summarizing the inscriptions, Dr Marie drew the following table to support the idea of an autonomous and specific effect of kola red on the muscles (see Figure 2.1): A: Normal – Slightly concave, regular decline; B: With coffein – High contractions in the first phase, rapid decline, more concave than the preceeding, C: With kola – High contractions, straight line, regular decline; D: With kola red – High contractions, S-shape, much longer than with caffeine. Endorsing these results, Heckel recomputed the enhancement effect in order to take into account the amount of energy provided by the various stimulants. He thus reinforced the contrast between kola and caffeine, leading to the idea that caffeine

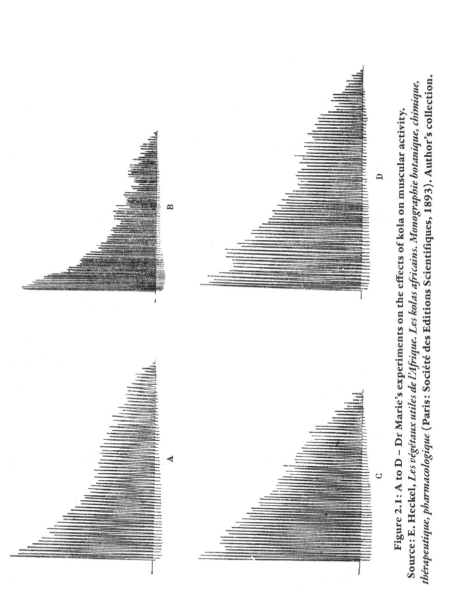

Figure 2.1: A to D – Dr Marie's experiments on the effects of kola on muscular activity.

Source: E. Heckel, *Les végétaux utiles de l'Afrique. Les kolas africains. Monographie botanique, chimique, thérapeutique, pharmacologique* **(Paris : Société des Editions Scientifiques, 1893). Author's collection.**

and kola red not only had different and parallel effects, but also that the whole powder could bring forth positive interactions and indeed synergies.

Ultimately, Heckel showed himself to be an industrious entrepreneur and a tireless promoter of kola: he actually managed to market a pharmaceutical specialty called '*Kola du Docteur Heckel*'. It was sold by a newly created company in which he seems to have had a direct financial stake.[13]

The introduction of kola into the Codex cannot, however, be explained solely on the basis of Heckel's research and the associated sales of kola preparations. To be adopted into the Codex, the drug had to exhibit promising effects. Furthermore, its mode of preparation had to be explained and a list of active ingredients and – eventually – the protocols for controlling composition and quality provided. Being a navy pharmacist and a colonial botanist working at the periphery of the main centres of pharmaceutical expertise, Heckel could hardly provide the requisite professional legitimacy. Kola's pharmaceutical *lettres de noblesse* were gained through the work of Emile Perrot and his colleagues at the laboratory of *materia medica* at the Paris Faculty of Pharmacy.[14]

Trained as a pharmacist and as a botanist (he completed a doctorate on the anatomy of plants from the *Gentianacea* family), Perrot started to work on kola after assuming responsibility for local courses of *materia medica* – replacing Prof. Planchon in 1900. Perrot's interest in kola originated in exchanges with the botanist Auguste Chevalier, whom Perrot had met during his botanical doctoral research. Chevalier was the foremost expert in colonial botany at the Paris Museum of Natural History, a specialist in plants from French West Africa, of their classification, as well as of their uses.[15]

Working together on the botany of kola trees, Chevalier and Perrot proposed a new classification that corresponded more closely with the categories used in West Africa. Their scheme was not based on the structure of sexual organs (as was customary in good Linean botany), but on the anatomy of the nuts themselves, distinguishing between kola trees having two as opposed to four or six cotyledons. One motive for such a classification was indeed that it matched the composition of the nuts, since – as Perrot documented – the caffeine content of trees with two cotyledons was much higher than that of trees bearing nuts with more numerous cotyledons, even if variability was quite high.[16]

There was more to this choice than mere analysis of composition. Perrot used the kola extracts as an exemplary case of what he called 'pharmacognosy', namely the integration of botany, pharmacology and chemistry in order to make new drugs out of plant resources, to optimize plant supply and to control the quality of extracts' preparation.[17] Thus, his laboratory didn't just investigate the composition of kola nuts, but also linked studies of composition with the development and standardization of kola conservation and extraction processes.

The main experimental output of the work performed by Perrot and his main collaborator, the pharmacist Armand Goris, was indeed the isolation of kolatin as a substitute for kola red. According to Goris and Perrot, the natural composition of active ingredients, i.e. the kola biological, was a complex comprised of caffeine and a phenol-derivative, kolatin itself. They claimed that kolatin was found only in fresh and well-conserved nuts, whereas what had been previously studied in aged and altered nuts was kola red, a less active by-product formed during the oxidation of the links between caffeine and the phenol component. In other words, kola red was kolatin without caffeine. The isolation of kolatin was a typical achievement of the pharmacists' extraction culture. As the Paris *material medica* experts wrote:

Fresh Kola nuts are opened, divided and kept in boiling alcohol (95°) for half an hour. This alcoholic solution is gathered while the kola nuts – in which the enzymes have been destroyed – are reduced to powder and treated twice more with analogous quantities of alcohol. The three solutions are gathered, filtered and distillated until one obtains a thick, sticky preparation ... This 'colature' is then introduced into a vial with chloroform. The latter dissolves the free caffeine, as well as a resinous substance. The operation is repeated three or four times until the chloroform no longer acquires a yellow colour. The entire extract is kept in a cold place for a few days until crystals appear floating on the surface and forming a dense white mass ... This cake is dried with sulfuric acid, turned into powder and treated with boiling chloroform to eliminate the remaining caffeine. It is then dissolved into boiling alcohol (30°) and left to crystallize in the presence of sulfuric acid.[18]

The complexity of kolatin was not perceived as a problem or a motive for further chemical inquiry and isolation. Instead, Perrot and Goris considered the combination as essential to the value of kola extracts. Replacing Heckel's human experimentation with laboratory animals, they concluded:

Kolatin is not a potent toxic. It may be injected in quantities as high as one gram per kilo without causing severe disturbances. In contrast to caffeine, its action on muscular contraction is nil: curves are not modified in shape or maximum level of muscular activity, even when high dosages are employed ... Its action on the nervous system does not result in well characterized reactions, one only notes longer periods of hyper excitability ... In warm-blooded animals, kolatin slightly slows their heartbeat, reinforces their energy and induces a slight increase in blood pressure. These phenomena last for varying periods of time, depending on the dosage ... This preliminary study was indispensable to a discussion of the combination of caffeine and kolatin. It is important to take into account that these two substances have partially antagonistic effects, both on muscles and on the central nervous system. It is worth noting that this antagonism may result in an inhibition of the violent contractions induced by a high dose of caffeine (especially affecting the heart) and which constitute the main contra-indication when using caffeine for therapeutic purposes.[19]

In other words, the value of the composition was not merely experimental; it also produced physiological effects and therefore affected both the definition of quality and the construction of a market. Focusing on kolatin's association with caffeine, Perrot began to argue that most nuts available on the French market and most extracts sold by pharmaceutical firms were actually without much value, both physiologically and economically, since they contained red kola rather than the combination.

The argument was a blow to kola producers. After the publication of Chevalier's and Perrot's book on kola, firms like Chalas started to advertise their preparation as 'Living Kola', alluding to the absence of oxidation and claiming that their '*Kolatinés*' were dissolved before any production of caffeine. Other producers, like Midy, did not adopt the idea of using only fresh nuts or talk about kolatin and its relation to caffeine, but instead began to advertise kola mixtures rather than pure kola red, advocating preparations 'containing ... caffeine, theobromine, tannin and RED KOLA, which is the most active ingredient in kola nuts and which is transformed into caffeine through the action of gastric juice'.[20]

Perrot and Goris not only provided the market with new facts about mixtures, they also sought to scale up and optimize the preparation using a standard protocol for sterilizing fresh nuts, a way of preserving the nuts' constituents by inhibiting the oxidation process.[21] The process involved two stages. The first stage was a simple sterilization at 110°C, which produced nuts that could be dried and powdered, thereby retaining their white colour, a decisive sign of their freshness and integrity. Although sufficient for most commercial preparation, this sterilization could – before industrial use (whether to make pills, syrups or kola wines) – be supplemented with a cold alcoholic treatment (a contemporary technique used in industry to stabilize plant extracts). This second step could also be used to isolate kolatin, benefiting from its binding with caffeine. As Goris and Perrot put it,

> The medical interest in this discovery is that kolatin displays the most interesting pharmacological properties as it antagonizes caffeine ... The action of the kolatin-caffeine complex remains to be studied, but one can already understand the action of fresh kola nuts. Although we cannot be sure to have prepared the complete active substance of the fresh nuts, we may state that the physiological extracts of kola (obtained by means of sterilization) are a decisive improvement over all pharmacological preparations in current use.[22]

The sterilization process was adapted to other plants by Goris and Perrot, who unified the two stages in a procedure using either aqueous or alcoholic vapours in a modified sterilization apparatus that avoided condensation on the inside upper surface. Perrot and Goris then published a series of articles presenting their innovation and discussing the production of pharmaceuticals using medicinal plants. The putative synergy of caffeine and kolatin was thus generalized:

Clinical and physiological observations on medicinal plants have for a long time shown important differences in their mode of action – differences that are related to the type of material employed, i.e. fresh or dried plants, complex mixtures or crystallized active principles extracted from the same plants. *Digitalis*, plants from the *Solanacea* family or Kola are among the best known and most often cited examples.

...

How can we explain such differences? Two explanations are conceivable: 1) The known and isolated active substances represent only a part of the global physiologically active component and one must admit that – in the course of preparation – other principles – important but unknown – have been discarded and left in the residues; 2) In the plant, the active principles are associated with other chemical substances, thus creating complex combinations with new physiological properties. It is not necessary that these other chemicals have themselves a therapeutic action, they may simply act by reinforcing or modifying the action of the principles considered to be the sole active ingredients.[23]

The protocol and the apparatus for the sterilization of fresh plants were patented and the *materia medica* laboratory granted a special license to the firm Dausse, with which Perrot and Goris had collaborated in generalizing the technique.[24]

Dausse thus became the main French producer of plant preparations. The firm had consistently argued that extracts were better than isolated substances and sought to develop a pharmacological and physiological understanding of the value of its own herbal extracts. Following the development and the industrial implementation of the Perrot and Goris process, Dausse changed the definition of its preparations, advertising the production of *intraits* rather than extracts.[25] This new promotional emphasis on the integrity of the plant material echoed Perrot's and Gori's own discourse on the general benefits of sterilization in the most straightforward manner. During the interwar period, Dausse published a comprehensive treatise on medicinal plants. This company-based pharmaceutical compendium was written under the guidance of P. Joanin, a colleague of Perrot. The general introduction explained:

If the present status of science only makes it possible to isolate dubious and unstable active principles, what is the actual meaning of extracts? An extract – if well prepared – is the sum of the active principles of a plant. Unfortunately, a whole generation of physicians has been accustomed to accept as self-evident the idea that isolated active principles are equivalent to the plants just because science has proven able to purify specific substances, sometimes crystallized, and granted them a formula and a structure. This type of chemical medication has replaced the use of extracts ... Such practice is perfect when seeking a very specific goal, the exclusive use of active principles, however, it impoverishes the physician's arsenal, excluding weapons of choice. It is current knowledge that digitalin does not reproduce the action of *Digitalis* extracts, that morphine does not reproduce the action of opium, that quinine does not replace cinchona extracts, that conicine does not calm pains the way a plaster of hemlock extracts can.[26]

Kola: A Colonial Biological

As mentioned above, kola was a colonial rather than a metropolitan product. One paradox of Perrot's deep interest in and engagement with the products of the kola tree was therefore the fact that he had never seen the tree, and depended either on Chevalier or the colonial products' market for his supply of nuts. How did this situation impact the Parisian knowledge of kola and the status of its preparations?

As Chevalier and Perrot constantly reported, kola nuts had been and were still used extensively by people in sub-Saharan and tropical West Africa. The knowledge used in transplanting the nuts to the Paris laboratory was not just botanical, but also ethnographic. Chevalier spent most of the years before the First World War as a botanical expert in French colonial Africa. His experience with local/indigenous knowledge played a central role in the botanical and pharmaceutical design of kola. The most obvious example of this is the classification of kola trees.[27] Chevalier investigated markets in French Guinea, Sudan and Sierra Leone. He learned that morphological differences between the nuts, i.e. having two or more cotyledons, correlated with sharp differences in quality, i.e. taste, duration and intensity of stimulation. He imported this grid into the classification of the kola species mentioned above, creating a strong hierarchy between *Cola nitida* and the other – newly defined – species.

A second, less obvious aspect of the colonial appropriation of indigenous knowledge pertains to the problem of combination and to the isolation of kolatin. Perrot and Goris not only took the fresh African nuts as reference material, but also mobilized the ethnographic observations made by Chevalier in order to stress and legitimize their choice. The monetary value of the nuts on the local markets was thus adopted as an indicator of their biological and pharmacological value. Thus, one strong argument in favour of Perrot's understanding of the oxidative degradation of kola nuts came from the experience of indigenous people, i.e. the great care with which African merchants preserved and transported the nuts:

> To be collected, the fruits must be twisted and pulled out. This must be done shortly before they acquire a green-brownish colour in order to avoid contamination by so-called sangara. A few days later the fruits are opened with a knife, taking care not to damage the nuts themselves, and left outside in a pile. The white-rosy membrane turns brown and disappears. The nuts are washed in order to eliminate the remains of this envelope. They are left three days in water or six to eight days in Orofira leaves. The nuts are then placed in baskets, forming beds separated by layers of Orofira leaves. These baskets are buried in the soil and regularly checked to remove the bad nuts. In this way one can keep good nuts from one harvest to the next and it goes without saying that these reserves are kept secret and carefully guarded by their owners.

For transportation in caravans, the nuts are placed in baskets with large openings, made of bout reed or Calamus stems. These baskets are opened on the top. They measure 60 to 80 cm in length and 25 cm in depth. They contain Orofira leaves, which are also used to separate the nut beds. Once full, each basket contains 25–30 kg of nuts and is carried on the head of a single man.

...

During the march, the baskets are opened every five or six days and the kola nuts are humidified with water that the Dioula men take in their mouth and spit over the nuts. Nuts which look too mature are removed and either discarded or immediately sold.[28]

The First World War radically transformed the status of kola as a colonial biological. During the war, the supply of pharmaceuticals became a strategic issue within the framework of a more general reorganization of the chemical industry provoked by the massive use of chemical warfare agents. In 1917, the government established a special 'office' for chemical products. It soon proposed the creation of a 'committee' in charge of improving the supply of medicinal plants. Established on 22 April 1918, the committee was led by Julien Constantin, professor of culture at the Natural History Museum, with Emile Perrot as the committee's vice-president.[29] The main tasks of the committee were to expand the collection of medicinal plants in the wild and to increase the production of rare cultivated species. Plant collection dominated wartime activities and involved the mobilization of primary schools, their students and teachers in parallel with the use of market incentives to boost the harvest. Although war emergencies vanished, the problem of medicinal plant supply remained part of the reconstruction agenda.

In October 1918, Emile Perrot issued a report of the committee, which stressed the threat posed by the overuse of plant resources and by the growing demand for and costs of imports.[30] The solutions he proposed in order to ease the supply crisis were twofold: improve the quality and the conditions of conservation in order to diminish the quantities used; promote research and experimentation in order to design cultivation protocols and to transform the most needed wild plants into domesticated species and agricultural products. The experience of Dausse was explicitly taken as a model for such industrialization: on the one hand, Dausse had generalized the use of sterilization; on the other hand, the firm had bought a large farm at Etrechy where it was both experimenting on new cultures and mass-producing plants like mint, *Belladonna* or *Datura*.

In 1919, the problem of medicinal plants was readily incorporated into the global modernization programme advocated by the Ministry of Commerce and Industry. A decree of 22 May replaced the wartime committee with a more ambitious, and industry-oriented, *Office National des Matières Premières Végétales pour la Droguerie, la Pharmacie, la Distillerie et la Parfumerie*, which was responsible for all non-food issues of plant supply and production. Emile Perrot was nominated as the Office's Director General.

The Office operated for most of the interwar period. It was officially closed in 1938 after the great depression led to its radical downsizing and transformation into a mere documentation centre in 1932. Under Perrot's directorship, it became a unique forum for 'science, commerce and industry' and defined itself as a 'Society for study, research and propaganda aimed at reorganizing the markets for plant raw materials and extending their production in France and the colonies.'[31] Financial support for the Office came less from the government than from business societies like the *Syndicat Général de la Droguerie*, the *Syndicat des Produits Chimiques* and the *Groupement des Producteurs de Quinine*.

Such partnership could have marginalized medicinal plants in favour of industrial raw materials such as lavender and other essential oils. But it didn't. During the first ten years, the Office promoted the production of medicinal plants in the field. Support for direct collection was abandoned and replaced with 'propaganda' about the main plants used in French pharmacies, their botanical traits and uses, as well as evaluations of need and market status. To these ends, the Office organized conferences, produced two films, distributed monographs on the flora of specific departments, and finally edited a series of posters and images to be distributed to teachers and students. Among the brochures' titles one finds: *Le Comité départemental de l'Aveyron aux ramasseurs de plantes*; *Faisons des plantes médicinales*; *Les plantes médicinales dans le département de l'Aude*; *Notice sur la récolte et la culture des plantes médicinales et à essences en Provence*; and so forth. The Office's publications also included monographs on specific products: *La Lavande*; *L'hydrastis canadensis*; *Les Menthes cultivées*; *Les plantes à thymol, Culture de la rhubarbe francaise*; to name but a few.

The Office's greatest efforts were actually directed toward the production of a dozen species, based on pharmaceutical, agricultural and market-based evaluations. The plants that were chosen already had records of cultivation and there was no attempt at radically new domestication. Instead, the Office supported assays designed to improve the yield and acculturation of species already in mass production, like mint, and sponsored the introduction of a new British variety. But Perrot concentrated his efforts on species in high demand and in danger of extinction, like *Aconite* or *Digitalis*, or which had to be imported, like *Hydrastis canadensis* or saffron. However, since the Office had no infrastructure of its own, the logic of the assays was strongly influenced by the proposals of firms, farmers and departmental committees. For example lavender, although it was not really a case that called for emergency intervention, became the target of numerous initiatives and experiments, beginning with the production of a major monograph that sought to evaluate and standardize culture methods. *Digitalis* represents another example of such local dynamics. Its cultivation was considered highly problematic because only a few varieties were fit for extraction and, more importantly, because cultivation seemed to result in an inevitable loss of active principles once the plant was taken out of its natural ecosystem. In the 1920s, *Digitalis* thus became a major topic of investigation within Perrot's service and prompted the Office to create its own *Commission de la digitale*. The Commission supported experimental cultures in the Alps that drew on Dausse's financial means to study the relationships between the use of fertilizers, the nature of the soils and the concentration of alkaloids in the plant material.

In the case of *Hydrastis canadensis*, a plant cultivated in the United States and used to treat inflammation and eye infections, and which had recently been introduced into the European pharmacopoeia, the Office estimated that

> there are good motives to encourage its cultivation and production since consumption is important and cultivation requires sophisticated procedures, which render the plants more costly ... The Office will therefore help all those who are ready to implement rational experimentation provided they start with a minimum of ten acres.[32]

In practice, experiments remained limited; the main promoters being Dausse and the Vilmorin seed company. The most innovative dimension of the Office's activities was its colonial policy. It was embedded in the Third Republic and its ethos of *mise en valeur*, which redefined the exploitation of plants in colonial Africa in terms of agricultural production rather than the nineteenth-century policy of collections and forest destruction. Accordingly, the Office promoted: (1) a more rational production of local varieties (especially those of commercial interest); (2) the introduction of European species where suitable, mainly in North Africa; (3) the introduction of tropical species that could be produced industrially on large plantations. In practice, not much was done in terms of office-based testing or production. A few experimental cultures, like that of saffron in Morocco or that of *Strophantus* in Cameroun, were launched; but most initiatives focused on writing monographs and organizing exploratory missions, for example to Egyptian Sudan in 1920, to Morocco, Tunisia and Algeria in 1921 and to West Africa in 1927.

This last mission to West Africa best exemplifies the practice of colonial pharmacy under the auspices of Perrot in his capacity as a representative of the central government and its industrial plants' office. The mission proper started in Timbuktu and was terminated in Conakry. Its aim was to evaluate not only the flora or plant resources, but more broadly the local agriculture, indigenous as well as European, its current practices and potential for 'development'. Perrot shared the view of colonial reformers in the 1920s that the first phase of colonization had been a military one, dominated by all forms of plunder and impossible to sustain in the long run. The adverse effects of this first phase derived not only from destructive harvesting and depleted forest resources (as best illustrated by the case of rubber investigated by Chevalier), but also from bad cultivation practices that exhausted the soil on poorly managed plantations. Such detrimental practices were, unfortunately, supported by greedy export companies looking for short-term profits and by incompetent or ill-advised colonial administrators.

Addressing the need for a proper choice of seeds for aromatic plants in the Guinean district of Kankan, Perrot thus noted:

> How difficult this choice is when big industry is the main consumer and seeks only to enhance its direct interest, looking for products obtained at the lowest price and pursuing only established habits. For this industry, the fact that human fools have ventured and lost themselves in the furthest reaches of the savanna, where they contribute to the national colonial enterprise and lose their health, is of no importance.[33]

Commenting on the measures taken by the local governor, who had promoted the use of ploughs, organized free distribution of a few dozens instruments to local chiefs and in whom he saw a model of the enlightened administrator, Perrot added:

> Why don't commercial houses follow a similar path of action? Is it because they don't believe in the truth? A few observations, which have been reported to me, support this idea. And yet it is not difficult at all to see the situation. It would be enough to send a few inspectors to the region of Kankan and to similar parts of Guinea to convince industry. They would see major opportunities for new and very profitable traffic.[34]

More generally, Perrot believed that agricultural reform could arise from a close alliance between local elites and French administrators, advised by competent experts like him. Such an alliance could preach by example and show the natives that it was in their own interest to: (1) adopt some aspects of European rational agriculture, beginning with the use of ploughs and fertilizer; (2) mechanize some aspects of their work; (3) commercialize part of their production and introduce industrial species that were in high demand.

Perrot's evaluation of the banana market is typical of this modernizing ethos. Dreaming of an expanded market in Europe, where bananas might become a routine part of the general population's diet, he argued throughout his 1927 report for a systematic policy of experimentation in public botanical gardens and for a policy favouring indigenous cultivation in villages rather than on large European plantations. Big commercial firms were among the major obstacles to the growth of banana production. Perrot remarked sarcastically that even after twenty years, those firms had still failed to solve the problem of transporting bananas to the metropolis.[35] Visiting Guinea, Perrot added:

> We arrived in Kebali ... Here the chief started drying bananas in the sun with excellent results ... One needs to repeat again the same old truth regarding the creation

of a special market. These new products are not going to be popularized by groceries specializing in colonial products. The core of the matter is no longer a question of snobbish sales, but a problem of routine normal business ... The cultivation of bananas has been imported from the West Indies and has been long practised by indigenous people. It is only in recent times that big plantations have been established. Numerous firms have been created, but too often under badly considered circumstances, with poor or no study of soil, irrigation and exposition problems. The administration started experimental trials, but with rather insufficient means. There is an official station in Camayenne collaborating with some plantation owners who have agreed to reserve part of their land for official trials and promised not to work on that part without approval from the station ... There are numerous small farms that could benefit from such experience; once the native farmer has understood, the question of banana production will be solved.[36]

Perrot thought differently about the rapid industrialization of kola production, but still devised various ways of enlarging the local market and securing larger amounts of quality nuts for European consumption. In particular, he recommended the development of kola cultivation in villages within the natural zone of kola growth, i.e. in Guinea and Ivory Coast. To achieve this aim, he encouraged the colonial administration to stabilize prices either by purchasing nuts and signing supply contracts with the *Office national des matières premières* or by providing tools (like ploughs) and technical advice. Perrot also relied on the authority of local chiefs, whom he viewed as the main intermediaries between tradition and modernity.[37] Furthermore, Perrot proposed a reorganization of the market in order to improve the quality of the nuts. He advocated: (1) the standardization of local transportation techniques based on indigenous practices (these techniques were actually supported by administrative circulars emanating from the Guinea governor); and (2) the introduction of sterilization in the main ports used to export kola nuts to European markets. Finally, Perrot hoped to revive botanical gardens that, as in Upper Guinea, had too often declined and that needed to become sites for the selection of kola trees as well as the development of cultivation guidelines.

As head of the Office, Perrot nonetheless remained cautious about the prospects of the European market:

Regarding European consumption (which is impossible to evaluate, even approximately), it would be better to employ stabilized (sterilized) nuts, since they alone retain the potency of fresh nuts. Before this becomes routine practice, however, one must wait for the time when the railway reaches the main production areas, when supply saturates the local markets and when prices are no longer prohibitive.[38]

The recommendations of Perrot, as colonial expert, do not seem to have triggered much transformation in West Africa. Judging by official reports, the most significant impact of the Office's investments on medicinal plants of colonial origins was their transformation into objects of experimental pharmacology and the publication of a stream of academic papers, theses and monographs.[39] This doesn't mean that the pharmaceutical and industrial development of kola remained a pipe dream. The interwar period witnessed significant growth in the number of specialized drugs – chiefly wines and tonics, but also kola extracts.[40] In colonial France, production was based on the local harvest and cultivation, rather than on industrial plantations, like those established in US-dominated Latin America. It is perhaps not too far-fetched to believe that such divergent modalities bear some relation to the French success of Coca-Cola and to the failure of Cola Coca, which was widely sold in metropolitan pharmacies in the 1930s.

Returning to Biologics

In the end, we can ask whether kola extracts were biologics. The question may be less obvious than it seems. Viewed from the vantage point adopted in the introduction to this chapter, that of the material origins of pharmaceuticals, kola extracts were definitely biologics. They were derivates of plants collected in nature. The notion of biologics is, however, less a problem of natural versus artificial ontology than a question of socio-technical order. As mentioned in the introduction, biologics were not just therapeutics 'made' out of biological things. They were technical objects both socially and culturally associated with nature and elaborated through industrial mass-preparation processes. Their importance was certainly linked to the therapeutic potency associated with the physiological properties of sera, hormones or enzymes, all 'new' products of nature bearing the aura of frontier science. But biologics also included 'old' (i.e. incorporated in European pharmacopoeia) as well as 'new' plant extracts, thus representing a boundary between the passing professional order centred on local preparations and the emerging industrial order centred on standardized specialties.

In this respect, kola extracts were typical. On the one hand, they were inscribed in the Codex; they were widely prepared with dozens of commercial products rooted in the culture of mixtures and galenic innovation; and they were associated with sales and marketing techniques based on reputation and name recognition. On the other hand, kola extracts were undoubtedly industrial specialties. They entered the catalogue of large companies like Midy, Clin and Dausse. They were widely distributed, mass-produced and subjected to factory-based controls of raw materials and output. The alliance of Dausse and Perrot's laboratory thus reveals general trends toward scaling-up, mechanization, standardization through biological testing and, not least, patenting. These trends have been associated with the making of other *material medica*-derived biologicals, from gland extracts to digital *intraits*.

Kola extracts were, however, biologics in the very special sense of them being colonial biologics. Perrot's trajectory is a paradigmatic example of the peculiar linkages between pharmacy, botany and industry that operated in the context of early twentieth-century French colonial enterprise. The circulations between the colonies and the pharmaceutical experts in the metropolis that had initially involved exploration voyages, inventories, botanical classification and writing pharmacopoeia eventually became a matter of productivity missions, agricultural experimentation, plantations and market organization. Perrot's late writings about kola therefore no longer focused on the physiological properties of the nuts. They addressed issues of mass cultivation by the natives, transportation from West Africa to France, commercial supply and demand from the middle and lower classes. Standardization thus acquired a different meaning that was unrelated to laboratory and/or industrial plants, but that centred on the problems of plantations and local agriculture, on the collaboration of experts and colonial administrators and on targets, including reference seeds, fertilization protocols, transportation and processing guidelines. The naturalness of industrial kola extracts was therefore as much rooted in their collection in nature or their preparation out of living entities as it was in the colonial dream of a progressive industrial regime that scientifically reordered the lives of African natives and their natural world.

3 STANDARDIZING THE EXPERIMENTAL SYSTEM: THE DEVELOPMENT OF CORTICOSTERIODS AND THEIR IMPACT ON COOPERATION, PROPERTY RIGHTS AND INDUSTRIAL PROCEDURES

Lea Haller

When British physiologist Ernest Starling introduced the concept of hormones in 1905, he assigned to organic chemistry the role of a basic science. He was convinced that once chemists had discovered the chemical structure of physiological substances that act like drugs within the body, medicine would be able to regulate processes of coordination in cases of hormonal imbalance:

> If a mutual control and therefore coordination, of the different functions of the body be largely determined by the production of definite chemical substances in the body, the discovery of the nature of these substances will enable us to interpose at any desired phase in these functions and so to acquire an absolute control over the workings of the human body. Such a control is the goal of medical science.[1]

For Starling, determining chemical structure and medical control went hand in hand. His unbounded belief in a glorious future for scientific medicine was based on the notion of imitation and copying. Notwithstanding the fact that, apart from adrenaline, no hormone had been isolated in pure form and synthetically standardized at the time, and that producing hormones was altogether a question of preparing biological material,[2] he was convinced that knowledge would automatically lead to power. He reduced the problem of standardization to one of refinement: the transformation of a natural object into a technological one. Henceforth, medicine would no longer experiment with treatments and drugs of unknown structure and effect, but would make use of nature's own remedies. 'A knowledge of the whole field', Starling wrote in 1908, 'would place us in command of the means employed by Nature herself'.[3] Glandular extracts would be tested physiologically to ascertain their effect, chemists would then provide the active principle in pure form, and eventually physicians would be able to control the bodily processes of stimulation and inhibition. Instead of being a repair workshop, medicine would become a control centre.

Starling could not anticipate the problems of standardization that emerged during the interwar period, when intensified cooperation between science and industry revealed the structure of most hormones. In this chapter, I will focus on the very process of standardization – understood as the transformation of a crude biological extract into a pure substance and finally into a standardized pharmaceutical product. I will argue that the problems engendered by this process were not due simply to the *biological* character of the hormones. Nor were the issues merely *technical*. Rather, they were linked to the cross-institutional and cross-disciplinary character of drug development and hence pertained to property rights, cooperation contracts, production processes, capital goods and the expected return on investment. In other words, I will examine standardization as a social and economic process that influenced both substances and protagonists, and consequently altered the entire process of research and development. Such an approach cannot be confined to the laboratory. It must focus on 'knowledge as circulating practices'.[4]

Science and technology studies generally emphasize the role of the experiment and of the laboratory in the transformation of a *natural* object into a *technological* one. The laboratory is conceived as a place where representations of nature are established with the help of different technologies and according to cultural patterns and epistemological traditions. We have a fairly good understanding of how nature is culturally shaped in a test environment and how the boundaries between the natural and the cultural, the normal and the pathological, and between the scientifically justifiable and the politically unacceptable are negotiated through these procedures.[5] We also know that the standardization process reflects more than just laboratory logic or the imposition of industrial norms on medicine. Recent studies in the field of pharmaceuticals emphasize the reciprocal exchange between clinics and industry – between bedside practices, evaluation procedures and the laboratory – in the standardization process.[6] The results of laboratory studies and of the recent history of pharmacology provide a guide for considering the broader social and structural implications of pharmaceutical standardization. My central questions are: how did the analysis and modification of biological substances affect the protagonists and their position? What was at stake in the emergence of new compounds? And what financial and process-related motives were at work in transferring chemical procedures from the laboratory to large-scale production? Answering these questions means focusing on the processes of communication in a heterogeneous network of different actors with different objectives. It is worth keeping in mind James Secord's observations on knowledge in transit: 'Struggles for access and control, however, are always at stake in any form of communication: to make knowledge move is the most difficult form of power to achieve'.[7]

The standardization process did not lead to a controlled access to nature or to pure, well-defined products. It did, however, disrupt and re-establish prevailing routines and arrangements. While in the narrow context of the laboratory or of a single discipline (for instance chemistry) a certain step might be hailed as a great discovery, it was paralleled by problems of property rights, agreements, trust and patents which forced a rearrangement of people and infrastructure. Put another way, the technological acquisition of a crude and undetermined extract by means of centrifuge and chromatography, precipitation, heating, dissolving and crystallization did not result only in chemically determined compounds and an expanding nomenclature. It also involved the repeated destabilization of the entire experimental system. To exemplify this argument, I will discuss three steps in the standardization of adrenal cortex hormones in the 1930s and their relation to the broader social, legal and trans-disciplinary context: first, the isolation of a variety of pure substances; second, the chemical classification of these substances; and third, a synthesis that led to an industrially produced hormone. The case is based on research carried out in the Ciba archives and on the records of the Swiss chemist Tadeus Reichstein.

Isolation

The adrenal glands are essential to life. Their destruction is followed by a fatal disease first described by Thomas Addison in 1855 (and subsequently named for him).[8] The isolation of epinephrine (adrenaline) from the adrenal medulla in 1901 – a hormone causing a rise of blood pressure – raised hopes that patients suffering from Addison's disease could henceforth be treated with it. The failure of this treatment, which followed Starling's conclusion by analogy, has long been cited as evidence for the inconsistency of the concept of hormones: apparently the pharmacological effect differed from the physiological function of the gland. The British physiologist Swale Vincent, for example, argued that 'the well-known value of adrenalin bore a very problematic relation to the function or functions of the adrenal body as a whole'. He rejected Starling's idea of a substitution therapy, which implied the similarity of physiological and pharmacological substances, and referred to the impossibility of curing Addison's disease by administering adrenaline: 'In Addison's disease adrenal preparations did not seem to be of the slightest value'.[9] It was only toward the end of the 1920s that it became evident that the adrenal cortex – and not, as expected, the adrenal medulla – produces a substance which is essential for life. This finding put things in another perspective.

Cortin, as the extract of the adrenal cortex was named, not only silenced the critics, but also led to chemical research designed to isolate the substance embodying the active principle. It was a laborious and expensive endeavour. Huge amounts of raw material from slaughtered cattle were required.[10] When the American chemist Edward C. Kendall announced in 1934 that he had isolated an adrenal-cortical substance in crystalline form, he compared the search for the one, chemically determined compound embodying the life-sustaining principle to a criminal manhunt: 'The police forces of the country may be called on to round up hundreds of gangsters. This, however, is an easy accomplishment compared to the capture of a specific individual'.[11] Kendall's analogy did not, however, take into account the main challenge, namely that there was neither an experienced team to conduct the research nor general agreement on how to identify a criminal subject, i.e. a purified substance, once it was '*arrested*'. Pharmacologists would have to develop biological tests to demonstrate whether the isolated substance was an active hormone or not.

Four weeks after Kendall's publication, on 28 May 1934, the Swiss chemist Tadeus Reichstein; his friend Gottfried Lüscher, the owner of Haco, a Swiss foodstuffs company supporting Reichstein's research; and Ernst Laqueur, a pharmacologist and co-founder of the Dutch pharmaceutical company Organon, met in Utrecht. On a previous meeting in Zurich, Reichstein, Lüscher and Laqueur had already discussed various fields of future cooperation. They now quickly agreed to investigate the cortical hormone. The agenda was simple: Organon was assigned to deliver the crude extract as starting material to obtain a crystalline hormone preparation, which, in case it exhibited physiological activity, would afterwards be prepared in quantities sufficient for Reichstein to establish its constitution and eventually to synthesize it.[12] With this agreement, a promising start-up programme was initiated, run by a raw-materials supplier, a financier and a chemist. Organon was among the pharmaceutical companies that had developed procedures to evaluate the activity of cortical extracts on test animals in the early 1930s. While the life-sustaining test was initially the standard method, different laboratories successively began to test the effects of cortical substances on different bodily functions.

At Organon's biology department, Ernst Laqueur assayed the substances isolated by Reichstein in the so-called Everse–de Fremery test, which was developed by two of the company's engineers.[13] In this test, the muscular fatigue of rats (one of the first manifestations of adrenal-cortical insufficiency) served as a criterion to ascertain the activity of isolated substances. It worked in a similar way to the dog test, which was mostly applied in the United States. The standard it produced was 'a rat unit' (analogous to a 'dog unit'), meaning the quantity of an isolated substance required to keep an adrenalectomized animal in a healthy condition. In 1936, Reichstein heard about a new glucose test developed by Fritz

Verzar, a Swiss physician. He was very interested in it and asked Organon if they would agree to send substances to Verzar for testing. Organon's representatives were less than delighted and suggested performing the test themselves instead of handing substances over to an outsider. Reichstein replied:

> My proposal to take advantage of Verzar's new test was of course not supposed to be a vote of non-confidence concerning the hitherto adopted methods ... However, all test methods seem to work particularly well where they were invented. I trust the dog test only when carried out by Dr. Pfiffner, just as you know best how to handle the Everse–de Fremery test properly. The same may be true of Verzar's new test.

Verzar indicated that he was able to test using only a tenth of the amount of substance required by the Everse–de Fremery method, 'which in my opinion', argued Reichstein, 'is reason enough to thoroughly consider the opportunity'.[14] Organon eventually agreed that substances be given to Verzar and paid for the additional expense.

Unravelling the raw material and isolating pure substances from cortin implied much more than talented chemists unlocking the secrets of nature. With every separation step the analytical uncertainty increased, and an enormous effort had to be made to obtain more or less reliable results with respect to the biological activity of the substances in question. In order to test the scarce material, the test animals first had to be standardized, a task which during the 1930s led to different test methods depending on the specific physical deficiency being evaluated. The question of which procedure was the most efficient and therefore should be applied could not be answered scientifically. It was a matter of diplomatic negotiation within existing cooperative settings, of know-how, of confidence and of economics.

Classification

In 1936, Reichstein declared that the isolated substances were probably steroids, which meant that they had a carbon structure of four fused rings and additional functional groups. An immediate consequence of this structural analysis was that it pitted Reichstein against his supervisor Leopold Ruzicka, the head of the Institute of Organic Chemistry at the Federal Institute of Technology in Zurich (ETH). Ruzicka worked in the field of sexual hormones – which are steroids as well – and he had an exclusive contract with the Swiss pharmaceutical company Ciba. The arrangement assured him considerable financial support and in turn allowed the company to exploit his findings.[15] Via Reichstein, knowledge about steroid synthesis could easily be leaked to others, even a foreign competitor, and so Ruzicka was risking a breach of contract. He would have preferred Reichstein to abandon his commitment to Haco and Organon completely. This, of course, was out of the question. The situation was so untenable that Ruzicka did not support the extension of Reichstein's employment at ETH. In 1938 Reichstein was offered a professorship in Basel, where he continued his adrenal cortex venture.

In 1936 it had become obvious that if Reichstein, Haco and Organon wanted to benefit from Ciba's knowledge, they had to enter into an agreement, particularly since Ciba, as well as Schering, held important patents on specific steps in the process of steroid synthesis. At the end of the year, negotiations with delegates from Ciba were initiated, proceedings that for a long time were overshadowed by mutual distrust. In May 1937 Ciba, Organon and Schering finally signed a contract for the so-called cortin field. Ciba acquired the right to exploit all of Reichstein's inventions in the field of adrenal-cortex hormones, whereas the company had to share 6 per cent of future revenues of any cortin-derived product with Organon. Organon retained possession of Reichstein's patents, and Haco received 25 per cent of gross profits of any product from the contract.[16] This agreement established minimum prices, shared licences and distributed markets, as commonly ascribed to a cartel. Moreover, as Jean-Paul Gaudillière has shown, such contracts regulated the management of anticipated intellectual property, i.e. of knowledge expected to accrue only in the future.[17] It stands to reason that the expectations fixed in the contract and the actual outcome of laboratory research might be at odds with one another and result in legally precarious situations.

The first compounds, which were not covered by the contract, were the aetio-cholanic acids. They served as an intermediate both for the production of cortin-like substances and for substances which went beyond the scope of the contract, namely progesterone and testosterone. The legal question was especially delicate because Reichstein had developed these intermediates in close cooperation with Ciba. Ciba claimed that the existing contract entitled it to file patents for the compounds. 'On the contrary', wrote Haco, 'it seems likewise evident to us that a process leading to a cortin-like agent belongs to Organon exclusively, even if this agent may be considered for other interesting therapeutic applications'.[18] This statement further clouded the issue. One week later Haco received another letter from Ciba, which read:

> To put it bluntly, the question we are interested in is, what happens with procedures which are not covered by paragraph two of article IIa, i.e., that were not developed with our help, but that could lead to either cortin, progesterone or testosterone, which of course is entirely possible?[19]

The chemical classification caused conflicts of loyalty, property rights and cooperation, and resulted in an expansion of the experimental system and a multiplication of participating members. Furthermore, the emergence of new, unanticipated compounds endangered and destabilized the well-balanced agreed-upon collaboration. To whom should the rights be assigned in the case of intermediates, which on the one hand led to contract products and on the other to completely different agents? In addition to the cortin contract, Ciba, Organon and Haco finally agreed on a pragmatic solution for such socio-technical monstrosities. The fabrication processes leading to compounds of the aetio-cholanic acid series were assigned to Ciba, which in turn paid Organon a one-off compensation.[20]

Synthesis

The third case to be considered concerns a test substance which Tadeus Reichstein and his assistant Marguerite Steiger had synthesized to prove the empirical formula of corticosterone, a hormone extracted from organic material. If their hypothetical formula for the biological hormone proved correct, the substance which they were able to synthesize would differ from it only by the lack of one oxygen molecule (hence it was called desoxy-corticosterone).[21] The synthetic compound was not expected to be of any value apart from structure determination of the other, active compound. Nevertheless, Reichstein sent desoxy-corticosterone to Laqueur who applied the Everse–de Fremery test to it. To the surprise of all, the synthetic desoxy-corticosterone not only proved active but was even more effective than the natural compound! It was the first substance with high hormone activity obtained by starting out with inactive material instead of adrenal-cortex extract. A synthesis feasible for large-scale production was suddenly within reach.

A total synthesis of the sterol ring system was not feasible. One had to start with a compound already containing it; the most common and the cheapest was cholesterol. At a medical conference in the Netherlands, Reichstein explained the procedure: 'First you oxygenate the whole cholesterol side-chain away in a rather brutal oxidation. It is a harsh and not very efficient reaction. The yield from one kilogramme of cholesterol is about ten grams of the required aetio-cholanic acid'.[22] From an economic point of view this was a very inefficient step. However, precisely this oxidation was already being carried out in the production halls of Ciba, though for a completely different purpose, namely to prepare progesterone. The required acid remained as a by-product. At a meeting of the sales department of Ciba in October 1938, one of the participants asked his colleagues whether it would be worthwhile to invest large amounts in producing desoxy-corticosterone given that very few patients suffered from Addison's disease. The answer was pragmatic. Although the field of medical indication seemed to be quite small on the basis of the existing test results, they affirmed that production should be commenced because it was linked with the production of progesterone.[23] In 1938 desoxy-corticosterone was tested in clinical trials, and in the same year Ciba launched the drug on the market under the trade name Percorten.

The only definite medical indication for it was the rare but deadly Addison's disease, caused by a lack of natural hormone production in the adrenal cortex. Nevertheless, Percorten was a product with a high profit margin, not owing to runaway sales but to its prestige. It represented successful cooperation between academic research and industrial production and hence stabilized the division of labour among 'pure' and 'applied' science, a rhetorical distinction which had emerged in the interwar period.[24] In an advertisement for the American market, Ciba promoted Percorten alongside the image of a Bunsen burner, the most important tool of the chemist. At the same time, the image recalled the iconography of the life-reform movement, which had an affinity for the hormonal body and for therapy that employed natural substances. The message of the advertisement was as clear as day: Percorten, a synthetically produced hormone, promised Addison's patients a vital force and a flame of life which would continue to shine even brighter.

Conclusion

When Organon considered producing desoxy-corticosterone in the United States for the American market, Reichstein was sceptical:

> I think that you completely underestimate the difficulties of the whole fabrication process. Even if you intend to relocate only the final steps of the synthesis, considerable preparation is required, as well as continuous control by an expert chemist experienced in the respective reactions.[25]

Even though the desoxy-corticostosterone formula was the same on both sides of the Atlantic, Reichstein was fully aware of the fragility of locally aggregated knowledge and knew that each transfer would bring about unexpected problems. Not that he would have judged this fragility as problematic in the sense of threatening his work. He knew that it was part of everyday business – a business as much concerned with chemistry as with diplomatic skill and strategies for handling the change typically involved in the process of standardization.

The history of corticosteroids revealed how much the standardization process depended on existing infrastructure, on patent infringements and on competitive interactions, and vice versa, how it influenced established forms of cooperation, the ways and means of exchanging material and the distribution of knowledge. Each analytical step produced uncertainties – not only scientific, but also social and political ones. Each successful step of standardization created a new situation, a starting point for establishing a new order with respect both to the object of investigation and especially to the conditions of cooperation, the legal situation, and technical and commercial aspects. Research and development did not precede the standardization process but developed simultaneously, or as Viviane Quirke put it:

> R&D was *invented* at a particular time and place, and ... the knowledge, practices and organisation involved in R&D were disseminated along with 'successful' products, such as antibiotics or the beta-blockers. R&D should therefore be seen as an innovation like any other, the result of a dynamic evolution, which has been time- and place-dependent, and has involved complex exchanges and circulations of norms, rules and regulations, within firms as well as between them, and between firms and regulatory agencies.[26]

Accordingly, I was not particularly interested in the inner-disciplinary debates surrounding a specific scientific problem, nor was I eager to write about the cultural, social and discursive conditions of the production of scientific knowledge. Instead, I have attempted to outline a history of knowledge and technology which goes beyond the laboratory and the geographical and disciplinary boundaries that often shape traditional science studies. If we view hormones as simultaneously industrial, scientific, legal, cultural and medical entities, we must necessarily consider the connections between completely different kinds of knowledge. This concurrent, interdependent production of knowledge, its disregard for institutional and disciplinary boundaries, its limits and constraints, and the changes it underwent, did not simply lead to a series of new pharmaceutical agents. To a large extent, it also shaped the modality of research and development, the process of pharmaceutical engineering and the way Western societies thought about drugs, health and disease in the first half of the twentieth century. Starling had annihilated the differences between organic and pharmacological substances. The standardization process of corticosteroids not only made them obvious again, but also revealed the social character of the transformation from one to the other.

4 CULTURES OF SUBJECTIVITY: COCA AS A BIOLOGIC AND THE CO-CONSTRUCTION OF DEVIANT SUBJECTS AND DRUG EFFICACY, 1880–1900[1]

Beat Bächi

Coca is a biological, psychotropic drug derived from a medical plant. The story of coca and cocaine has been told many different times. Recently, Bettina Wahrig analysed the narratives in coca research and focused on the history of coca leaves and cocaine in the second half of nineteenth-century Europe. The first coca leaves came to Europe from South America in the 1750s. More than a century later, in 1859/60, Albert Niemann isolated the active components of coca leaves in Friedrich Wöhler's laboratory in Göttingen. He baptized this new alkaloid *cocaine*. The isolation of the active substance in these 'miraculous leaves' was important not only for the chemical purification and standardization of this biologic. It also provided the substance with a new potential of becoming a drug 'looking for diseases'.[2] Reports focusing on the 'miraculous effects' of the Indian plant started to circulate in the European medical press just as cocaine was isolated from the leaves. Notably, the Italian physician Paolo Mantegazza published on this topic after returning to Italy from a stay in Argentina in 1859, henceforth transforming the Andean coca leaves into an 'Italian cure-all'.[3]

But coca and cocaine, respectively, were never conclusively stabilized. These substances and the narratives that attached meaning to them and their effects travelled through numerous networks and across quite different contexts and fields of interest. There was also much hype surrounding coca and cocaine in both popular culture and the beverage industry, especially since the 1880s. A very popular coca wine had been produced and sold commercially since 1863 under the name of *Vin Mariani*. Pope Leo XIII and Queen Victoria were but two of many public figures who wrote a thank-you letter to Angelo Mariani for a free sample of *Vin Mariani*. The letters and pictures of these persons were used by Mariani to promote his coca wine. But Mariani's product was just the most popular among many other coca wines in the 1880s. In the US city of Atlanta,

John Smith Pemberton had made a name for himself as a producer of a prosperous coca wine and several remedies. Confronted with laws on prohibition, he had the idea of creating a beverage that would boost power and prevent headaches. Hence, he concocted a soft drink out of coca and cola nut extracts mixed with syrup and water. This new drink would later be sold in drug stores under the name of Coca-Cola. Around the same time, Sir Arthur Conan Doyle's famous detective, Sherlock Holmes, also began consuming cocaine in *The Sign of the Four* in order to enhance his thinking and acting. And it was not just human beings who began using cocaine to increase their performance – racehorses too were 'doped' with cocaine.[4]

Purifications: From an Andean Plant to a European Chemical Compound

What does coca's history tell us about biologics? Coca is a prime example of the processes of purification and standardization. On its way from the Andes to Europe, this biologic was purified and standardized not just chemically, but also culturally. An important step in the naturalization of coca in Europe after its transformation into a purely chemical substance involved the use of new devices and techniques designed to demonstrate its effects. In describing cocaine's cultural purification during the 1880s, this chapter follows the traces of this miracle drug from the Andes to Sigmund Freud in Vienna, to the Swiss Alps, and ultimately to Turin, where Ugolino Mosso (the brother of the well-known physiologist Angelo Mosso, who invented fatigue research) experimented with it and where the forensic anthropologist Cesare Lombroso (1835–1909) was exploring deviant subjects in Italian society. The study of cocaine's effects developed its own trajectory, as simple self-experiments with cocaine were gradually replaced by laboratory settings, where its subjective effects were mediated and documented by (scientific) instruments. In connection with this, another shift occurred in the production of evidence of cocaine's effects. Initially, its agency was described in terms of self-awareness. But by the middle of the 1880s, this narrative of verification gave way to the mathematical precision of measurement. Numbers, tables and the graphical method were used to detach cocaine's effects from human subjects and their accidental dispositions. Hence, this chapter demonstrates the impact of biologics on the creation of bodily concepts and shows that coca was an ambiguous substance, since the desired effects changed and could switch to become deleterious ones.

At the fin-de-siècle, the scientific world was, according to Sigmund Freud, literally obsessed by cocaine. Plenty of new applications came to be discussed and adopted, for example the use of cocaine as an anaesthetic in eye surgery. Furthermore, cocaine began to be produced on an industrial scale, which made scientific research on its physical properties much easier. In 1885 in Detroit, the US manufacturer Parke-Davis & Co. sold cocaine in various forms. The company promised that its cocaine products would 'supply the place of food, make the coward brave, the silent eloquent and render the sufferer insensitive to pain'.[5] In Germany, the pharmaceutical company Merck in Darmstadt also began producing and selling cocaine in the 1880s. Nevertheless, cocaine's acculturation into the Western world remained precarious and would require further acts of purification.

The writings of Sigmund Freud on coca from 1884 onward played an important part in this (cultural) purification process.[6] While studying coca's *stählende Wirkung* ('steeling effects'), Freud became interested in coca's potential as an 'energy-saver' or 'nerve nutrient' (*'Spar-Mittel'*). These substances were believed to make the energy use of food more efficient. They were the object of much discussion throughout the 1860s and 1870s and included coffee, tea, alcohol, tobacco and coca.[7] These 'energy-savers' seemed to threaten the first law of thermodynamics. But, as Freud stated, the potential of 'energy-savers' did not 'necessarily' contradict the first law of the conservation of energy.[8]

For Freud, as a trained physiologist, the form of coca used in Europe was not coca leaves, but rather cocaine in its pure alkaloid form. This distinction between coca leaves and cocaine had already surfaced in the title of the first of his many publications on coca: 'Coca Leaves in Europe – Cocaine'. Regarding coca's transfer to Europe, Freud's most striking remarks concerned the presumptive association between coca's effects and the 'Indian race'. In this respect, Freud states that reports from travellers like Tschudi and Markham had proven that the effects of coca leaves was not limited to the 'Indian race'.[9] This observation was an important prerequisite for coca's acculturation to modern, Western forms of scientific method and instrumentation. The first prominent way to apply statistical methods to study the effects of cocaine was, as so often, to study soldiers. The army provided lots of well-controlled subjects for physiological experiments. Consequently, the most important experiments that led Freud to take up his own research on cocaine were a series of trials to test the effects of cocaine on performance in the army. Theodor Aschenbrand had conducted just such experiments and published them in the *Deutsche medizinische Wochenschrift* in 1883.[10] Unlike Aschenbrand, Freud did not recruit a huge number of probands, but just a single, individual body to establish the effects of cocaine with 'mathematical precision'.

After Freud's first publication on coca, Merck offered to pay Freud to experiment with the cocaine derivative *Ecgonin* in October 1884.[11] Freud accepted the offer from Darmstadt. When he began his experiments, he first of all had to derive and distinguish the notion of 'work' from the work of the Indians. In an environment that prized productivity and where idleness had become one of the most castigated vices, 'work' became transformed into a numerical relationship between input and output. Freud's object was to measure scientifically the effect of cocaine on abstract manpower. He wanted to objectify with mathematical precision the impact of cocaine on muscular work. For this purpose, the most promising instrument to objectify cocaine's effects with mathematical precision was the 'dynamometer'. It weighed about one kilogram and consisted of an oval steel clasp, a measuring plate with a dual scale (in myriagrams and kilograms), a pointer, as well as a multi-pieced rig from which to hang the apparatus. This made it possible to accurately measure both tension and pressure, be it from humans, horses or even machines.[12]

Accidental Personal Dispositions and the Dynamometer's Subjectivity

Regarding Freud's uses of the dynamometer, Albrecht Hirschmüller (who has also conducted research on Freud's relationship with the pharmaceutical company Merck) has done pioneering work.[13] Further important contributions to this topic have come from Christof Windgätter, who studied the dynamometer's uses in anthropology, the clinic, the office, 'the text' and the factory.[14] It is difficult to overestimate the enthusiasm surrounding the dynamometer at the turn of the nineteenth to the twentieth century. In the hands of anthropologists, this device travelled widely during the nineteenth century, for example to the 'Creoles', 'Timorese and Papuans', 'Mozambique negroes' and the 'Sandwich Islanders'.[15] It also circulated within societies and different fields of knowledge, thus initiating and bringing together discourses from hitherto separate areas of research. Hence, one can literally describe the dynamometer as a boundary object, connecting and transforming different fields of knowledge production.[16]

The discourses on coca and the dynamometer revolved about the concept of fatigue. In his inspiring work on 'Energy, Fatigue, and the Origins of Modernity', Anson Rabinbach has analysed the emergence of a new ideology of productive work and the transformations of the 'human motor'. Rabinbach concludes that in the context of the laws of thermodynamics, a new view of fatigue came to prevail: whereas the pre-modern concept of fatigue was structured by caution, the modern concept of fatigue (emerging according to Rabinbach in the last third of the nineteenth century) sees exhaustion as the limit to productivity. Furthermore, in its modern form fatigue is a quantifiable, objective, impartial and normative benchmark, but not a fixed limit.[17] It seems that cocaine's energy-saving potential was one of the main reasons for Freud not just to describe the effects of the drug in the simple prose of self-awareness, but also to 'portray' ('*darstellen*') coca's enhancing effects in an 'objective' way.[18] The dynamometer hailed from a tradition that Lorraine Daston and Peter Galison have called 'mechanical objectivity', a form of objectivity that had emerged as a dominant scientific ideal with the spread of new techniques of mechanical reproduction and image-making in the mid-nineteenth century.[19] Freud wrote that one of the central characteristics of such an 'objective' instrument was that it showed 'regularity' ('*Gleichförmigkeit*') and not 'accidental, personal dispositions' ('*zufällige(n) persönliche(n) Disposition(en)*').[20] Freud was obviously in search of the average man – in his individual body – and his quest was reminiscent of the mathematician, astronomer and social statistician Adolphe Quételet (1798–1874), who was an especially avid user of the dynamometer designed by Regnier. Quételet was the inventor of the *homme moyen* ('the average men') and the field of *physique sociale* or social physics. In his studies, Freud speaks of two dynamometers, but we only know the origin of one of them, namely the one designed by the French neurologist Victor B. Burq (see Figure 4.1), who had constructed at least two different apparatuses.[21]

Freud recorded the results of his dynamometer trials on the influence of cocaine and transformed them into tables (see Figure 4.2). The left-hand column of the table depicted in Figure 4.2 listed the time of the trial. The right-hand column contained notes on the subjective state of the proband ('tired', 'euphoric', etc.). The intermediate columns contained, from left to right, the readings taken from the dynamometer, the maximum values and the average values.[22] Freud not only transformed his private office into a laboratory, uniting the experimenter and the test subject in one person, but also – more importantly – adjusted his plot to accommodate his methods of measurement and accompanying forms of numerical notation.[23] Ultimately, this numerical notation made the border between the normal and the pathological, as well as the one between health and illness, permeable. Nevertheless, Freud's overwhelming use of the word 'normal' without scare quotes seems to indicate that, at the time of his research with coca and cocaine, he still perceived the normal to be a rather stable point of reference.[24]

Freud not only experimented with cocaine as a stimulant for muscular work, but also studied its effects on psychic reaction times. He conducted these experiments with Sigmund Exner's (1846–1926) *neuramöbimeter*. Freud describes this device and the experiments he performed with it as follows:

> The *neuramöbimeter* is comprised mainly of a metal nib, calibrated to 100 oscillations per second. The proband disrupts its vibrations as soon as he hears the sound generated by the release of the compressed spring. The time from the moment the sound is heard until the nib is lifted is the reaction time, which is directly recorded in hundredths of seconds as the number of oscillations of the nib.[25]

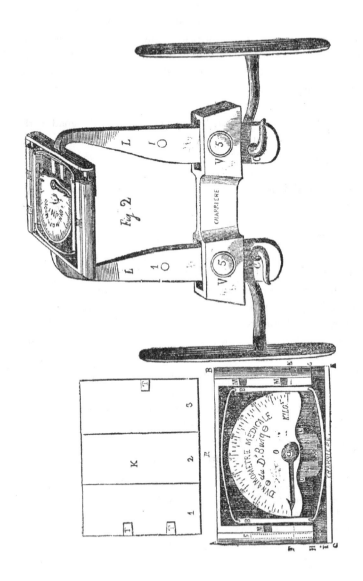

Figure 4.1: One of the dynamometers Freud used was designed by the French neurologist Victor B. Burq.[26] Source: V. B. Burq, 'Dynamométrie médicale', *L'union médicale: Journal des intérêts scientifiques et pratiques du corps médicales*, 106 (1895), pp. 460–2, on p. 461. Author's collection.

Zeiten	Drucke	Maxima	Mittel	Anmerkung
8 Uhr Früh	60	60	60	müde
10 „ „	73—63—67	73	67·6	nach Visite
—	darauf eine geringe, nicht bestimmte Menge Cocaïn			
10 Uhr 20 M.	76—70—76	76	74	heiter
10 „ 30 „	73—70—68	73	70·3	—
11 „ 35 „	72—72—74	74	72·6	—
12 „ 50 „	74—73—68	74	70	—
2 „ 20 „	70—68—69	70	69	—
4 „ — „	76—74—75	76	75	normales Befinden
6 „ — „	67—64—58	67	63	nach angestrengter Arbeit
8 „ 30 „	74—64—67	74	68·3	etwas müde
—	darauf 0·1 Cocaïn. mur.			
8 „ 43 „	80—73—74	80	75·6	Aufstossen
8 „ 58 „	79—76—71	79	75·3	—
9 „ 18 „	77—72—67	77	72	Gefühl von Leichtigkei⁴

Figure 4.2: Table from Freud's study on the knowledge of cocaine's effects on efficiency. Source: S. Freud, 'Beitrag zur Kenntnis der Cocawirkung', in *Schriften über Kokain*, ed. A. Hirschmüller (1885; Frankfurt/Main: Fischer, 1996), pp. 87–98, on p. 93. Author's collection.

Regarding his experiments with the *neuramöbimeter*, Freud noted that the results were less clear than the ones performed with the dynamometer. Nevertheless, the observed effects were 'similar'. 'I often noticed that my reaction times under the influence of cocaine were shorter and more regular than they were before I had taken cocaine'.[27] It is remarkable that uniformity seemed to Freud an important sign of scientific proof. The notions *'direkt gegeben'* ('directly given') and *'Gleichförmigkeit'* ('regularity') are strongly associated with each other and suggest that Freud's notion of objectivity involved aesthetic criteria. Furthermore, the detailed description of the diagnostic device is part of his theatre of evidence. Consequently, the tables and numbers produced with the dynamometer and the *neuramöbimeter* convinced Freud that he had 'portrayed' (*'darstellen'*) the effects of cocaine with 'mathematical' precision.

With or Without Cocaine? New Topologies of Work and Subjectivity

A lot of researchers experimented with coca and cocaine at the end of the nineteenth century. Philipp Felsch's research on the topology of work and fatigue suggests that these substances fascinated mountain climbers.[28] A telling example is E. Kraft's report on his experiments with cocaine in the Swiss Alps in 1886. Kraft had the opportunity to test cocaine's effects when he made a trip to the *Schilthorn*. He had reached its summit, once with and once without cocaine. His experiences convinced him of cocaine's effectiveness in aiding alpinists. In the same volume of the *Pharmaceutische Zeitung* in which E. Kraft published his findings on cocaine's advantageous effects, another article on cocaine and mountain climbing appeared as well. Here, too, the enhancing effects of cocaine were much acclaimed. The author finished his report on experiments conducted during an excursion of the Biel chapter of the Swiss Alpine Club to the *Sulegg*:

> And whereas my colleagues only reached the top of the mountain, the *Sulegg*, at half past five in the morning, I was able to hoist the flag I'd taken with me one hour earlier. The weather was wonderful that morning and the view of to the terrific Alpine scenery, especially the *Jungfrau* ('virgin'), was amazing.[29]

While I don't want to over-interpret the sexual associations evoked by the term *Jungfrau* here, it doesn't seem to be mere coincidence.

Another interesting actor in coca and fatigue research was Ugolino Mosso, the Turin-based physiologist. As previously mentioned, Ugolino was the brother of Angelo Mosso, the 'Galileo' of fatigue research, as Rabinbach has called him. Taking Freud's experiments as his point of departure, Ugolino Mosso produced so-called 'fatigue curves' ('*Ermüdungskurven*') using (quite likely his brother's) ergograph in the 1890s. The ergograph, or ergometer, was developed in 1884 by Angelo Mosso and was comprised of two parts (see Figure 4.3, top image):

> a positioning apparatus, with a supporting plate for the arm and metal tubes, which keep the index and ring finger still, as well as a recording device with a metal pin and goose quill that moves via a tension wire with leather band, weight and pulley. The strength of the middle finger is measured as the subject moves his finger, either on his own at a given tempo, supplied by a metronome, or as the finger contracts in response to electric stimuli.[30]

Regarding this new mode of knowledge transcription, Christof Windgätter has remarked: 'Of particular importance is that, with the ergograph, measurements no longer needed to be read off and then transcribed into tables. Instead, a diagram is drawn in real time'.[31] Bodily functions were transferred into images (see Figure 4.4). At the end of the nineteenth century, graphic interfaces emerged between the body and its numerical values. This new fusion of writing, numbers and images was supported by a strong belief in balance, regularity and averages.

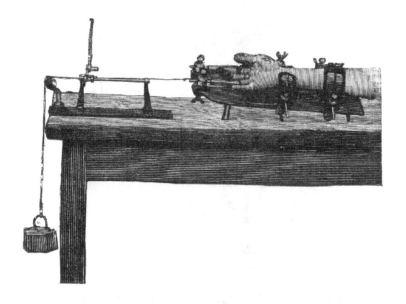

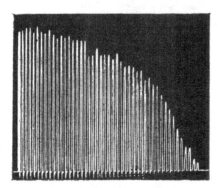

Figure 4.3: Ergograph of Angelo Mosso. This instrument was used to produce 'fatigue curves' (see this figure, bottom image). Source: A. Mosso, *Die Ermüdung*, trans. J. Glinzer (Leipzig: Verlag von S. Hirzel, 1892), pp. 90–1. Author's collection.

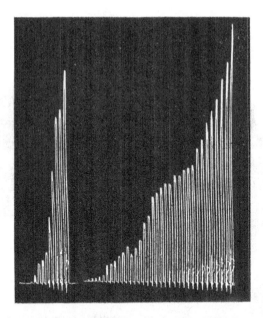

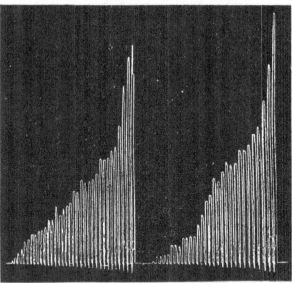

Figure 4.4: Fatigue curves used by Ugolino Mosso to demonstrate as scientifically as possible cocaine's power to boost performance. Top image: muscle contraction without cocaine; bottom image: performance after cocaine consumption. Source: U. Mosso, 'Ueber die physiologische Wirkung des Cocains. Eine experimentelle Kritik der Arbeiten über den Mechanismus seiner Wirkungsweise', *Archiv für die gesammte Physiologie des Menschen und der Tiere*, 47 (1890), pp. 553–601, on p. 580. Author's collection.

For Ugolino Mosso, it was obvious that the 'graphical method' served to produce 'sociotechnical evidence'.[32] In the concluding remarks about his research
on cocaine's favourable effects on simultaneous walking and reading, he wrote:
'The measurements made with the ergograph have confirmed, in the most beautiful way, the results already produced by empirical methods and conventional
observations'.[33] In Mosso's argument, aesthetic criteria quite naturally played
a major role.[34] Accordingly, he applied the graphical method to a variety of
other phenomena, such as respiration following a dose of cocaine. In his experiments, Mosso used the pneumograph, a device invented by Etienne-Jules Marey
(1830-1904), one of the pioneers of photography.[35]

Mosso was clearly most impressed by cocaine's effects on a special form of
work. With respect to cocaine's acculturation in Europe, one part of Mosso's
experiments with cocaine is especially remarkable. Mosso writes:

> At twenty past nine I set off for Chieri and walked without pausing for fourteen-
> and-a-half kilometers, four kilometers of flat terrain, six kilometers uphill, and
> four-and-a-half kilometers downhill, all the while reading scientific journals and
> books, before returning to the laboratory at a quarter to four.[36]

Unfortunately, we do not know how he managed to carry so much scientific literature. Nevertheless, here we have the European form of the sublime effects of
cocaine. The Indians, admired by European travellers because of their unlimited
power to work and carry (the colonizer's) things, were replaced by a bourgeois
scientist, reading and walking in Italy. Not only the substance had been transformed – its effects were also manifested in a completely different way.

Both cocaine and the dynamometer have their own trajectories. In fin-de-
siècle Europe and without cocaine, the dynamometer was an instrument in
search of a deviant subject. Whereas Friedrich Nietzsche, as far as I can see, only
wrote about the dynamometer, Cesare Lombroso actually used this instrument
to locate foreign elements within society, to locate a subject that came to be
known as '*uomo delinquente*'. Following the traces of the deviant subject, Lombroso found muscular strength to be one of the '*stigmata degenerationis*'. With
the help of measurements taken with the dynamometer, he attempted 'objec-
tively' to elicit the signs characterizing degenerate subjects. He believed that it
was possible to draw conclusions about the nature of the soul based on physical
attributes and vice versa.[37] From this point of view, both coca and the dynamometer softened the demarcation line between the normal and the pathological
and established a new threshold between moral and criminal subjects.

Conclusion: Biologics and Cultures of Subjectivity

Biological substances played a decisive role in the creation of new representations of the body. These new representations and the instruments used to derive them were powerful means of transforming the Indian way of consuming coca – chewing coca leaves – into a measurable effect on the modern, working body – incorporating chemically and culturally purified and standardized cocaine. In this perspective, the switch from coca to cocaine and the new cultures of subjectivity also produced new deviant subjects and a new understanding of drug efficacy.

To release its power in Europe, cocaine had to be cut off from its Indian origins, albeit without forfeiting its mythical and utopian potential. To naturalize coca in an industrialized world that placed a premium on productivity and objectivity, it became purified from its natural, biologic origin and chemically standardized as cocaine. The biologic and hence variable and diverse coca plant had to be transformed into a precise, stable substance for concise experiments. Its utopia was thus moved from the Andes to the Swiss Alps, the factory and the study of deviant subjects. Coca's biologic origins lived on in cocaine as a promise of mythical power. That cocaine could promise to transgress the laws of thermodynamics in the twentieth century was rooted in coca's capacity to embody the utopian power of plant substances that originated outside civilization. Hence, the isolation of the alkaloid was only the first in a cascade of events that transformed coca as a biologic derived from Andean leaves into a European chemical compound. First of all, proof was needed that the effects of coca leaves were not limited to the Indian race. Once this process of cultural purification had isolated the biologic from its contextual origins, cocaine became more and more detached from its herbal substrate. A further step in the naturalization of coca in Europe involved industrial manufacturing and the production of new indications. Thus, cocaine became cheaper and distributable in a standardized form that had none of the disadvantages of coca leaves for scientific experiments, namely their natural variations and the potential loss of their active compound.

To demonstrate cocaine's effects on work with scientific, 'mathematical' precision, work had to be transformed into a measurable – and ever increasable – entity. Central to this transformation was the concept of fatigue. The emerging modern concept of fatigue saw exhaustion as the limit of productivity. In its modern form, fatigue was a quantifiable, impartial and normative benchmark, but not a fixed limit. To produce scientific evidence for cocaine's and its users' potential to transgress the limits of power, both had to become entangled in a network of diagnostic instruments like the dynamometer, the *neuramöbimeter*, and the ergograph. Here we can observe important changes in the cultures of objectivity as well as subjectivity. Shifts in diagnostic instruments are connected with transformations in conceptions of healthy bodies, both physiological and political ones. By using the average man as an ultimate yardstick, diagnosis produced and still produces thresholds and normal ranges, differences, degenerations, as well as deviant and (a)moral subjects.

Notwithstanding these continuities, at the end of the nineteenth century there was a shift from an initial prose of self-awareness to an objectification of physiological effects using measurement, numbers, tables and then curves. Here we can see the roots of a new theatre of medical evidence. The dynamometer still represented the tradition of mechanical objectivity. Likewise, the ergograph, as a self-recording device that produced fatigue curves, was still rooted in this tradition. Nevertheless, these curves were harbingers to the future importance of visualizations of the organisms' expressions. With this new aesthetics of proof, the Indians chewing coca leaves and thereby symbolizing, in the eyes of European travellers, unlimited power, were replaced by bourgeois scientists conducting experiments in their laboratories, climbing mountains or walking through northern Italy and reading scientific journals. On its way from the Andes to Europe, not only had the substance itself become transformed, but the narratives and the forms of demonstrating its effects had also changed profoundly. New cultures of subjectivity emerged by using and chemically objectifying pure cocaine in Europe. Nevertheless, its (biological) origin in an *other* culture proliferated new deviant subjects as cocaine was naturalized in Europe. From the mysterious Indians and their wonder drug, associated with wilderness and nature, coca became in late nineteenth-century Europe a chemical, demystified and industrialized means of becoming a permanently productive subject – a subject that could control its potential deviance from the laws of productivity by objective scientific means.

5 VITAL REGULATORS OF EFFICIENCY: THE GERMAN CONCEPT OF *WIRKSTOFFE*, 1900–1950

Heiko Stoff

The German compound word *Wirkstoffe*, combining agency (*wirken*) with materiality (*Stoff*), is hard to translate. The English term 'biologically active substances' as well as the Dutch *actieve substantie*, the Spanish *sustancia activa*, or the French *substance active* fail to capture its full meaning. While it had not been widely used before the first decade of the twentieth century and then mostly in the sense of a specific fabric or as synonymous with an initial power, it gained prominence in the 1930s as a biochemical concept uniting a new physiology of effective substances and the industrial production of pharmaceuticals with a life-reform discourse on a pure and strengthened body.[1] Well into the 1950s, the term *Wirkstoffe* exclusively referred to enzymes, hormones and vitamins as chemical agents that, although minute in quantity, showed profound physiological and biological effects. These biologically active chemical substances were vital to the organism due to their capacity to regulate the metabolism and the functioning of tissues and cells; but as standardized biologics, defined by their ability to compensate for deficiencies, they were also pharmacological actors, agents that promoted healthy and efficient bodies.

Research on and development of these strictly speaking hypothetical substances, at least in the first third of the twentieth century, was far from a German speciality. Indeed, interest in them extended to all transatlantic countries, notably the US, Canada, Great Britain, France, Switzerland, Spain and the Netherlands. To this day there exist national historiographies of hormones and vitamins, mostly linking them to political, economic or cultural contexts, such as war research in Britain, consumer society in the US, the pharmaceutical industry in Switzerland or the Dutch colonial empire.[2] But it was only in German-speaking areas that these compounds were subsumed under the single name of *Wirkstoffe* because of a conjunction of so-called natural product chemistry (*Naturstoffchemie*), the pharmaceutical industry and life-reform discourse.

While not much was known about the chemical identity of these substances and their actions in the animal body until the late 1920s, they nonetheless enabled new forms of representation of the organism, new ways of intervening in fundamental bodily processes, as well as providing new options for bodily perfection and human betterment. Well before biochemists, biologists and the pharmaceutical industry began cooperating to produce effective molecules out of raw materials collected in hospitals, slaughterhouses, police barracks and fruit farms; there were already long lists of characteristics organized around certain problematizations that rendered the existence of biologically active substances necessary.[3] In a kind of 'chronological reversal' (Culler), the path from social, political and scientific problems (as well as intriguing biological effects) to chemical identity involved various stages of institutionalization, regulation, standardization and activation.[4] To quote Bruno Latour, I'm interested in what transforms a substance into what it requires to subsist as part of 'a complex ecology of tributaries, allies, accomplices and helpers'.[5] Active substances seemed to be well-qualified to solve many pressing problems of the first third of the twentieth century: sex, gender, aging, degeneration and inefficiency. This response to the crisis of modernity comprised part of their attributes, just like the effects measured in bioassay animals, chemical structures and their crystalline form. *Wirkstoffe* were as much political as they were chemical.

In pledging to produce efficient bodies and protect consumer rights to fitness, health and youthfulness, hormones and vitamins were part of – and in some respects – a catalyst of modernity. Alfred Kühn's metaphorical definition of *Wirkstoffe* as vital regulators of efficiency ('*Regulatoren des Leistungsgetriebes*') perfectly illustrates the expectations associated with these chemical, political and self-technological agents in Germany, Switzerland and Austria.[6] From the 1890s, a remarkable manifestation of this new concept of high performance gained widespread popularity in these countries and influenced both political and scientific actions. Modernism, either as an affirmation of new lifestyles or as a critique of civilization, was interconnected with a discourse on life-reform that focused on the body politics of youthfulness, sexuality, purity, nutrition, nature and health.[7] Hormones and vitamins were affiliated with new technologies of the body, its reshaping, regeneration and rejuvenation, as well as with the very bodily deficiencies that had come to define the risky situation of modern human beings in an industrial civilization.[8] In this essay I will examine the reciprocal implications of efficiency and deficiency that determined the concept of *Wirkstoffe* and show how it enabled associations between physiology, the pharmaceutical industry, the life-reform movement and the modern state's concern for the quality of its population. *Wirkstoffe* were efficient actors of regulation, they were institutionalized as pharmaceutical and political tools, stabilized by industrial-scientific methods and activated for therapeutic, preventive and optimizing purposes. They combined a discourse on purity, naturalness and effectiveness with the inventiveness of biochemists and the productivity of pharmaceutical companies. But in a strange twist, the effectiveness of these chemical agents also turned them into potential actors of toxicity and carcinogenicity. The very idea of *Wirkstoffe* was thereby rendered precarious.

Efficient Actors

In the late nineteenth century, the German anatomist and embryologist Wilhelm Roux, founder of the 'Developmental Mechanics of Organisms' (*Entwicklungsmechanik der Organismen*), connected the analysis of developmental processes to the experimental technique of teratology. Defects, deformities and deficiencies produced in experimental animals – together defined as a lack of agency and materiality – served to highlight an organism's 'normal modes of reaction'.[9] In associating visibly deficient symptoms with invisible causes, the experimental production of defects generated new knowledge about the internal environment and established new agents of vital bodily functions. Developmental biology adopted the concept of physiological constancy, but concentrated on the relation of deficiency and efficiency. The organism as a stabilized internal environment was contingent upon chemical agents of internal secretion that could be activated for purposes of prophylaxis, therapy and enhancement. Claude Bernard's concept of internal secretion and Roux's experimental techniques – the production of deformations and the visualization of invisible processes – both shaped the life sciences in the late nineteenth and early twentieth century by redefining diseases and enabling new therapeutic practices. Until the 1920s, the experimental systems of Developmental Biology shaped the constitution of chemico-physical laws, i.e. the ongoing search for the chemical causes of biological development and its control.[10] Deficiency was a feature of the terrifying plasticity of the animal body, which manifested itself in those *monstrosities* that could be observed, produced and abolished. The experimental production of teratogen effects facilitated new knowledge about the factors that regulated normalcy. Subsequent to Roux, those trials attempted experimentally to form living beings 'at our will'.[11]

The science of internal secretion succeeded spectacularly when in 1889 the 72-year-old physiologist Charles-Édouard Brown-Séquard, Bernard's successor at the *Collège de France*, injected himself with animal testicular extracts and afterwards claimed that he felt strongly revitalized. In his report, Brown-Séquard attributed this bodily transformation to the efficiency of certain substances produced by the sex glands. Above all, he sublimely promised rejuvenation through improved performance and increased male virility.[12] Two years later, Brown-Séquard's controversial 'organotherapy' was validated by George R. Murray's successful therapeutic treatment of *myxoedema* with an active substance from the thyroid gland of sheep. The substitution, grafting or reimplantation of glands with internal secretion substantiated the curative efficacy of certain unknown substances. As the historian of science Chandak Sengoopta remarks, with his 'embarrassing but prescient self-experimentation' Brown-Séquard inaugurated a clinical revolution, but also, I would add, a radical pharmacological, industrial and body-political change.[13] The long list of deficiencies – aging, impotence, acromegaly, Addison's disease, myxoedema, cretinism – corresponded to the utopian promise of a vital, productive and efficient *new man*; a strengthened modern body, the exact opposite to the nervous and degenerated body of the nineteenth century.[14] Notably, testicle and ovarian extracts were defined and used as agents of efficiency and sexual enhancement. In the 1910s the Austrian Physiologist Eugen Steinach institutionalized sex hormones as normalizing actors of sexual variation and rejuvenation, and of sexual consumerism. He did so in the famous experiments he performed on the masculinization of female rats, the feminization of male rats and the rejuvenation of rodents and men at his laboratory in the Viennese biological research institute.[15] Steinach's claim about hormonal rejuvenation lost its persuasiveness during the 1920s, due to its scientific untenability and a moral critique of artificial rejuvenation during the world economic crisis. But as Steinach wrote triumphantly to his colleague Harry Benjamin, nobody would get the 'rejuvenation germ' ('*Verjüngungsbazillus*') out of sex hormones again.[16] Hormonal and organ therapy not only promised therapeutic innovations, but also a utopia of human perfection; it was both a sign of quackery and a new clinical practice.[17]

The histories of hormones and vitamins have been written independently of each other, but for contemporaries these substances seemed closely related.[18] The successes of organotherapy in the 1890s also influenced research on diseases that could not be sufficiently explained by germ theory. The idea of an accessory food factor, which when it was lacking could cause deficiency symptoms, was manifested in an endemic disease of nervous disorders, which in Indonesia was known as beriberi. The Dutch physician Christiaan Eijkman, who under the auspices of the Dutch colonial administration was commissioned to research the illness, resisted the microbe dogma every step of the way and interpreted the phenomena as a dietary deficiency.[19] Nutrition experiments, carried out by Frederic Gowland Hopkins, Elmer McCollum and Wilhelm Stepp amongst others, subsequently proved that a diet including all known necessary substances was insufficient to correct specific deficiencies. For food also contained hitherto unknown substances that were essential for the efficient functioning of the organism; and when lacking in an otherwise adequate diet, they disrupted bodily equilibrium and resulted in diseases of deficiency like beriberi, scurvy or pellagra.[20] Some organs and nourishments seemed to contain factors that were necessary for the well-being of animals and so active substances like hormones and vitamins were considered to be *substitutive* and *curative* agents.

When in 1905 Ernest Starling coined the term 'hormone' and seven years later Casimir Funk recommended that the term 'vitamin' replaces the awkward phrase 'accessory food factors', they both introduced perfect, albeit splendidly ambiguous notions.[21] From the first decade of the twentieth century onward, hormones and vitamins came to be related to political problematizations: they provided a vocabulary to critique industrialization, urbanization, as well as civilization in general. Hormones in particular have been rightfully described as agents of prosthetic modernity and gender policies. They elucidated the crisis of modern bodies while at the same time designing new bodies to solve biopolitical problems.[22] Diet became a central element in reform movements, connecting both self-technologies and science with vital natural forces. Vitamins soon became one of the main conditions of health, efficiency and vitality. Popular discourse was replete with stories of their success and utopian promise. Scientists were likewise working to both constrain and exploit the miraculous potentials of these biologics. The path from an efficient *specifica* to an omnipotent *panacea* was short.[23] In 1931 the highly respected German pharmacologist Walther Straub concluded that both vitamins and hormones were dead matter – chemicals that were being constantly produced in small amounts by the life processes in plants and animals. But even these small doses were capable of provoking the most drastic and even, he seemed to hesitate, miraculous effects in human and animal organisms.[24]

Standardizing Efficiency

At the end of the nineteenth century, compounds derived from every organ with internal secretion and used for every conceivable therapeutic purpose circulated on the pharmaceutical market. At that time, gland extracts were mostly aqueous extracts, while twenty years later they could be extracted with organic solvents and further purified.[25] In the early 1920s, no active substance besides thyroxin and adrenaline had been isolated and chemically defined. The market for hormones was dominated by hormonal and organ-based extracts of dubious quality. While the reputation of male hormonal preparations was tarnished because of their use as remedies against impotence, follicle hormone preparations promised to control the reproductive functions of the female body. The effectiveness of ovarian extracts in the treatment of sterility, menstrual disorders and climacteric dysfunctions was supported by clinical evidence and both scientifically accepted and politically desired.[26] Pharmaceutical companies like Hoffmann-La Roche in Basel, Merck in Darmstadt, Engelhard in Frankfurt/Main, Freund & Redlich in Berlin or Knoll in Ludwigshafen produced vast quantities of these extracts.[27] But by 1922 the gynaecologist Bernhard Zondek had warned against the exaggerated expectations aroused by the practical successes of organotherapy in the field of gynaecology. He even posed the heretical question of whether any such thing as substitution therapy existed at all. According to Zondek, the compounds were much too diverse and impure. Their biological effects depended on the mode of production and the procedures used to examine those effects were prone to error. In addition, it was unclear whether any of these preparations contained sufficient amounts of an active biological substance.[28]

Until the mid-1920s, the traces of an experimental and clinical situation and the effects of biophysiological experimental systems constituted qualities and properties of specific competencies. Roux's former assistant, the pharmacologist Ernst Laqueur, explained that organ preparations were nothing but the sum of unknown ingredients. And while the dosage and dispersion of any substance were crucial in achieving biological effects, the first step toward standardization involved enhancing the quantity of known ingredients in a preparation.[29] The same held true for vitamins. As one science popularizer summarized in 1921: all knowledge about vitamins was purely physiological. Only the effects were well known and needed to be understood as actions of unknown substances.[30] Two preconditions were necessary for the successful chemical processing, purification and clarification of active substances: the chemist needed accessible biological source material and a specific quantitative assay to measure the concentration and purity of any compound. Hormones and vitamins had to pass standardizing procedures to finally succeed as autonomous and efficient substances.[31]

In 1931 the pharmacist Joseph Herzog wrote an article about successful drugs that had been developed since the turn of the century. After discussing Antipyrin, Pyramidon, Aspirin, Veronal, Novocain and Salvarsan, he concluded that – unlike biology – chemistry was losing its relevance as a pharmacological tool.[32] Herzog considered vitamins and hormones to be natural products that could be obtained from animal organs and tested in animal experiments. But even if the biological raw material was standardized using biological assays, characterizing these substances was still a chemical procedure. The development of biologics involved in equal measure both a biological discovery and a technical invention.[33] According to Fritz Laquer from Bayer, the biological analysis constituted the basis for chemical research and therapeutic application. Pharmacology in the 1920s was characterized by the biological production of chemicals and the chemical production of biologics.[34] In the first third of the twentieth century, research on biologically active substances and the mass production of biological compounds depended on the organization of cheap raw materials and the development of biological assays to stabilize their effectiveness. In 1932 Carl Oppenheimer even spoke of an 'age of standardization' ('*Epoche der Eichungen*').[35] Hormones and vitamins demonstrated their potency and usefulness by way of specific bioassays that relied on laboratory animals: the growth of a cockscomb, oestrus growth or vaginal cornification in rodents, the disappearance of symptoms of diseases like scurvy or beriberi, as well as the tests designed to treat and prevent them.[36] But biological usefulness, objectified in rat and mouse units, didn't necessarily correlate with a specific chemical structure. Similar compounds could produce very different effects, and the same effects could be produced by very different chemical substances. This opened up a huge field of activity, helping to establish new markets and ultimately to provide those markets with new drugs. Stabilized substances that had proven their usefulness in a bioassay could also be used for other therapeutic aims and more marketable purposes. Furthermore, a slight alteration of the chemical structure could produce an even more efficient agent. The mere ability of active substances to pass a bioassay revealed nothing about the therapeutic value and marketability of these substances as pharmaceutical drugs, as biologics.

The industrial and ontological production of the invisible determinants of efficiency involved a complex network of biochemists, physiologists, clinicians, pharmaceutical industrialists, health politicians, consumers and the media. In this assemblage of molecules, discourses and interest groups, the contested differences between health and disease, curing and strengthening, active substance and drug, biocatalysts and commodities were finally eroded. Biologically active substances constituted a new definition of health and illness, an 'ultrachemistry' and an 'ultrapharmacology'.[37] The modern body, a controllable flexible system regulated by active substances, was never absolutely healthy, but always potentially sick and weak.[38] In this regard, hormones and vitamins gained the status of both natural substances and pharmaceuticals. In 1927, Walter S. Loewe coined the phrase 'medicine chest of the organism'; and Hermann E. Voss called hormones 'the body's own pharmaceuticals' (*'Eigenarzneien des Körpers'*). According to the pharmacologist Max Dohrn, hormones exercising a chemico-physical influence on the living cell should be compared to drugs. Joachim Kühnau concluded that vitamins were nothing but drugs that had the special quality of being active in minute amounts and functioning preventively. To keep the organism in good health, they should be taken for a lifetime. Straub ultimately maintained that only those humans were healthy who had the right, optimal and balanced chemical volume of vitamins.[39] From the 1920s onward, every human subject was obliged to secure its health and fitness through hormone and vitamin therapy. But the specific effectiveness of active substances in curing specific deficiency diseases corresponded with a much broader crisis, or rather, state of urgency. Vitamin D, for example, not only cured rickets, but also seemed to ameliorate the evils of capitalism, urbanism and civilization, such as poor hygienic conditions, faulty nutrition, dark and dreary rooms, and insufficient air and sunlight. Vitamin D became a tool of the caring and provident state, good education and rational science.[40]

Germany's science-based pharmaceutical industry was actively promoted by the ambitious German Empire and was an international leader until the First World War. But in the depressing post-war years, just as scientists the world over started to compete in developing hormones and vitamins, Germany's once famed biological and chemical science was in crisis. In 1921, much to the discontent of some politicians and representatives of the pharmaceutical companies, German scientists lost out to their Canadian colleagues in the race to develop insulin.[41] But as a result, the newly founded German Research Foundation in concert with pharmaceutical companies like Schering, Merck, IG Farben and a new elite of biochemists like Adolf Butenandt, Richard Kuhn and Adolf Windaus mobilized all their resources to isolate and synthesize sex steroids (Butenandt between 1929 and 1935), vitamin D (Windaus in 1927) and vitamins A and B2 (Kuhn in 1933 and 1934). The main task of biochemistry was to isolate active substances, to elucidate their chemical composition, and to work on developing further active derivatives. The coalition of natural-substance chemists and pharmaceutical companies was exceptionally successful in this regard and produced a vast amount of biologically active molecules. All three biochemists were rewarded with Nobel prizes; the cooperating pharmaceutical companies developed brand-name products like Progynon, Vigantol and Betaxin; and the State acquired the tools needed to advance its public health policies and biopolitical agendas.[42] These remarkable successes gave the chemistry of natural products, which already had a tradition stretching back to the early nineteenth century, the special status of an independent discipline combining a new physiology with the activation of pharmaceuticals. Until the mid-1930s, the isolation of natural substances from animal organisms and the synthesis of bioactive molecules was the main purpose of the highly productive cooperation between life scientists and the pharmaceutical industry. Synthesis didn't so much replace isolation, as acquire the status of a sometimes cheaper alternative, such as in the production of ascorbic acid. Then again, Schering, owing to its collaboration with Butenandt, achieved the systematic production of semi-synthetic analogues. Dehydroandrosterone, which was used to manufacture steroid hormones, functioned, according to Jean-Paul Gaudillière, as an industrial and molecular platform – a technical-epistemological object of both metabolic and industrial value.[43]

Endangered Regulators

Around 1900, the old physiology of a body regulated by the nervous system, as Edward Schaefer concisely formulated, had been replaced by a new physiology of chemical regulation. According to Hans-Jörg Rheinberger, Bernard's idea of an internal environment was a localized epistemological break, but the concept of biological regulation was ubiquitous.[44] In the first third of the twentieth century, the term biocatalyst gained prominence and was associated with the regulation of processes in the cell as well as the organism. From then on, catalysis meant regulation. The concept of regulation united society and organism, political practice and physiological experiment, forming an assemblage of new techniques, new things, new questions and new problems.[45] As Christina Brandt has explained for the history of gene expression, the use of metaphors like regulation, catalysis and control was not unique to the information theory of molecular biology in the 1950s, but was an integral part of the *Wirkstoff*-concept that had been around since the 1920s.[46]

The concept of *Wirkstoffe* specifically came to mean the reaction of hormones and vitamins with the catalytic properties of enzymes. In contrast to hormones and vitamins, which were defined in terms of their biophysiological effects, enzymes were chemical agents and products of an experimental discourse on the chemistry of life.[47] While the history of enzymes, discounting their biotechnological place in the history of brewing, is written in relation to debates about vitalism and mechanism, the interplay of regulation, specificity and catalysis is crucial to the concept of biologically active substances. The nexus of catalysis and specificity, first formulated by Louis Pasteur, was determined to be a chemical reaction in 1894 by Emil Fischer. His famous and momentous analogy, which constituted the relationship between enzyme and substrate in terms of a lock-and-key model, established the principle of complementarity as a highly productive hypothesis for enzymatic reactions. The axiom of catalytic specificity linked structure to efficiency.[48] According to Alwin Mittasch the main theoretician of the concept of catalysis in Germany in the 1920s, specificity and selectivity meant the reduction of a certain substance to a certain performance. The best example for this specific catalysis was the differentiation of labour between various enzymes in their role as 'constructive specialists in the metabolism' ('*schaffende(r) Spezialisten im Stoffwechsel*').[49] Biological specificity, as Lily Kay has shown, was interwoven with other sociotechnical constructions of modernity, like organization, differentiation, specialization, cooperation, stability and control.[50] This discourse not only made modern genetics and molecular biology possible, it also fostered the materialization of specific regulating substances. The concept of *Wirkstoffe* resulted in the conjuncture of enzymatic specificity with hormonal and vitamin efficiency. In the words of Oppenheimer, the 1920s and 1930s were shaped by a concept of 'tremendous consistency of all fundamental processes in the living substance'. He further spoke of an awed amazement with regard to these over-refined regulation processes that controlled the cellular gearbox called life and that dictated the laws of growth, metabolism and formation.[51] Mittasch again remarked that a substantial stimulation effect, which had been described for hormones and vitamins, could also be found in enzymatic processes: wide-ranging effects even in minute amounts; highly disparate effects of chemically related substances; the inversion of tendency through a slight shift of the double bind; similar or identical effects of chemically extraordinarily different bodies; an over-additive interaction of simultaneously present substances; impressive synergisms and antagonisms. The sole but important difference was that hormones and vitamins, unlike enzymes, affected processes of formation and development.[52]

The intervention into bodily processes and the control of metabolic processes wasn't possible until both a concept of an organism controlled by chemical agents had been constituted and active substances standardized. Cancer research, genetics, reproductive medicine, nutrition science and the medicine of metabolic diseases all changed dramatically in the first half of the twentieth century. But the system of chemical regulation also established the means for ensuring control over the body, an alignment of the organism to the norm, and a politics of normalization in which each aberration was necessarily a state of pathology.[53] While Georges Canguilhem's much cited lineage from Bernard's internal environment to Walter B. Cannon's concept of homeostasis and Norbert Wiener's cybernetics rightfully underscores the importance of the concept of an organism that is, due to chemical self-regulation and adaptation, able to cope with the external environment, it also ignores the fact that in Germany in the first decades of the twentieth century a concept of self-regulated equilibrium existed in its own right and had been commonplace since the 1920s.[54] In November 1928, Dohrn attributed all processes in the animal organism to a chain of adaptations to the external environment and a steady interplay of organs within the organism itself, a subtly regulated physiological process, a harmonic equilibrium of all forces and processes, which if disturbed would result in pathological conditions.[55]

In September 1938, the pharmacologist Hermann Druckrey, in a letter to Butenandt, proposed a model for organisms that incorporated new knowledge from biochemistry: accordingly, *Wirkstoffe* had to be differentiated into exogenous chemicals, like pharmaceuticals, poisons or vitamins and the body's own substances, like catalytic enzymes, which in turn reacted with vitamins. The regulation system functioned through the interactions of different chemical, humoral, physical and nervous agents as mediated by hormones.[56] The relationship between internal and external environment plays a major role in the concept of *Wirkstoffe*. Physiological experiments in the 1920s were preoccupied with organisms threatened by external attack, with regulatory systems weakened and irritated as a consequence of war, hunger and urbanity, and with the threats posed by so-called poisons of civilization, like alcohol, nicotine and caffeine.[57] This rhetoric of foreign threats and the need for bodily self-defence – most clearly expressed in Emil Abderhalden's speculative 'defence enzymes'

(*Abwehrfermente*) – was already in use in the 1920s, but it gained momentum in the 1930s and 1940s.[58] Social hygienic and biopolitical problematizations were connected to biochemical questions; the physiological body and the body politic stood in more than just a metaphorical relationship to one another. In this regard, the concept of a regulation system based on biologically active substances converged with the discourse on healthy and powerful bodies that were endangered by modern life, its foreign matter and poisons. The critique of civilization came to be materialized in the concept of *Wirkstoffe*.

Activators of Efficiency

In the twentieth century, the efficient-deficient body, controlled by active substances, was integrated into a system of therapeutic regulations. The concept of biologically active substances thereby not only connected the clinic, industry and the laboratory, but also involved the biopolitical interests of the state, a new consumer culture based on self-technologies, and a new concept of nutrition informed by the life-reform movement and by notions of a strengthened as well as purified body. During the 1930s, *Wirkstoffe* combined a new physiology of internal regulation and external threat with the natural chemistry of efficient substances and in so doing featured prominently not only in textbooks, but also as themes of political mobilization.[59] *Wirkstoffe* helped to elaborate Nazi concepts of the body, as well as their public health and nutrition policies.

A global market for vitamin and hormone products existed in the 1920s. The talk of 'vitamania' (*'Vitaminrummel'*) and the 'rejuvenation craze' (*'Steinachrummel'*) permeated the transatlantic world.[60] The chief aim of these fads was the promise of enhanced performance. The clever marketing strategists of pharmaceutical companies like Hoffmann La Roche in Switzerland adapted their products – specific molecules like antiscorbutic vitamin C – so as to accord to this promise.[61] Although these developments transpired in liberal-democratic and consumer-oriented societies that relied on individual rights and self-government, the notion of enhancing individual and collective bodies using active substances also fit perfectly well with the ideology and martial aims of the National Socialist regime. The goals of rejuvenation, dietary reform, health care and enhanced performance were all easily transformed into Nazi policies.

Sex steroids played a major role in the biopolitics of sterility treatment, mostly in relation to menstrual disorders like amenorrhea and hormonal sterilization, which by the 1920s had already become the object of experimental research. This culminated in Carl Clauberg's vision of a 'research institute for reproduction biology' (*'Forschungsinstitut für Fortpflanzungsbiologie'*) combining positive and negative eugenics in one single institution. The obstetric hospital, which he hoped to see incorporated within Adolf Hitler's Schutzstaffel (SS), was supposed to be affiliated with a concentration camp. The clinic was to treat infertile women of desirable stock with hormones, while those deemed reproductively unworthy would be sterilized, not surgically, but by means of hormonal manipulation.[62] Clauberg was a respected scientist and devoted Nazi who worked for the SS in concentration camps, forcefully and brutally sterilizing Jewish women. His project sought to radicalize a gynaecological programme that was for the most part shared by his colleagues in Kiel, Berlin, Heidelberg and Munich.[63] Once again, vitamin C was highly important for Nazi food policies because, thanks to Hoffmann La Roche's marketing efforts, it promised to combine health policies with enhanced performance and prevention with optimization. Merck, which specialized in the production of vitamin C derived from fruits and plants, couldn't satisfy the demands of the Nazi state and so during the war huge amounts of ascorbic acid were bought from the Swiss company.[64] By order of the Wehrmacht, candy containing ascorbic acid (so called V-drops) were produced and transported to the front in hopes of enhancing soldiers' health and military effectiveness. The vitaminization of food became an important aspect of nutrition research and food engineering. From 1940 onward, vitamins C and D were provided to infants, children and pregnant women, as well as to soldiers and indispensable workers. Delivering the optimal quantity of vitamins to people (be it for mere survival or for productive work) was a wartime necessity. Both endocrine gynaecology and nutrition science, practised by young scientists born around 1900, boomed during wartime. Hormones and vitamins were seen as effective agents of Nazi policies.[65]

But just when Nazi policies aimed at the immediate activation of efficient substances came into force, a debate on the complexity of the regulation of internal environments began and contradicted these ambitions. A regulation model was compatible to Nazi policies as long as it was combined with a chemistry of natural substances like Butenandt's and Alfred Kühn's '*Genwirkketten*', which were introduced 'to characterize chemically identifiable products of genic [!] action endowed with the capability of controlling chemical or morphological developmental processes' and which later came to be seen as a forerunner of molecular biology.[66] While in this case, regulation meant a causal relationship that could be explained by and produced with the experimental systems of developmental physiology, at the same time new knowledge had been generated about highly complex chemical reactions and interactions in the organism. As Butenandt summarized, chemistry had become increasingly important for the solution of biological problems. The isolation of biocatalysts was the main biochemical task of the 1920s and 1930s, but this knowledge also raised new questions about the structural, chemical and physiological connections and relations of *Wirkstoffe*.[67] The interactions between biologically active substances, i.e. a system of antagonistic or synergistic reactions, couldn't be ignored, even though the Jewish scholars who comprised a large portion of the vibrant community of German biochemists were forced into exile, even though Otto Warburg's work at the Kaiser-Wilhelm-Institute for Cell Physiology was marginalized, and even though National Socialist research policy, hell-bent as it was on producing hormones and vitamins, showed no interest in replacing the lost talent. One might even speak of a crisis of the concept of causal specificity in the 1930s and 1940s, when more and more scientists warned that the activation of pharmaceuticals had to consider unforeseeable antagonistic and synergetic reactions.[68]

This debate arose just as the Nazi state began mobilizing all of its resources for war. In particular, the controversy over artificial or natural vitamins was linked to the new paradigm of interdependent actions of active substances in the organism. In a seemingly paradoxical way, the antagonist-synergistic discourse highlighted the belief that, despite their effectiveness in bioassays, no substance could itself cause biological or physiological effects. German advocates of dietary reform like Werner Kollath from the Hygienic Institute at the University of Rostock criticized the use of industrially produced biologically active substances as surrogates. Kollath was an outspoken opponent to the doctrine that an isolated vitamin was the sole reason for deficiency diseases. In this regard he was also an enemy of the exceedingly successful chemistry of natural substances that had spawned close collaboration between biochemists and the pharmaceutical industry.[69] Kollath himself relied heavily on the concept of vitamins, but he emphasized a complex and synergistic system of vitamins' physiological actions and other vital substances that would evoke antagonistic and pathological effects if any one single vitamin was missing or misplaced. In this regard, avitaminosis was simply a consequence of lopsided physiology. According to Kollath, the highest degree of health would be ensured not by supplementation but by an optimal mixture of all vital substances.[70] In Kollath's differentiation, synthetic vitamins couldn't produce 'absolute health' ('*Übergesundheit*'), as Hoffmann-La Roche and other companies had promised. Vitamins, he stated, only have a physiological effect when reacting with auxiliary substances like aromatic substances and enzymes; a healthy diet had to consist of 'wholefood' ('*Vollwertkost*'). Deficiency diseases, again, were simply the outcome of failing food production and improper food preparation.[71]

There was indeed an ongoing debate about the pros and cons of synthetic versus natural substances: could the total synthesis produce the asymmetry of a carbon atom? Did similar physiological effects refer to identical substances? And finally, were synthetic substances as effective and efficient as natural substances?[72] Vitamin research demonstrated, according to the expert Hermann Schroeder, how necessary it was to understand nutrition in holistic terms.[73] Other scientists, like the paediatrician Hans Rietschel, doubted that isolated or synthesized ascorbic acid really was physiologically equivalent to vitamin

C, because to his mind it lacked the complexity of the latter.[74] In 1942, Wilhelm Alter simply characterized synthetic vitamins as non-effective imitations, as 'vitaminoids'.[75] Chemists were not amused and vehemently opposed this critique in their professional journals and even called it a declaration of war against Germany's chemical industry.[76] Alter's and Kollath's rebellion was an attack on the wartime policy consensus on vitamins and nutrition shared by industry, science and the state. In 1942, Kollath's views provoked the leading vitamin experts of the day, Abderhalden and Carl-Arthur Scheunert, to angrily denounce them as 'fanciful' ('*fantastisch*').[77] When Alter again dismissed as worthless the so-called Cebionbonbons, which Merck produced as tablets containing ascorbic acid, Abderhalden reacted aggressively, accusing Alter of undermining military morale, which naturally was a dangerous accusation during the Nazi regime. For Abderhalden, it was irrelevant whether or not a substance that could pass a bioassay or any other test was part of a foodstuff, isolated from biological raw material or artificially produced, because in terms of metabolism the molecules functioned in exactly the same way, even if they, as Abderhalden admitted, interacted with enzymes and were unable to activate vital processes outside of a living substance.[78] Karl Maier feared that this debate would revive the old notion of an enigmatic life force at a time when the synthesis of organic compounds should have eradicated the old difference between natural types and artificial products.[79] Ultimately, Stepp and Schroeder underscored the importance of synthetically produced natural substances for public health.[80]

This fierce debate in the middle of the war exemplifies how strong the discourse on *Wirkstoffe* as natural substances that safeguarded a powerful, healthy and pure body had become. While nutrition experts and biochemists flatly rejected Alter's intervention, arguing that in a state of emergency synthetic substances were simply indispensable, they also emphasized the fundamental or even moral superiority of natural substances. The defence of chemical research and productivity was not a eulogy to artificiality or haphazard vitaminization. Wholewheat bread was always better than white bread plus vitamin B1, proclaimed Abderhalden, fruits and vegetables better than vitamin C pills.[81] Nazi dietary policies were marked by the internal contradiction of biohygienic nutrition physiology and chemico-pharmaceutical productivity. Both sides had their place in the Nazi system, as can be seen in the coexistence of synthetic and natural products in the wartime economy. Indeed, the industrial production of biologically active substances coexisted with the identification, culling, testing and manufacturing of fruits like rosehips, all sorts of apples, paprika and even gladiolas.[82]

Foreign Matter and Vital Substances

The notion of *Wirkstoffe* was altered by the introduction of more and more chemical and physical assays for enzymes, hormones and vitamins in the late 1930s and the problem of antagonist and synergistic reactions. There are two ways in which the concept was transformed in the 1950s. In general, the concept of *Wirkstoffe* was subsumed under an overall chemicalization of life processes. The biophysiological discourse about efficient, but miraculous active substances had already been relativized by research on the macromolecular protein structure of enzymes and insulin in the 1930s. In the 1950s, due in part to the internationalization of scientific discourse, *Wirkstoffe* were transformed into chemical agents regulating biosynthesis, processes of metabolism and gene expressions in complex forms of representation like cycles, chains, cascades and systems. Hormones, vitamins and enzymes were still efficient agents for efficient bodies in a highly productive society. But their narrow definition as *Wirkstoffe*, laden with scientific, industrial and political interests, was no longer needed to satisfy their respective objectives.

Wirkstoffe were biochemical agents that seemed to possess regulating and controlling powers, pharmacological tools that could be activated for manifold purposes. But what if these central agents of growth, development and constitution went astray? Synthetic active substances, mere chemicals, had in this respect lost the quality of *Wirkstoffe*. The more chemical these substances were (like steroids), the more suspicious was the public, the media, and some scientists themselves. The end of *Wirkstoffe* in the late 1940s also marks the beginning of an ongoing discourse on dangerous *Fremdstoffe* (foreign matter) contaminating the human body.[83] The intense debate about natural and artificial substances in the early 1940s coincided with a dispute about the potential carcinogenicity of steroids or toxicity of certain vitamins. These potent and autonomous chemical agents, generally seen as magic bullets against cancer, were also unpredictable; their proven status as useful actors of growth and development made them precarious.[84] In 1940, Butenandt introduced an exhaustive new definition that classed as cancer all malignant and atypical tumours that didn't fit holistically within the organism, that eluded its regulative and configurative authority, and that achieved autonomy from it through growth and metabolism. Significantly, however, it remained an open question as to whether cancer could be caused by qualitative or quantitative effects, by the structure of molecules or by their dosage. While Butenandt was collaborating with Schering, he was certainly interested in vindicating the steroid structure of oestrogens from the charge of carcinogenicity and instead blaming carcinogenic effects on the dosage.[85]

But the dismissal of *Wirkstoffe* as precarious and dangerous *Fremdstoffe*, as foreign intruders into the holistic system of biochemical processes, also provoked the new concept of *Vitalstoffe* (vital substances), consolidating the life-reformist aspects of *Wirkstoffe*. In 1954 Hans-Adalbert Schweigart, a former official in charge of Nazi nutrition policies, founded the International Society for Vital Substances (*Vitalstoffgesellschaft*). In the following years, the society organized numerous conferences that aroused great interest in the public and the media. Beginning in 1956 he also published his own journal called *Vitalstoffe. Zivilisationskrankheiten* (Vital substances and Diseases of Civilization). The society counted Kollath and Scheunert amongst its many members. Albert Schweitzer acted as president emeritus from 1956 to 1965 and his successor was Linus Pauling. The society was a powerful counter-organization to the pharmaceutical and foodstuff industry. The rise of *Vitalstoffe* correlated with the prohibition of *Fremdstoffe*. The society's general goals of health, purity and naturalness, as well as its fight for a new German food law, were favourably received in the contemporary media. Schweigart spoke out against all food additives, colourants and antibiotics in food, against irradiation and the use of nearly all chemicals, while simultaneously promoting Kollath's wholefood nutrition. This was a highly attractive standpoint for anyone dissatisfied with health, ecology, dietary policies and modernity itself. At the same time, however, the organization was also a shelter for former activists of Nazi food policies who, in redefining the concept of nutrients and poisons, resumed highly political discourses on purity and contamination. According to Schweigart's definition, vital substances (enzymes, co-enzymes, vitamins, hormones, exogenous-essential amino- and fatty-acids, principal- and trace-elements, aromatic substances and flavour enhancers) were constituents that functioned in the organism as biocatalysts. But their synergistic interactions were always endangered by industrially produced substances from steroids and synthetic vitamins to azo dyes.[86]

While from the 1950s onward *Wirkstoffe* simply meant all biologically active substances in an organism, the ambiguity of the concept of *Wirkstoffe*, a notion which was so important for biological and chemical policies in the first half of the twentieth century in the German-speaking areas, was finally divided into two strictly separated entities of *Fremd-* and *Vitalstoffe*. This concept again fostered a new transatlantic discourse on vitality and devitalization, established a highly profitable industry of nutrients and constituted a regime of self-governmental techniques that both strengthens and defends the efficient body of today.

6 THE DETACHABILITY OF REPRODUCTIVE CELLS: ON BODY POLITICS IN SPERM AND EGG DONATION[1]

Sven Bergmann

In her study on organ transplantation, medical anthropologist Linda Hogle refers to the constant context-dependent ambiguity of human biological material as 'entities that are simultaneously precious human remains, technological artefacts, waste products, and therapeutic tools'.[2] According to the definitions listed by the editors in the introduction, such bodily detachable human entities and fluids can be conceptualized as biologics. This essay is about a particular kind of human material: gametes (or germ cells), reproductive substances which are needed for procreation and that are differentiated into sperm and oocytes. Gametes can be termed biologics because they mostly originate from living organisms; in addition, in some cases post-mortem sperm retrieval is performed.[3] Reproductive treatment relies on gametes as a natural resource that cannot be synthesized. Like other biologics, the regulation of gamete donation, their storage and the standardization of these processes pose several legal problems. Therefore the aim of this essay is to show why gametes are a particular kind of biologics, given that they cannot be standardized like other biologics and that their very use calls into question their ontological status. Furthermore, the ways in which they are made available from the body are quite differentiated and rooted in gender dichotomies, depending on whether sperm or oocytes are involved.

In contrast to other types of biologics like vaccines or vitamins that are designed for preventive or therapeutic use, gametes are used for reproductive treatment (as a means of substitution). Gametes of a third party (usually described as the donor) do not cure infertility in recipients, but they are used to trigger reproductive processes in a recipient. Consequently, donated gametes can be regarded as replacing dysfunctional gametes and as intervening in and enhancing bodily processes of reproduction. There are also some gendered assumptions about other bodily effects of gametes, mostly about effects of sperm in female bodies[4] – but in this essay I will concentrate on the main role of gametes as a means of reproduction and heredity. Like other bodily detachable material, sperm plays a role in forensic DNA testing: on the one hand it can be extracted and detached from a body (and therefore found at a crime scene), but it can also be traced back to the person where it generated because it is attached with genetic information. But in contrast to other body cells like in human hair or tissue, gametes can fuse with other gametes and therefore generate a pregnancy which may result in the birth of a new person. The ubiquity of detachments and attachments of reproductive substance is constitutive of what I will call the very paradoxes of detachability: even in cases of anonymized gamete donation, these bodily separated substances remain assembled with attachments. Anthropologist Kaushik Sunder Rajan reminds us that living material has 'a separate social life, but the "knowledge" provided by the information is constantly relating back to the material biological sample'.[5] As a result, forms of doing kinship with anonymously donated gametes complicate legal situations. Donated sperm or oocytes are seen as natural substances, but their use in the reproductive processes of other people is sometimes seen as contrary to nature.

Drawing on empirical material, this essay explores the relation between the body and its reproductive substances in the context of assisted reproductive technologies (ART). First, I will present an overview of different processes used to deal with reproductive substances in relation to two kinds of gametes: sperm and egg cells (ova/oocytes). Then, I want to show how they are detached from the female and the male body, how they are selected, treated and classified in the laboratory and how they are stored and marketed. The conclusion will take into account the specifics of gametes and why they seem to resist standardization – much more so than other biologics in this volume do. The examples I use draw on ethnographic fieldwork in two infertility clinics in Spain and the Czech Republic, both with large egg donation programmes for mainly foreign patients. Furthermore, I include material from visits to two expanding Danish sperm banks and data from internet research. Written by an anthropologist with an interest in Science and Technology Studies (STS), this essay differs from the majority of chapters in this book in that it does not adopt a primarily historical perspective on gametes[6] or reproductive technologies,[7] but rather an ethnographical one. Regarding the locations of data collection, this essay is mainly concerned with (largely Christian-secular) Euro-American perspectives on kinship and substance.[8]

Gametes, Detachability and Technologies for Standardization

What makes gametes so different from other bodily cells? From a biologist's perspective one can say it is their different mode of cell division through meiosis. During meiosis, the genome of a diploid germ cell (two sets of 23 chromosomes = 46 chromosomes) passes through DNA replication followed by two rounds of division, resulting in four haploid cells. Each of these cells contains one complete set of 23 chromosomes (half of the genetic content of the cell it originated from). If meiosis produces gametes, these cells must fuse during fertilization to create a new diploid cell before any new growth can occur – in other words, the creation of new entities or human beings. Because of their divided chromosome sets during meiosis, gametes bear some sort of biogenetic 'kinship device': heredity in multiple forms of combinations.

In spite of ongoing experiments designed to create spermatozoa from adult stem cells in mice and that might someday unlock the possibilities of parthenogenesis, two different kinds of haploid germ cells are still needed for human reproduction.[9] What has changed is that, with in vitro technologies, procreation can also be placed in the laboratory. In assisted reproduction, Bruno Latour's allusion that 'we live in communities whose social bond comes from objects fabricated in laboratories',[10] has deep implications: embryos are made in the laboratory using sperm and egg cells detached from human persons, later they are re-transferred to a female (human) body. In vitro fertilization (IVF) enabled the fusion of egg and sperm outside the body in a Petri dish and a body-temperature incubator in the laboratory. In 1978, the first in vitro procreated human being, by then popularized as the first test-tube baby, was born in the UK. In the 1980s, third-party reproduction using ova provided by another woman was successfully performed.[11] The impact of this technique (usually labelled 'egg donation') has challenged the long-standing Roman law principle *mater certa semper est* by detaching ova from women's bodies (donors) for the first time and implanting them in another female body (recipients). By contrast, sperm has always been considered detachable from the body and therefore fatherhood has always been more invisible; in contrast to uncontested motherhood, paternity had 'to be symbolically or socially constructed'.[12]

In contrast to egg cells, human semen has a longer history as a substituting and experimental tool. In the eighteenth century, Spallanzani's experiments with 'spermatic animalcules' are the most noteable, although he neglected the significance of sperm for procreation.[13] It was not until the 1880s, a hundred years later, that scientists agreed procreation was the fusion of two distinct cellular entities, egg and sperm, and understood how that fusion was used as a biological foundation for modern gender difference.[14] Accordingly, sperm is now (even in some biological textbooks) regarded as an active entity, whereas the egg cell is conceived as being rather more passive.[15] As a consequence of conceptualizing sperm as vital and mobile, at the end of the nineteenth century other elements in seminal plasma, like spermine, a polyamine which is contained in human semen, was marketed for organotherapy as a 'fountain of youth'.[16] In the twentieth century, sperm was used to experiment with cell manipulation in vitro. These experiments benefited from sperm's easy detachability: that it can be obtained without invasive procedures through a single sexual activity. Due to its easy detachability from the body, sperm has been a well-used research substance for experiments that involve freezing living things. Their ability to survive in the freezer of the laboratory was proven by thawing them to reveal live sperm, which Hannah Landecker in her history of cell culturing has described as the onset of cryobiology.[17] In 1949, Christopher Polge and colleagues from the National Institute for Medical Research accidentally discovered the protective qualities of glycerol in freezing chicken sperm.[18] With efforts in cryobiology, the linear lifespan of cells could be halted and reactivated. This has become one of the central dialectics of what has become known as biotechnologies: the tension between 'animation and cessation'.[19] The controlled stopping and restarting of linear lifetime was first used in the post-Second World War industrialization of cattle reproduction; and the first commercial US sperm bank which used cryopreservation technology to freeze human sperm opened in 1972. Nevertheless, artificial insemination with fresh sperm in vivo has a much longer history – whether it is done with the 'assistance' of clinicians or with 'do-it-yourself technologies'.[20] The 'turkey baster' (as a medium for DIY insemination at home) is still a metaphor with 'symbolic power in lesbian reproduction'[21] and it illustrates that substances that are so easy detachable, like sperm, cannot be fully regulated by medical authorities. Beyond that, these instances show that actors sometimes circumvent regulations and medicalization and even actively engage in their own objectification. The pathologization and technologization of infertility is not always a one-sided product of the biomedical regime, but instead a much more ambivalent choice of patients as empirical studies of assisted reproduction demonstrate.[22] In the following section, I will show how the delivery of gametes is performed and what this is saying about gender performativity in reproductive medicine.

Applied Detachability: Procurement of Gametes

How are gametes (in assisted reproduction) detached from the body? What treatments do donors have to go through? The European Union Tissue Directive from 2006 defines 'procurement' as the 'process by which tissue or cells are made available'.[23] The procurement of egg and sperm are quite different. The following scenarios will highlight differences in the egg and sperm on the day of procurement.[24]

Scenario 1: An operation theatre in a private infertility clinic in Barcelona. Seven people from the clinic and I, the ethnographer, are inside, standing. On the table is the anaesthetized body of an egg donor. Debora, the operating gynaecologist, sits in front of the woman's spread legs.[25] Ovas are removed by transvaginal ultrasound guided aspiration (an ultrascan with an attached aspiration needle that is injected through the bladder into the ovary). Gemma, the surgeon's assistant, is watching the tube of the catheter, the end of which is fixed to a battery of test tubes. She is calling: 'sale' (it comes) when fluid is flowing and 'para' when it stops, so the surgeon moves to the next filled testicle. During the operation, Gemma shows me a test tube with four red points at the bottom: 'This is what we are looking for'. After all follicles are extracted, one of the assistants gets an adhesive label for the test-tube box and immediately takes the test tubes to the IVF laboratory which is on the same floor. In this case of an egg donor, the eggs will never return to her body, she will instead receive €900 as compensation for the procedure. In the case of conventional IVF, two or three selected eggs will return about three to five days later, fertilized with sperm, to the patient's body via a catheter (embryo transfer).

Scenario 2: A Danish sperm bank located in an office building in Aarhus from where frozen sperm is shipped to many international destinations. In the middle of the department is a small waiting room from which one can see two doors with digital entry signs. When the light turns green, a sperm donor can enter a room that is decorated with a poster of a half-naked woman and equipped with heterosexual softcore and hardcore magazines and porn DVDs. He closes the door behind him. Sperm donors collect their ejaculate in a little vessel and afterwards hand it to the laboratory employee over the counter. There it will be prepared and afterwards put in straws to be frozen in cryo-containers in liquid nitrogen (at -196°C). In the Danish sperm bank, donors get about €20 for one sample. At another sperm bank in Copenhagen, sperm donors can also get a video clip with their own sperm sample under the microscope if they provide a USB flash drive.

Whereas egg delivery occurs in an operation theatre with anaesthetized bodies, without agency and intimacy and where a lot of people are entering and watching, including non-medical researchers like me, sperm delivery is done actively and alone by masturbation: a sexual action that has very rarely been observed by ethnographers.[26] Although the equipment of masturbation rooms with (heterosexual) porn as therapeutic tools is commonplace in the literature,[27] it underlines sperm donation as some form of sexual work with the objective of producing a sample of a good volume. Interestingly, the 'cum shot' (live ejaculation) in the average heterosexual hardcore porn movie is also termed the 'money shot' because some directors pay their actors extra money for a successful cum shot.[28] Nevertheless, the procurement of sperm is restricted to a short sexual action after 48 hours of sexual abstinence which – according to current research – produces the best donor sperm and results in the best pregnancy rates.[29] Short periods of abstinence – natural phases of regeneration – serve as the best vehicle for the quality of this biological material and no special diet or athletic programme is required. Instead, recent studies show that environmental influences affect sperm quality much more than tobacco, alcohol or marijuana.[30] To my knowledge there is no use, nor even research on, hormonal stimulation of human sperm.

In contrast to sperm delivery, egg donors are involved in a strict regime of medical compliance with regards to hormonal stimulation, sexual abstinence and clinical visits for ultrasound scans that culminate in the surgery described above. Until now, there have been few studies on the long-term risks of high stimulation in IVF donor cycles.[31] While hormonal stimulation circumvents the nature of ovulation by bringing more than one egg to harvest, sexual abstinence mimics cultural techniques of self-control. Compliance is required in both cases, while the female case is much more medicalized. Because its passiveness is not contaminated by sexuality, egg donation is often far more closely associated with altruism, while sperm donation is merely seen as a job for students.[32] If, in a Danish sperm bank, donors can get a video clip of their own sperm sample on a USB flash drive, then gendered symbols of substance still matter in procurement and detachment of gametes: the image of the active motile sperm versus the passive waiting egg.[33]

Substituting Nature in the Laboratory and Tasks of Classifying Substance

After alienation from the body, how is substance enacted in the laboratory? How is reproductive material classified, selected and prepared? After gametes are extracted from the body and brought to the laboratory, they traverse through purification, preparation and classification procedures; therefore the laboratory and some technologies are seen as either simulating natural environments or halting the gametes' lifespan by freezing them. Culturing and storing of cells in the laboratory was not so much a question of origins, but of conditions, 'of what makes it possible for these biotechnical things to exist in these detached, transformed ways'.[34] Culture media helped to externalize internal processes by substituting particular bodily functions like asepsis (laboratory), fluid (culture medium), structural support (e.g. oil for embryonic culture) and warmth (incubator).[35]

In the laboratory, sperm must be separated from seminal plasma; eggs must be quickly and efficiently separated from blood and nurturing follicle cells for use in IVF.[36] Washed and classified, sperm ends up in frozen straws in liquid nitrogen, while egg cells are separated from surrounding cells, put in an artificial nurture medium and then immediately fertilized on the day they are harvested, because IVF cycles with frozen eggs still deliver poorer results.[37] Between fertilization and embryo transfer, fertilized eggs remain in the laboratory for between two and three days in a nurturing medium and a body-temperature incubator. 'We treat every embryo like a little patient' is a slogan of a Spanish clinic's marketing DVD. Nevertheless, embryologists in this clinic explained to me that the best place for eggs would always be in the uterus, that's why they referred to the incubator as 'the womb'. While sperm is immediately sent on a cold pathway, eggs are cared for in a body-temperature atmosphere. Because embryologists see the laboratory as a brief artificial simulation of a natural environment, they try to reduce the time spent outside the incubator to a minimum. Once, Nuría, an embryologist in the Spanish clinic, wanted to show me an egg cell before performing intracytoplasmic sperm injection (ICSI) under the microscope. But I, the stubborn ethnographer, wanted to ask some scientific question first, so she instructed me: 'Hurry up, time is running out'. In fresh IVF cycles with donated eggs, there is also a certain time constraint for the recipients. While sperm can be frozen and thawed, a fresh IVF cycle has time constraints and spatial fixes; it requires that recipients be synchronized with the donor and at the disposal of the clinic at a certain time for embryo transfer – otherwise fertilized eggs would have to be cryopreserved for a frozen cycle that has lower rates of success.

A large part of the laboratory work involves classification. As Geoffrey Bowker and Susan Leigh Star have noted, regardless of whether classifications 'become standardized', they are 'both material and symbolic'.[38] In IVF clinics, sperm is categorized using WHO reference values to assign normal classifications like *Normozoospermia* (average sperm count) or pathological classifications like *Oligozoospermia* (low sperm count) or *Azoospermia* (meaning an absence of sperm cells in semen) as indicators for male infertility.[39] Semen analysis was introduced as '*Spermiogramm*' during the Nazi regime by the German physician Hans Stiasny in Berlin.[40] Subsequently, sperm and male fertility were measured with a standardized scheme still in use today, where motility and form are employed to distinguish between normal and pathological sperm.[41] Whereas regular semen analysis appeared to me (during participant observation) to be an endless and boring task of counting and calculating cells, the qualification process for ova seemed a much more visual task that mobilized categories like beauty. Egg cells and embryos are always qualified and selected via their morphological structure; but sperm only rarely require morphological selection under microscopes with very high resolution, for example in cases involving the newer technique of IMSI (Intracytoplasmic *morphologically* selected sperm injection).[42] During fieldwork in the Spanish laboratory, one of the most common phrases that embryologists used while watching oocytes under the microsope was 'estos son bonitos' ('these are beautiful ones'). As I learned during my research, beauty is not foremost an aesthetic valorization; instead, oocyte and embryo selection via morphological structure is considered best practice in IVF laboratories. But in recent papers, this simple evaluation by appearance is devalued as a 'beauty contest'.[43] Morphological evaluation is orientated towards an oocyte's or embryo's potential for development: as a study in 2012 has shown, morphological selection of oocytes seems to enhance results in fertilization, but there is no evidence suggesting that it effects the further development of the embryo.[44] As embryologists told me, a beautiful embryo can also exhibit a genetic disposition. Only invasive techniques such as pre-implantation diagnosis (PGD) can provide evidence on the chromosomal level. It remains significant that while a sample of sperm is mostly evaluated by quantitative standards, each oocyte is qualified by notions of attractiveness. Besides these Aristotelian binary classifications, such semantic differences also point to biological variations regarding the production of gametes, i.e. to their natural economy. Regarding male and female gamete production, there is a striking disproportion in quantity and reproductive age. According to WHO criteria, an ejaculate containing a minimum of 39 million sperm cells is classified as normal.[45] In contrast, in a female menstrual cycle about 10–20 follicles mature, from which normally only one follicle ovulates. While male and female bodies can be reproductive in old age, in most females the production of reproductive substance declines around menopause. In reproductive medicine quite often the shortage and scarcity of egg donors is lamented,[46] echoing Levi-Strauss's linkage of sexuality, reproduction and economy.[47] The binary division between variety and scarcity certainly regulates the selection of sperm and egg donors.

Different Models of Selection of Egg and Sperm Donors

In the case of egg donation, reproductive medicine in the laboratory relies on two kinds of gazes: first, the gaze of the clinicians or staff regarding the reproductive capacity and health status of donors as assessed by anamnesis and the bodily and mental impression that donors make during consultation; second, the gaze of the embryologist with regards to the morphological status of a substance once the biological material has been donated. Hence, while staff in the laboratory handle the biological material itself, in the clinic or sperm bank employees deal with the supplier of gametes. From the perspective of most IVF practitioners, the most persuasive sign of a good egg donor is the presence of an earlier pregnancy, regardless of whether it resulted in a live birth or an abortion. Aside from standardized screenings for sexually transmitted diseases, some sperm banks and IVF clinics also screen for certain genetic diseases or examine the karyotype. But other factors in the recruitment and selection of egg donors lie somewhere between estimation, experience, common sense and best practices. Therefore, these practices differ a lot between different IVF clinics and result in the recruitment of quite different groups of donors.[48] Most of these tacit and visual activities have become silently embodied in the built environment and in notions of good practice. Nonetheless, what I observed in these two European clinics was that nearly all egg donors who passed the screening were recruited by the clinics because of the scarcity of this reproductive material.

By comparison, the evaluation and selection of sperm is much more about numbers, curves and quantities. Even though social behaviour and staff impression can also exclude a sperm donor, it is not so much his phenotype but his sperm count under the microscope that counts in ranking him as a 'straight shooter'[49] and finally recruits him for the programme. In addition to other criteria, motility also counts as an important factor in determining fertility. According to interviews with two Danish sperm bankers, about 95 per cent of their clients have normal sperm (according to WHO standards), but from the aspirants in this group they recruit only 10–20 per cent. Bjarke Mortensen, a Danish sperm bank director, explains this discrepancy as the difference between 'sperm for house use' and 'crème de la crème':[50] while average, normal sperm is sufficient for DIY use, for use in ARTs sperm banks want to sell a 'product' that is about much more than the average.[51] Because of that and in contrast to the recruitment of egg donors, many applicants for sperm donation are refused, not because they are infertile but because they are only average. So sperm donor recruitment initiates a process of coping with the heterogeneity of possible aspirants. The daily work in sperm banks involves negotiating these standard values and can result in scrutinizing and challenging a donor's virility: 'You will get half a metre higher when you get a sperm donor. It's a nice feeling to ... Men have something like that, I think.'[52] Jesper Lindberg, director of another sperm bank in Copenhagen, stresses that it is important to let the applicants know in advance that most of them will be rejected, but that (in most of the cases) the rejection does not mean they are infertile. But he admits that for some of his clients this is something they do not expect before approaching the sperm bank, because it is not included in their own perception of their masculinity and virility. False conclusions deducing fertility from potency or sexual activity are legion among the myths of reproductive masculinities (for example the misconception that identifies sperm with ejaculate). Sometimes even marketing for sperm donors promotes these allusions, such as when a Californian sperm bank advertises with the slogan: 'U. C. Men, Get Paid for Something You're Already Doing! Call the Sperm Bank of California.'[53]

In contrast, egg cells cannot be tested in advance; the result is determined solely on the basis of medical and fertility history, staff impressions and counting criteria for egg donor selection. According to Spanish and Czech gynaecologists, an average egg donor cycle produces about twelve to fifteen oocytes which are used for one to two recipients. According to information from Dansperm, an average sperm sample (taken from one masturbation session) results in six to seven straws (flexible tubes for cryopreservation storage). For one insemination, one to two straws are used.

Sperm donor recruitment and marketing mirror the dichotomy variety/scarcity in gamete donation. While most egg donors become accepted, only a few aspiring sperm donors are recruited. Because of the easy detachability and naturally higher quantity of sperm, sperm donation has become, in its own right, a branch in assisted reproduction that sells above-average material. Out of a *quasi-*

natural surplus economy, sperm bankers have succeeded in recycling a substance which, under other circumstances, would be disposed of in a tissue or in the gutter. In an interview which lasted one and a half hours, sperm banker Jesper Lindberg used the term 'product' eight times when referring to sperm. While referring to 'our product' he speaks in his role as a broker or agent between sperm donors and recipients. In referring to the 'end product', he stresses that sperm banks are not only selling human substances, but are primarily purifying, preparing, grafting and enhancing the former waste product (ejaculate) for its new trajectory as a biological with its own biovalue (money, drugs, kinship).

Hereditary Traits Attached to Biological Material

What is contained or concealed in a gamete provided for a third party? Linda Hogle observes that 'information management is a by-product of human materials technology, further influencing work and social arrangements'.[54] As a result, the body of the donor is re-inscribed into representational data, like a 'data double',[55] an identity without a body registered in a database. In most European countries, only physicians or clinics can order sperm samples, whereas in the US customers too have access to some donor databases. Bjarke Mortensen from Dansperm told me an ironic detail about their database for US customers:

> We figured we could make it by alphabetic [codes] instead of numbered [codes] and then we give them [the donors] a name, Scandinavian name with four letters. And then it turned out to be a good marketing point because American females find it cute and more personalized than a number. A lot of American sperm banks [laughs], they would have preferred to have such a system themselves.[56]

This narrative shows how 'sperm as a technoscientific commodity is given cultural meanings in practices of consumption'.[57] Gametes which are detached from the bodies of (in most European cases) anonymized donors are loaded and attached with meaning and allusions.[58] Consequently, they are transformed into imaginary bodily markers shifting between their former owner, the proper body as origin and a set of chromosomes packed with phenotypical markers, e.g. when Mortensen talks about his 'products': 'Redhead is quite difficult to sell, except to Ireland'. What still remains attached to the substance are some of the donor's or his ancestors' bodily traits, e.g. blue eyes and brown hair as phenotypic resemblance markers. Accordingly, in some cases gametes have become highly radicalized and gendered commodities: sperm from Danish sperm banks is a top seller in the US; marketed as 'Viking' or 'Nordic' sperm, it is a symbol of pure continental whiteness and 'hyper-masculinity'.[59] In most European countries, recipients cannot choose the sperm by catalogue; clinics match only a few phenotypical markers (this is obliged by state law in Spain). But these few parameters are seen as highly important in imagining a child with some kind of resemblance to his parents. In other words, donor/recipient matching should prevent too much non-similarity: the child should appear as though it had been conceived naturally. Matching eye, hair and skin colour should establish the social legitimacy of the relationship between parents and the children created via donation. In Euro-American kinship, reproductive substance is given special prominence: it is assumed that 50 per cent is inherited from the mother and 50 per cent from the father. Therefore gametes are conceived as containing information, traces and ideas of origin.

Economies and Temporalities of Kinship Technologically Assisted

Reproductive cells are precious, sold and marketed like gold or diamonds. Why is that? The marketing and consumption of human gametes is expanding in countries like Spain and the Czech Republic, where by state law donation must be altruistic and non-commercial and where the compensation rate can be seen as a source of additional income for students and migrants (Spain) and poorer women from rural regions (Czech Republic).[60] In more liberalized markets like the US, 'Ivy League Donors' sell their eggs for thousands of dollars. Otherwise, in daily life, substances like menstrual blood or ejaculate that contain reproductive cells are mostly regarded and treated like waste products. They are disposed of in tampons, condoms or tissues and finally end up in the gutter or the trash bin. They are not usually seen as having something like a personal reference to their owner or human source. But in reproductive medicine this connection exists: gametes, even though separated from the body, are thought of as somehow related to their progenitors and can be characterized as 'inalienable possessions'.[61]

For sperm and/or oocyte transactions, two different economic systems evolved: sperm banks and IVF clinics. With regard to modes of production, sperm banking has more in common with mass production and consumption (Fordism) than does fresh egg donation in IVF clinics. Thanks to cryobiology, sperm can be easily stored, documented and standardized as an (information-laden) technoscientific product. Even though the choreography of a donor cycle with a recipient has something in common with the just-in-time-production invented by Toyota in the post-war era, the procurement and delivery of ova is, by contrast, more closely associated with natural resources and natural cycles. For that reason, industrialized agriculture ('egg harvesting') and, most notably, mining serve as metaphors. Unlike the large quantities in sperm production, oocyte stimulation and extraction involves a maximum of (reproductive) work to extract minute quantities of scarce and non-renewable resources, just like mining rare materials such as gold or diamonds.[62] While sperm banking has become a standardized storage technology, dealing with ova is still a much more precarious practice – at least until better results can be garnered from frozen eggs, which current studies suggest can be expected soon.[63] If oocytes were stored like sperm, sperm banks would develop not just according to the blueprint of businesses that *store* reproductive cells, but also according to the blueprint of businesses that *deposit* people's own gametes. In the case of some male cancer patients, depositing sperm is still a common medical procedure. In addition, if infertility is a likely outcome of one's profession or illness, sperm cells can be deposited and used in the future, prolonging an individual's reproductive age.[64] If storing reproductive substances at a younger age could solve the problem of later infertility (caused by declining quantity and quality of gametes), then donation by strangers would be restricted to cases of primarily infertility. Subsequently, freezing of oocytes at younger ages for oneself could be characterized as a donation to oneself that crosses temporal boundaries, but not bodily ones.

Cryobiology has already overridden such natural continuities. Embryos have been successfully transferred after years of storage.[65] This has been presented as proof that length of storage does not affect frozen cells. Cryopreservation and thawing are technologies that enable transformation. From the perspective of reproductive futures, one possible development would be that egg donation might dissolve and present itself, in hindsight, as a transitional phase. IVF egg donation is still one of the most successful methods in assisted reproduction because it separates hormonal stimulation and embryo transfer as actions in two different bodies (donor/recipient). In spite of this, however, the potential health problems and inconveniences for egg donors resulting from such (transnational) stratified division of labour are often ignored by IVF practitioners.[66]

Nevertheless, egg banking challenges the actual practices of IVF clinics. In sperm donation, the majority of clinics do not rely on their own sperm banks, but instead cooperate with a few (mostly US and Danish) sperm banks selling their product internationally. It is worth noting, however, that compared to sperm donation (a process that requires no medical assistance), the preparation and stimulation required for egg donation is – at least to date – a genuine clinical activity: gynaecological examination, ultrasound scans, control of medication and finally oocyte extraction in the operation theatre. At present, oocytes are all too precarious and complex materials: their quantity is finite and they are not easily extracted from the body of their progenitor. Egg cells cannot be ordered and shipped like cryopreserved sperm. By contrast, sperm is easily and amply obtainable from a body. With appropriate laboratory arrangements, sperm can easily be tested and classified under low sterility conditions. A reliable pool of donors provides sperm banks with high-quality sperm to meet the demands of increasing numbers of customers all around the world. Although sperm donors are not as easy to recruit as many people might think,[67] sperm banking has become a standardized and industrialized business. One reason for this has to do with the great number of sperm cells in one ejaculate, alongside cryogenic technology that allows for easy storage and shipping. Standardization and competition will enable a small number of big sperm banks to dominate the whole market for cryopreserved sperm.

Nevertheless, while the procedural technology and transactions become more standardized, the tiny sperm cells themselves are not considered candidates for standardization because this would contradict the demands of their recipients (I will return to this thought in the conclusion). Therefore, marketing sperm as a 'product' entails a rather prosaic symbolism: for it contrasts sharply with the more 'sacred' ova, which before IVF was never seen as being detachable from the female body in a way that separated female generativity from gestation. By contrast, male generativity depends upon the detachability of a male substance from the male body.[68] Because of sperm's 'natural' detachability, fatherhood has always been the more insecure position. The act of substituting a husband's sperm is mentioned in documents dating back to the late eighteenth century.[69] Furthermore, in the twentieth century sperm donation has often been associated with adultery,[70] whereas egg donation lacks this cultural analogy. It was only after IVF made ova detachment outside the body possible that oocytes were recognized as detachable biologics. This technological breakthrough has threatened motherhood at the end of the twentieth century. For precisely this reason, the 1990 German Act for the Protection of Embryos[71] tries to ensure that the old Roman law principle *mater semper certa est* serves as one of the major arguments for the prohibition of egg donation in contemporary Germany: fragmented or 'split motherhood'[72] should be avoided. Reproductive heterosexuality and its norm of a nuclear family (with two parents from different sexes) is still conceived to be the most natural form in many European laws and medical texts, although it becomes contested via non-normative and queer use of reproductive technologies and new forms of kinship.

Conclusion

Donated gametes can substitute and trigger reproductive processes in bodies whose reproductive cells no longer function. In the case of IVF with a person's own gametes, it is not the biogenetical material of the gametes themselves that can be enhanced (they can only be tested, selected and discarded), but rather their preparation and purification. The quantity of oocytes can be multiplied with hormonal stimulation and embryologists can select the morphologically best-looking egg cells and the most motile sperm. This indicates how conditions of procreation can be understood as therapeutic tools in the context of assisted reproduction: procreation is detached from the body and takes place in the laboratory, under the microscope, in the incubator. Thanks to cyroprotectants and freezing containers, gametes have become technoscientific products. The freezer made it possible to 'stabilize and standardize living research objects that were by their nature in constant flux',[73] such as sperm. The products derived from egg donation require a larger reproductive work force and more expensive enhancement technologies (hormonal drugs). Their (bio)value is regulated by their scarcity and contingency (compared to sperm). It is not only the amount of labour needed to produce them that differs markedly, but also the imaginary (hetero)sexual metaphors and dichotomies that underlie the fertilization in vivo and in vitro.[74]

Unlike other cell lines, sperm and egg cells (because of their haploid chromosome set) do not multiply and their cytoblasts need to fuse to activate the first mitosis of an embryo. Although other substances can be transferred to other bodies without presupposing any biogenetic relation, gametes endow genetic information: they preserve genetic material of the prior, the current and possibly of the next generation as a symbol of kinship in Euro-American culture. As a consequence, forms of biological and symbolic relatedness remain intact, either in genealogical traces, or in resemblance markers like phenotype, or in the notion of substances circulating through time and space: gamete donors 'pass' both literally and metaphorically 'through' several persons and they thereby do make relations as the incorporated parts of 'others' bodies'.[75] While other biologics or therapeutic tools made of human substance or tissue are viewed from the perspective of detachability, making them 'thing-like' and 'non-self',[76] gametes still have a dual structure: they are detachable (sperm) or can be made detachable (oocytes). But even if they cross bodily boundaries, they always remain attached to genealogical information as long as Euro-American conceptions of kinship and origin are still mediated through (genetic) substance.[77] On the other hand, and as demonstrated by new efforts in cryobiology, the freezing of living material has already challenged and mediated (new) relations between self, the body, age and time.

These instances constitute the paradox of technologies like sperm banking, that are very standardized, and their 'product', which eludes standardizations because of customer demand for difference. Unlike biologics such as vaccines or vitamins that can be produced industrially from assays of biological organisms, gametes are genuinely (re)produced by the bodies of their originators. Indeed, in the case of oocytes, where there is much concern about scarcity, the quantitative production is technologized by means of hormonal control. And in any case, the individual gametes by their nature cannot be standardized, because each gamete – even those from the same person – is different due to chromosomal crossover during meiosis; each gamete is attached to something unique: a recombination of its originator's genome. While people certainly require a standardized vaccine and standardized screening for blood as well as sperm donors, no one desires standardized sperm cells, because standardized or replicated gametes would produce quite similar, indeed much too similar outcomes. That is why in some countries the regulation of sperm is still informed by the discourse on incest.[78] As in biological heredity, the aim in kinship is to (re)produce variety and every new kin should be unique (although some resemblance to ancestors is culturally desired). If we imagine sperm to be like some kind of pharmaceutical drug, for example if sperm would be promoted as an anti-depressant,[79] then replicated cell lines could be taken into consideration. But in reproduction, every gamete is non-identical with another gamete – and that differs from notions of cloning that so often pervade the discourse about assisted reproduction. In reproductive medicine, nature is not replaced, but rather assisted.[80]

In this chapter, I have shown that processes involving the donation, extraction, preparation, storage and transfer of gametes are standardizable, but that the gamete itself is not. The reason for this is that, in assisted reproduction, gametes are not just a therapeutic tool (as are most other biologics), but also a reproductive means. While other bodily material can more easily acquire the status of a thing, gametes are problematic due to being constantly attached to their originators. Whereas tracing sera, vaccines or urine back to their biological origins is more closely related to immunological problems (contamination of assays), in the case of organ transplantation and human reproduction there remains the unresolved cultural problem of an ongoing but non-traceable 'relation' to the originator of the biological material. Therefore, in the area of human reproduction, 'the difference between persons and things is particularly difficult to define, defying all attempts at drawing a simple line where there is a natural continuum'.[81]

7 HUMAN TISSUES AND ORGANS: STANDARDIZATION AND 'COMMODIFICATION' OF THE HUMAN BODY

Sophie Chauveau

The human body provides fluids, tissues and organs to medicine: these materials may replace a deficient organ, tissue or physiological function or be processed into medicinal substances and assume the role of drugs. Due to extensive scientific research and surgical innovations, the uses of the human body have expanded greatly since the end of the Second World War. These scientific and technical innovations would not have materialized without the organized collection of human body parts such as organs, tissues, fluids and especially blood.

The materials in question are inserted into frameworks of standardization, and their status changes from an integral part of the human body into 'something that is consumed'; hence, they are comparable to drugs, but differ in that they are of human origin. This may explain why these products can be considered 'human biological materials' or 'biologics'. Just like other biologics, the criteria of standardization (purity, safety, efficiency and dosage) are essential to the production process. When we examine human body products, we must consider both the means and consequences of standardization.

A number of preliminary remarks are necessary, the first of which concerns the specificity of human body products. Biologics are usually understood to be (non-chemical or non-artificial) products and substances that are provided by nature. They consist mainly of plants, vitamins or hormones and refer broadly to the idea of 'naturalness'. In national and European legislation on medicinal substances, biologics comprise one of several categories in the classification of therapeutic agents. While therapeutic agents derived from blood are subjected to drug legislation, human body parts are not considered therapeutic agents of the same category: transplanted organs replace deficient ones, and so human body parts are more akin to *living things* than to products derived from living bodies, i.e. biologics in the narrower sense. Nonetheless, I will argue that human body parts can be subsumed under the general framework of biologics.

There are three general types of material of human origin: fluids, tissues and organs. The fluids are blood, milk and sperm. I do not intend to analyse anew the case of products derived from blood; their standardization is distinct from that of drugs or biologicals.[1] But in the course of this chapter I will draw on some aspects of this type of standardization, because it offers a general framework for our discussion. Tissues are taken from human bodies and include the skin, corneas, bones and cardiac valves to name but a few of the most important examples. Corneas have been collected and distributed by organizations in the US and Europe since the 1930s and 1940s. For a long time, cardiac valves and bones were considered to be surgical waste or *res nullius*, although this did not prevent their collection for surgical or therapeutic uses (replacement of cardiac valves, bone grafts). Since the 1980s, several firms have begun packaging and standardizing these tissues. Indeed, packaging has changed the status of these human tissues: they are no longer considered *res nullius*, but instead are products for use in surgery or other therapeutic settings. Finally, the most important organs are the kidneys, liver, heart, lungs and pancreas. The development of transplantation techniques and devices for these organs began in the 1950s. Since the 1980s, transplant surgery has benefited from the use of immunosuppressive drugs, to the point that transplantation surgery has almost become routine surgery, although the supply of organs is insufficient to meet demand.[2]

I would like to analyse the ways and means of the standardization of human biological materials. The increase in the use of human body parts was accompanied by an elaboration of the rules that regulate the extraction, processing and distribution of those materials. Some of the rules concern the preservation of human dignity, others deal with the safety of the human products, still others regulate the distribution to patients, etc. These rules are part of the standardization of human body parts. Broadly, I consider that standardization is a process of change: human body parts are transformed into products like drugs or surgical materials. This change is a complex process: standardization is a 'technology of trust'[3] that involves not only the establishment of knowledge but also of authority. The trust in question here relies on both cognitive and social orders. The cognitive order is established through a consensus regarding the control of the collection, processing and distribution of human body parts and tissues. The social order is constituted by physicians, donors and recipients on one hand, and hospitals and organizations like donors associations or procurement networks – that taken together we may call a 'transplant community' – on the other. Developing the use of human body parts relies on standardizing processes within these respective cognitive and social orders. The knowledge and the know-how that makes the use of human body parts and products possible derive from different disciplines such as immunology, surgery and biotechnology. The establishment of authority depends not only on the elaboration of rules and the enforcement of laws, but also on recognition of the networks of physicians, patients, donors and public authorities that are involved in the whole process and embodied in national agencies, donor associations and policy agendas (organ donation, increasing transplant surgery).

Another preliminary remark concerns the way in which the standardization of human body parts is connected to the transformation of these living things into commodities. Shall we consider the standardization of human fluids, tissues and organs as qualifying these medical products to be economic 'resources'? In the specific context of analyses of the controversies about organ transplants and blood transfusion, the word commodification is frequently used to describe the appearance of a market for products derived from the human body or its parts. Human body parts are transformed into drugs or therapeutic agents or objects of scientific research by the process of commodification.[4] Some authors argue that commodification creates markets that are more effective at maximizing resources (human body parts). However, it may also create inequalities between producers and consumers of spare organ parts.[5] I would like to use 'commodification' in a broader sense as the particular, specific and original (unusual) way of standardizing the human body using knowledge, authority and rules. I distinguish between three major aspects of the commodification of human body parts: the technical change, the creation of a new economy and the use of different categories. Only with regard to this last point, the question of categories, am I referring to Wahlberg and Bauer.[6] In other words, the framework of commodification helps us to understand how the organs, considered as gifts, are changed into resources.

Technical change allows the commodification of human body parts. Blood is changed into products derived from it, or growth hormones are extracted and packaged for injections. Commodification requires scientific knowledge and technological innovation. The technical devices are sometimes very expensive and subject to high tariffs rather than normal market forces. Technical change also involves a means of 'recovering' human body parts. Commodification creates a new economy of human body parts. It's not only the high value of such products that justifies the high prices, but also the intervention of commercial and industrial firms in the production and packaging of some human biological materials. Those firms contribute to the emergence of an original market. In addition, the promise of such products increases the demand for them, insofar as demand relies on patient expectations. Furthermore, the physicians who conceive of the uses of human body parts also create demand. This demand challenges the organization of the collection and distribution of human body parts. We need to ask whether or not the management of collection and distribution by non-profit associations can be analysed in terms of market forces. Questions about the consent of givers (posthumous givers) and the compensation provided to them suggest the importance of commodification. In the search for resources, we should also give due consideration to the practices of 'death productivisation' (i.e. of increasing the output of dead bodies and hence the number of the organs removed).[7]

There is a legal dimension to commodification. When human body parts are changed into drugs, they can be sold or patented. If they prove to be harmful, the producer may be sued for damages. The law may help to protect recipients and to define the rules by which human body parts can be collected and distributed. Finally, the conception and the definition of the human body are challenged by commodification.

We must underscore the fact that the transformation and growth of the activities of organ and tissues transplantation have influenced theoretical analysis about the provision of organs. During the 1970s and early 1980s, as the success of transplantations was still uncertain, social scientists insisted that organ procurement be characterized as the 'gift of life'.[8] Since the end of the 1980s, the use of the immunosuppressive drugs has contributed to the success of organ transplantation surgery, and the demand for organ procurement has increased. The rhetoric of commodification has become one of the most popular ways of describing this change in transplantation activities. In brief, the development of contested categories (or markets) has been justified by a new framework of analysis and new concepts.[9] As historians, we not only observe the transformation of transplantation surgery, but also seek to understand how it has created tensions and to explain changes in organ and tissues procurement.

In the following chapter I will analyse the standardization of biologics, especially of body parts that are deemed to be 'resources' and involved in a process of commodification (commodification being the specific way in which human biologics are standardized). This means that I will describe some of the rules and practices that contribute to the work of classification and that at the same time enhance therapeutic devices and applications. I will focus on the problems that evolve from the acquisition and collection of human body parts, paying particular attention to the question of safety. I will describe the controversial management of the distribution of human body parts as a dispute over rules; I will examine the map of therapeutic uses to which standardized human body parts are put; I will describe the status of these living things; and I will emphasize the fact that physicians, patients and public authorities are all involved in the very standardization of human biologics that enhances their commodification.

First, I will analyse changes in the criteria governing the collection of human biological materials; second, I will stress the different economies of human body parts and their reliance on specific and changing organizations; and finally, I will describe the emergence of new categories. Some of the examples analysed here are taken from work in progress on the history of organ and tissue collection and distribution in Parisian hospitals from the end of the 1960s to the early 1990s.

'Harvesting' Human Biological Materials: The Manufacture of Human Resources

When they describe the procurement of organs, 'surgeons frequently employ the expression "organ harvesting", viewing this as an unproblematic way to underscore the act of reaping life to assist others in need'.[10] In this description, the donor is no longer a human person. The collection of human body parts raises many questions about the procurement of organs, tissues or fluids and the availability of these products.[11] I will first revisit the change in the standards of collection by way of a discussion about the definition of death; then I will show how technical devices may help in acquiring sufficient human biological materials and in changing some of them into human resources.

The definition of what we are used to calling 'brain death' was a crucial step in the standardization of the production of body parts. It contributed to an optimization of death, thus helping to collect more organs. In France, irreversible coma (*coma dépassé*) was defined as a reliable criterion for death at the end of the 1950s.[12] The decree promulgated by the French Health Ministry in April 1968 stated that irreversible coma is characterized by 'the irreversibility of injuries incompatible with life'.[13] In 1968, an ad hoc Committee of the Harvard Medical School published a report entitled 'A Definition of Irreversible Coma', introducing irreversible coma as a new criterion for death.[14] Irreversible cessation of cerebral function had to be confirmed by a flat EEG. A brain-dead donor is like a living cadaver. Before 1968, physicians took organs from living donors: only kidneys were transplanted, since people can survive with one kidney. Kidneys removed from living donors were expected to work normally. Compared to transplants from living donors, kidneys that had been taken from a patient whose blood circulation had ceased were less reliable. The resumption of diuresis was less certain in the latter case: the criterion of irreversible coma reduced this uncertainty. Nowadays, brain death is the phrase commonly used by physicians, whereas irreversible coma refers to a state of unconsciousness characterized by the failure of vital signs.

Thus, the brain-death criterion not only raised hopes of acquiring better organs, but also created new opportunities and helped increase the number of organ transplantations. The transplantation of other organs like the heart or liver was performed experimentally with some success during the 1960s. At the same time, changes in lifestyle during the 1950s and 1960s, such as growing individual mobility, resulted in an increase in the number of automobile accidents that helped to boost the 'harvest' of organs. But new problems appeared very soon. Physicians and surgeons had to decide whether someone was dead and whether his/her body - on account of its organs - could be used or exploited to extend or to give life to other patients. In 1968 in Japan, Professor Wada was accused of having dubiously diagnosed brain death before he performed the first heart transplant in Japan.[15] Prior to the 1980s, Japanese society refused to consider brain death as a valid criterion for death: the family first had to accept the death, making its determination first and foremost a social and familial event.[16] In 1997, the Japanese government declared brain death to be equivalent to the death of a human being, thereby paving the way to the first heart transplant with a brain-dead donor in 1999.

The gradual acceptance of brain death as a decisive criterion of death allowed for the optimization of death, i.e. an enhancement of the 'output' of dead bodies as measured by the number of organs and tissues that could be removed from one body. It contributed to a change in the status of human body parts. In the transplantation regime regulated by brain death, explanted organs and tissues enter into a time span between their removal from the dead donor and their transplantation into recipient patients. Since the 1980s, it has become commonplace to remove several organs from one patient: kidneys, liver, heart and cornea. This multiple organ removal can be viewed as a 'productivization' of death.[17] This pattern of operating on dead donors can be compared to the increased resource recovery observed earlier in blood collection: ever since the fractionation of blood became feasible, several products have been derived from it.

In order better to understand the mechanisms involved in the productivization of death in the case of organ transplantation, I will provide a short overview of how other body parts, namely blood and tissues, are dealt with. In general, technical devices have helped to refine the collection of human body parts. One main difficulty has been the preservation and storage of blood or tissues. In the case of blood, the addition of chemical substances and the choice of an appropriate temperature has allowed it to be conserved for several days. During the 1930s, the first successful devices for conserving blood supplies were developed, allowing them to be stored and managed. Later, in the 1950s, the fractionation of blood and the desiccation of plasma divided the original blood resource into several derivative products that could be kept for several months before use.[18]

The case of tissue collection provides additional insights into the entanglement of technical procedures and rules of practice. Since the end of the 1930s, physicians and surgeons had been responsible for managing the collection and distribution of blood, organs and tissues. The first eye bank (for corneas) was founded in Philadelphia in 1938; in 1944, the first national eye bank in the US joined together nineteen hospitals. In France, an eye bank was established at the hospital *Hotel-Dieu* in Paris in 1949. The bank was promoted by the physician and deputy Bernard Lafay, who had been inspired by the US 'Eye Bank for Sight Restauration'. In addition, the French Parliament passed legislation in 1949 that legalized the collection of corneas from dead people, provided they had given their consent.

Hence, after 1949 and, as was the case with blood and other organs, cornea grafts depended on the consent of the donor. By contrast, cardiac valves, bones and surgical waste were for a long time classified as *res nullius*; their medical use did not depend on the explicit consent of 'donors'. During the 1990s, the status of these human biological materials changed. Several surgeons investigated the status of explanted hearts and cardiac valves, since this human biological material could be used for other medical purposes. Each of these materials presented problems of their own. For example in the case of bones, the safety of the product was problematic: physicians' correspondence collected for a report ordered by the *Direction des Affaires Médicales* of the *Assistance Publique-Hôpitaux de Paris* illustrates that some surgeons wrote to their patients expressing concern about the risks of infection (by Creutzfeld-Jakob disease, otherwise known as mad cow disease). Some even wanted to obtain the consent of patients before using 'surgical waste'. The rise of tissue banks prompted many questions about the rules of procurement and the status of these human body parts.[19] Similar problems characterized the collection of cord blood.

The specific situation varied from one 'human product' to the next. In France at the beginning of the 1990s, 25,000 to 40,000 femoral heads were collected each year from old women who had fractured their femurs, 10,000 saphenous veins – used in coronary bypass surgery – were held in storage, approximately 27 m^2 of skin were stored and 10 m^2 were cultivated, and between 3,000 and 4,000 cornea grafts were performed each year. Some of these human tissues were reworked abroad: French surgeons sent them to the US where commercial firms performed the storage and packaging operations (cardiac valves, bones and skin). In the late 1980s and early 1990s, the processing and trade of human tissues developed into a lucrative market. That is why French officials sought to establish a *dispositif* governing the organization and moral regulation of tissue processing.[20] Debates on tissue economy dealt with issues of profitability, the traceability of the products and the donations' origins.

The head committee of the *Assistance Publique-Hôpitaux de Paris* initiated discussions on these topics in 1989.[21] A committee responsible for transplantation activities was established in March 1989, gathering together surgeons, anaesthetists and hospital managers. Discussions about the tissue economy reveal the changing status of body parts. For example, the heart was considered to be merely a solid organ, procured by donation and used for transplantation. But how was one to assess an explanted heart that became a collection of tissues with various uses? Parisian surgeons agreed that an explanted heart should be treated as a donated organ: the patient's consent was a prerequisite for the medical use of the explanted heart. In these debates, physicians understood an *explanted heart* to be the heart removed from a patient designated to receive a transplanted heart. The explanted heart remained useful for its cardiac valves and blood vessels.[22] The storage and the packaging of human tissues also raised other problems. Since American firms dominated the market, discussions on the agreements reveal that it was difficult to verify the origins of the tissue (especially whether it had been donated or sold). The *Comité d'Ethique des Hôpitaux de Paris* recommended avoiding commercial firms, unless they offered products that could not otherwise be provided.[23] This rule was also observed in the case of products derived from blood. Finally, before the vote of the bioethics law in 1994, the *Direction des Affaires Médicales* required in 1993 that the use of human tissues for medical or research purposes accord with the principle that the human body not be marketed.

To sum up, surgeons and physicians have 'invented' human biological material since the 1960s, thanks to changing principles (brain-death criteria) and the development of new technical devices, such as the processing of blood and tissues and the conservation and transplantation of organs. The 'harvesting' of organs and tissues changes the original, body-derived materials into medical resources: human body parts replace their 'damaged' analogues in a patient, and one 'brain-dead' person may even become a tool for the recovery of several other patients. Physicians and surgeons have defined a number of standards to ensure the 'quality' of organs: the donor's health, the way he died, and the life he lived are some of the criteria included in the standardization rules of organ procurement.[24] The transformation of human biological material into a medical resource offers numerous arguments in favour of voluntary donations and 'gifts of life', because human biological material remains a scarce resource. This scarcity has played an important part in the development of the economy of human body parts: of course it is a scarcity that is proportional or relative to the increasing use of this biological material. In this new context, the rhetoric of a 'gift of life' is intended to enable the mobilization of organs and tissues donors and, ultimately, changes the 'gift' into a 'resource'.

Economy of Human Biological Material: Procurement, Distribution and Allocation

In 2003, Jesica Santillan, a young girl aged 17, died after an organ operation in which she received the heart and lungs of a patient whose blood type did not match hers. She was Mexican and had been hospitalized at Duke University Hospital in Durham (North Carolina). Human errors caused her death. But the story of J. Santillan helps us understand some of the characteristics of the economy of human biological material.[25] She and her family were illegal immigrants. The young girl had pulmonary hypertension and physicians recommended lung transplantation. With the help of churches, the family began to raise funds and in 2002 the young girl was registered on the waiting list for organs. On 7 February 2003 she received a heart-lung transplant. But it was only after the operation had been performed and while she was receiving immunosuppressives that the surgeon learned that the blood groups did not match. The matching of the blood groups of patient and donor, which should have taken place when the allocation was decided upon, had simply been forgotten, and at that time no provision was made to double-check the match before the operation. J. Santillan received a new transplant thirteen days later, but her condition deteriorated and she died two days after the operation. This story provides insights into the American health-care system and the situation of immigrants. It also reveals that there is a gap between 'transplant haves' and 'transplant have-nots'. This story illustrates the problems involved in the procurement, distribution and allocation of organs and tissues in the US. The success of a transplantation depends on high quality-standards and a high degree of organization and monitoring, both of which seem to have been lacking in this case. In many countries where the collection of organs relies on voluntary donation, the organization of transplant activities is a mix of donor and market economies: this mix is the specific economy of human biological materials. We have to take into consideration the emergence of this new, specific type of economy that involves the exchange of organs, tissues and fluids, or roughly, human biological material. We have to ask how the organization of this material – and the rhetoric that sustains it – encourages the emergence, affirmation and development of a category such as resources that challenges the 'gifts'.

As the case of Jesica has shown, the use of human biological material requires better management of its collection and distribution.[26] But difficulties also arise from the specific character of biological material. As I have mentioned before, organs and blood collection rely on voluntary, unpaid donors. Yet money plays a decisive role in all aspects of recruitment, conservation, distribution and allocation. The whole organization of the procurement of body material relies on financial means and seems very businesslike. Money and payments are necessary, for instance, in order to transplant organs and to manufacture products derived from blood. Business companies perform some of these processes. Two models of exchange coexist: one is based on donations and another on the evaluation of patients' needs and the cost of therapy. The second is much more like the economy of commodity exchange than the first.

The first successful transplantations during the 1960s posed several difficulties related to the collection and distribution of organs and tissues and later to the prohibition on paying donors. Physicians and surgeons had to meet several requirements that involved securing enough organs (or blood) to satisfy demand and ensuring safe handling procedures. Very soon, organ collection organizations were forced to juggle the priorities of medical need and geographic proximity when selecting recipients. These organizations assumed responsibility for decisions about which patient on a waiting list would receive a specific organ, thus partly relieving physicians and surgeons of their responsibility to decide issues of life and death. These organizations also established standards for both organs and their recipients. In cases such as liver transplants, which are frequently a question of life or death, the emergency medical condition was deemed paramount; in others cases, geographic proximity was considered more important, since transporting organs increases the length of ischaemia and spoils the material.

Organizations for collecting organs were established at the end of the 1960s. In the US, the Southeast Organ Procurement Foundation (SEOPF) was formed to coordinate transplants amongst its members. Ten years later, the SEOPF implemented the first computer-based organ matching system called the 'United Network for Organ Sharing' or UNOS. In 1982, the SEOPF established the kidney centre for round-the-clock assistance in placing donated organs. The UNOS separated from the SEOPF in 1984, becoming a non-profit member organization in accordance with the National Organ Transplant Act (1984). The UNOS coordinated the Organ Procurement Organisations (OPOs), which managed organ collections at the local level, in close cooperation with hospitals.[27]

In France, the collection of organs was managed by France-Transplant (FT), a non-profit association under the law on associations of 1901.[28] Jean Dausset, who discovered the Human Leukocyte Antigen (HLA), founded the association in 1969 and headed it until 1989. FT is located at the Saint-Louis hospital in Paris. FT was mainly interested in kidney transplantations, and nephrologists and biologists exercised the greatest influence over the association. FT produced tests and sera used for matching HLA groups between donors and recipients. The association also collaborated with the donors' associations (*Associations pour le Don d'Organes et de Tissus humains* or ADOT) founded in 1969.[29]

The UNOS and FT defined rules for the distribution and allocation of organs. The management of human biological material was similar to the allocation of resources and the rules these organizations established have contributed to the emergence of standardized practices. As human body parts became resources, it was necessary to respect the rules of *distributive justice*. But *resource management* remained under the control of physicians and surgeons who were more concerned about their own reputations and interests: for a long time, physicians and surgeons headed the organizations for organ or blood collection. Some of them tried to secure organs for their own patients and by doing so enhance their reputations as transplant surgeons.[30] Because all of these organizations relied on voluntary donors, they also promoted a rhetoric about the 'gift of life' that could hide the complexity of the rules for the allocation of organs and tissues – and in the French case even hide some abuses. For example, the close relationships between France-Transplant (the organization that manages the resources) and France ADOT (the organization that collects from voluntary donors) have facilitated the development of arguments promoting donation and gift.

Public opinion has not criticized the functioning of those organizations: the public seems to trust the ideal of donation. For their part, patients waiting for an organ are confident that the gift and its management by non-profit organizations ensure a trustworthy and reliable system, as shown by several anthropological and sociological inquiries.[31] In France, neither the donors nor the recipients would admit that the whole organization is governed by an economy that mixes gift-giving and financial transactions, where the human body parts are considered as resources and the allocation of these scarce human biological materials is subject to standardized and routine practices.

What are the practices of procurement and distribution? What could we learn from the testimony of physicians, donors or recipients? Healy argues that in the US the procurement organizations have elaborated accounts of donations that help donors and recipients to interpret their actions in terms of a gift-giving relationship. The absence of face-to-face transactions helps to reinforce this discourse. According to Healy, 'What makes a gift is the relationship within which the transaction occurs'.[32] But I argue instead that 'What makes the resource is the manner in which the organ or tissue is used'. Physicians, surgeons and organ procurement organizations are all intermediaries that are situated between donors and recipients and that help change the organ or the tissue into a resource.

People involved in transplantations not only manage the collection of organs and tissues and the allocation of these resources, but also, and importantly, they manage the daily routines of procurement and distribution of these human materials. An analysis of these practices helps in understanding how organs and tissues are changed into resources. The archives of the *Assistance-Publique Hôpitaux de Paris* hold much information on the history of transplantation in Paris since the mid-1970s that helps describe some routines and demonstrates that the establishment of rules and organizations contributed to a kind of standardization.[33] The nephrologist belongs to a nephrological medical service and sometimes performs a kidney transplantation as a member of a transplantation team. The rule is the same for the procurement of organs: there are no original teams for such a task. Organs and tissues are first considered as resources by surgeons and physicians.

The management of organs relies on the registration of prospective recipients and their being matched with resources. In France, prior to reforms that reorganized the whole procurement and distribution process in 1992 (the government established a national agency to manage collection and distribution in place of associations that seemed too beholden to private interests), little heed was paid to the rules governing organ distribution and many transplantation teams tried, sometimes successfully, to bypass the rules of distribution. For example, when kidneys were removed from a deceased donor, nephrologists usually kept one kidney for their own patients and gave the other one up for donation. Indeed, sometimes both kidneys were kept. The exchange of organs throughout the entire country based on rules designed to establish priority also reveals the transformation of organs into resources. Organs are not just resources that save patients' lives, but also resources that enhance the reputation of physicians, the more so given their great scarcity. In the 1980s, the number of organs removed each year by Parisian medical teams was quite low: at most one or two per month per team. Such scarcity also impeded ambitious attempts to standardize the practices.[34]

In the US, the principles of organ distribution and allocation have also changed since the 1970s. In the 1960s and 1970s, anyone needing an organ received it, regardless of health insurance. No discrimination in the access to the most advanced medical devices or surgery was recognized. How to prioritize allocations became the object of intense bioethical and academic debate. Which patient was to be prioritized? A patient whose life was in danger? One who could recover faster? One who had been waiting the longest? According to the National Organ Transplantation Act (NOTA, 1984), the Federal Task Force on Organ Transplantation and the American Society of Transplant Surgeons were responsible for developing guidelines that stipulated that 5 to 10 per cent of the organs collected would be provided to foreign patients living in the US. Surgeons who disregarded the ethical rules were threatened with the revocation of their licences to practice. At the same time, the high cost of transplantation surgery – and the cost of the immunosuppressive drugs prescribed to organs recipients throughout their lives – provoked discussions about the choice between transplantations or dialysis for people suffering renal failure. During the 1980s, the American Health Administration promoted the Diagnostic Related Groupings (DRG), which influenced the choice between dialysis and transplantation. And in 1986, the Task Force on Organ Transplantation ordered the selection of some transplantation hospitals based on patient survival rates, the quality of equipment and the number of transplants performed.[35] Hospitals were allowed to maintain their transplantation facilities based on their performance. As a result, the number of transplantation hospitals decreased and it became easier to enforce the rules and to promote standardized practices.

In France in 1992, the Health Ministry promoted a reform of the procedures used in organ procurement and transplantation.[36] The roots of the reform can be traced back to several events: a number of scandals involving tainted blood were exposed in 1991 and 1992; the *Affaire d'Amiens* saw several organs of a young man removed without the full consent of his parents; 'French organs' were being distributed to foreign patients treated in Parisian hospitals; simultaneously, questions about the status and uses of human tissues had grown in number.[37] After 1987, the Health Ministry repeatedly asked physicians and surgeons to increase the number of transplantations and encouraged organ donations. In 1988, the Huriet–Serusclat law defined the informed consent required of people participating in clinical trials. Also, the reform of transplantation activities in France was linked with the elaboration of the first bioethics law of 1994. By the beginning of the 1990s, patients and the public were more informed than ever about organ collection and distribution in France, and the media denounced abuses in the management of transplantation activities. Public opinion took an active interest in questions about organ procurement, donation and distribution: the impact of the public health crisis involving tainted blood, the suspicion that the procedures were being abused and more generally the threat to public interests help to explain the heightened public awareness.

The reforms in the US and France aimed to rationalize the whole activity, to promote transparency in the criteria used to register patients on waiting lists and to harmonize transplantation practices. The reforms have contributed to the emergence of a specific organization responsible for the procurement and distribution of organs and tissues and of transplantation activities. The human biological material is now managed like a non-ordinary resource: that means that the standardization of collection and distribution has given birth to new categories of human body parts.

The reforms in France and in the US promote organizations that manage organs and tissues as 'resources'. But at the same time, politicians continue to refer to the 'gift of life': the tensions between the real economy of biological material and the rhetoric one remain vivid.

Categories: The Disjunction between Gifts and Resources

Human biological materials are both donations and resources. And for that reason it remains difficult to consider these products as being standardized. On the one hand, because human biological materials are procured by donation (or as a gift), they remain 'personified objects' of human origin and cannot be classified as objects to be used and consumed. On the other hand, human biological materials are reworked to be used in surgery and changed into resources. For these reasons, human biological materials are illustrative of contested categories. I refer here to the idea that 'the practical stabilization that routines, regulations, codes of conduct or laboratory protocols afford is never shielded from contestation and negotiation, for example, through clinical encounters, mediated 'public understandings' or informed consent processes'.[38] Their dual quality, as both gifts and resources, places limits on the process of standardization, but at the same time demands the elaboration of rules and guidelines to prevent potential abuse.

Whereas transplant recipients are encouraged by hospital staff to depersonalize their new organs and speak of them in terms that can sometimes even approximate car repair, procurement staff regularly tell donors' relatives that transplantation enables the donor's essence to persist in others who are thereby offered a second chance of life. These competing messages offer evidence of what I refer to as a form of 'ideological disjunction',[39] meaning the tension between the rhetoric of a 'gift of life' and the economy of biological materials as 'resources'. This disjunction allows organs to be considered as both resources and gifts. The donor is anonymous (a deceased giver) and it would be unbearable for the recipient to imagine the donor as a man or woman named X, with a family, a job, and so on.

Gift and resource: these two categories have influenced the delineation of rules and practices. Human biological material is objectified as it is transformed into products for therapeutic use. Furthermore, it is subjected to safety requirements. These transformations rely on particular institutions, including blood and organ collection agencies, the legitimacy of which is based on arguments about donation and gift-giving, as well as hospitals, biotechnology firms or pharmaceutical enterprises that provide, manufacture and package the biological materials.

Since the 1980s, transplantation surgery has become routine, although uncertainties, mainly about organ procurement, continue. Because the criterion of brain death is generally not questioned in Western societies, issues involving the consent of a deceased donor are of greater concern. Do the families accept the removal of multiple organs from their beloved, recently deceased relative? What attitudes should surgeons adopt when families refuse organ removal? Decisions are made more difficult by the fact that most cases of brain death are caused by severe automobile accidents.[40]

As mentioned above, cornea donation in France has been regulated by law since 1948. In 1976, a French law promoted by the radical-socialist politician H. Caillavet established the principle of 'presumed consent'. This allowed surgeons to extract organs once family members had been informed and consulted, provided the deceased hadn't expressly objected to organ donation during his lifetime. Families can refuse to allow organ removal on several grounds (cultural, religious, sentimental, etc.), but it seems that the way the gift is described and justified by the team of surgeons and nurses involved in transplantation activities can have a decisive impact on families' decisions.[41]

In the US, the National Organ Transplantation Act (NOTA, 1984) outlaws organizations from profiting from the sale of solid organs. Organ transplantation must rely on voluntary donations and may not be pursued as a commercial venture. The Secretary of Health and Human Services (HHS) collaborates with the non-profit Organ Procurement and Transplantation Network (OPTN) in maintaining the national transplantation network. In accordance with the HHS, UNOS administers the OPTN.[42] OPTN has established a national register of individuals needing transplants and matches it with available organs. NOTA promoted organs as national resources and UNOS is responsible for defining the criteria by which patients are listed on the national register. The executive committee of UNOS is comprised of physicians (50 per cent), families and patients (25 per cent) and non-physicians (25 per cent).[43] NOTA was designed to 'insure equitable and timely access to the lifesaving procedures'.[44]

In France as in the US, governments have passed laws on organ donation in order to prevent abuses. The US law in 1984 and the French law in 1994 prohibit the marketing of organs and seek to ensure that everyone has an equal chance of receiving an organ transplant. What matters most is the management of the resource and its collection. In France, the 'presumed consent' helps surgeons to avoid blame. In Parisian hospitals, physicians have become used 'to not desperately trying to find evidence for refusing an organ donation'.[45]

The latest developments reflect this conception of human biological materials as resources, but as resources that remain outside mercantile economies. Bioethics laws offer protection to organ donors in France. The French laws in force since 1994 define the rules governing donor consent and limit the use of human body parts. Laws have become necessary because the procurement of organs challenged the development of organ transplantation.[46] The bioethical debates turn on a number of issues: the removal of multiple organs from one unique donor and the implicit notion of an 'optimization of death', as well as the mobilization of living donors (for kidneys, livers and lungs).[47] The enactment of the bioethics laws in 1994 has answered several questions about the use of human body parts. The main principle is the inalienability of the human body: no one is allowed to sell parts of his body and no one is allowed to patent body parts or stem cells. Several articles in these laws deal with medical activities (prenatal diagnosis, assisted reproduction devices) and research agendas.

In the US, the regulation of transplantation has also changed during the 1990s. In particular, NOTA has been criticized on a number of points: patients have complained about differences between the states; UNOS has been seen as being not sufficiently supported by HHS; and there were no satisfactory standards adopted for liver transplants (the only case of 'super urgency'). But new regulations were adopted in 1998. The allocation of organs is now based on urgency and not on geography. The same medical criteria are supposed to be followed throughout the country: the allocation of organs favours the sickest patients and those with the best chances of survival. The number of organs collected in a hospital is no longer a criterion for the number of organs received. The opponents to these regulations have argued that HHS wasn't qualified to regulate transplants, but advocates maintain that the HSS does a better job than UNOS. Since 2000, new policies have been promoted based on algorithms related to medical urgency and the likelihood of survival. These policies decreased the number of patients who died while waiting for transplants, while still maintaining a very high level of success.[48] The public has played an important part in changing US regulations and has considered government to be a helpful partner.[49]

As hospitals and more broadly the health-care system have been increasingly subjected to the market economy over the last two decades, it has become more difficult to evade the laws of the market when collecting and distributing human biological material. Given this new context, two alternatives have emerged. The first one promotes markets for organ transplantation. Given the scarcity of human body parts, a market for them would help avoid traffic and normalize exchanges: the collection and distribution of human biological material would be managed 'like a business', with all the attending costs of exchange and manufacture.[50] The second alternative adopts a mercantile perspective on organ transplantations, accepting notions of supply and demand, while prohibiting the sale of organs and ensuring their distribution according to principles of optimally effective and fair allocation of the resources. This perspective also calls on ethicists to provide arguments that undergird management decisions, for example decisions that pit emergency cases against geographic proximity. The new organization of organ collection and distribution in France since 1992 is partly influenced by this second alternative. The *Agence de la Biomédecine* manages organ collection and distribution as a scarce, but public resource. Organs are characterized as medical assets to be used in support of public interests and as social goods; they are a national resource.

Human biological material is both a gift and resource: it belongs to both categories. This specificity is a consequence of the commodification of human biological material. This dual character also explains why we cannot consider these biologics exclusively in terms of standardized objects (they show up the limits of standardization, for one cannot classify something of human origin, i.e. a unique and personified object, as a standardized object). As a resource, this material can be subjected to classifications, safety rules, market pricing, and so on.[51] As a gift, human biological material can be brought within several discourses that argue in favour of the 'gift of life'.[52] This may help to make acceptable the removal of organs and tissues – since removal in itself is not a gift.[53]

Conclusions

The development of the uses of human body parts has required the elaboration of rules and guidelines with the aim of ensuring safety, efficiency and respect for ethical principles. This in turn has helped to increase the number of transplant surgeries and to make them more commonplace. But the economy (collection, procurement, distribution, allocation) of human biological materials relies both on donations and a market: the contested biologics – some of which are transformed into drugs (products derived from blood) or surgical objects (cardiac valves) – are also contested categories. 'Bodies that are materially implicated in each other through tissue donation and transplantation are also socially implicated, and medical systems that exchange and circulate tissues are also social systems'.[54]

The analysis of the controversies surrounding the use of human body parts (organs and tissues) can help to describe the moral economy governing uses of the human body and more broadly the hopes and expectancies associated with therapeutic agents (drugs, biologicals, human biological material). This perspective encourages us to examine health-care systems in terms of how they exchange goods and services, of their norms and obligations, of their values and ethics and of how they are organized in social relationships.[55] Since the standardization of human biological material involves a process of commodification, it appears to be linked with economic, social and political interests.[56]

Finally, social scientists have defined several models for allocating organs. The first one is the gift economy. It remains a theoretical model because constraints imposed on transplantation activities – such as the costs of organ and tissue procurement, conservation, control, etc – don't allow for the existence of a pure gift economy. The second one is a 'resource economy' in which human materials are obtained by donation and regulated by state management of allocation, cost controls on transplantation surgery, safety rules, etc. This second economy is a pure economy in which organs and tissues are sold on a market. The model of a resource economy, with some differences as far as the regulatory role of the state is concerned, is the most common. This model is necessary in order to understand how human organs and tissues are standardized.

8 THE SCIENCE OF MEASURING VITAMINS: QUALITY CONTROL AND COMPETITION IN THE DUTCH VITAMIN INDUSTRY BEFORE THE SECOND WORLD WAR

Pim Huijnen

No doubt few things had more impact on the academic field of biochemistry in the interwar period than industry's involvement in the production of vitamins and other pharmaceuticals. Hendrik Westenbrink, who worked as an administrator in one of the most important scientific laboratories for vitamin research in the Netherlands in the 1920s, harked back nostalgically to the time before the Great War, when 'university laboratories were the only places where scientific activities could unfold and where researchers could work on the most topical subjects with the help of modest resources'. In a paper published in 1938 Westenbrink added that:

> Nowadays different branches of industry are so interested in developing biochemistry in certain directions, that the mighty industrial research laboratories as well as the university laboratories funded by industry have taken the lead. All because of the large sums of money needed for human resources and instruments ... The expenses for the rapid purification [of vitamins] are commonly only covered by those who expect to make a profit in the short or long run.[1]

What Westenbrink described here had far-reaching consequences for university scientists. The more academic vitamin research grew dependent on commercial funding, the more scientists had to cope with the pressure and influence of industry. It was, after all, industry that produced pharmaceuticals and drugs and it was the companies that had an interest in new and potentially profitable areas of research. Most universities could not muster the large sums needed for this type of research.

As several historians of science have shown recently, these circumstances led to close cooperation between industry, medical scientists, biochemists and others involved in the research of vitamins. Harmke Kamminga, for instance, has focused on the 'interconnected interests' of scientists and industry in the search for the chemical structures of vitamins in this period.[2] Sally Horrocks has pointed out that the industry more often profited from the assistance of academic researchers than vice versa. For example, companies made use of the authority of their academic advisors in their advertising campaigns.[3] The fact that vitamins formed such an innovative field of research underscores essential characteristics of the history of the entwinement of academic and industrial research from the 1920s onward.

Both Kamminga and Horrocks have illustrated their theses with case studies from Great Britain. Others have dealt with aspects of the industrial, political and/or social dimensions of scientific vitamin research in the United States, Germany and Switzerland.[4] In this essay, I aim to show how tightly scientific vitamin research and industrial vitamin production were interwoven in the Netherlands before the Second World War. In particular, I intend to demonstrate the central role of calibration and standardization. After all, it was only by creating standards and by calibrating preparations using such standards that scientists could distinguish the products they supervised on behalf of certain companies from other products, like traditional cod liver oil, produced without scientific consent. Naturally, this form of quality control had great marketing potential. Companies started using the names of their academic advisors and their standards more and more in advertising campaigns.

This is all the more interesting because in the literature it is often assumed that the establishment of standards in commercial vitamin production did not take place in this period – that is, before the chemical structures of vitamins were known, before they became synthetically reproducible, and before the vitamin levels of industrial products were uncontested.[5] In reality, however, science-based quality control, standardization processes and marketing were already heavily entangled by the late 1920s and 1930s.

The point to be emphasized is that the fact that pharmaceutical companies produced biological – and not synthetic – vitamins as drugs was central to the emergence of this intertwinement. The role of scientific authority in vitamin production and standardization was all the more crucial before the synthetization of vitamins, precisely because of the lack of uncontested standards in this period. Jean-Paul Gaudillière has elsewhere defined biologicals not as being opposed to chemical drugs, but as being 'more complex, more difficult to handle, and less standardized' than chemicals.[6] These ambiguities were not necessarily problems that had to be overcome. Particularly in matters concerning the use of standardization as a tool for competition and strategic management, as will be elaborated upon below, these characteristics could also be turned into benefits.

Organon and the Introduction of Vitamin Preparations in the Netherlands

The notion that nutrition was comprised not only of proteins, fat and carbohydrates, but also of new nutritive elements called vitamins only emerged during the First World War. In the 1890s, beriberi research in the Dutch Indies had supported the view that malnutrition could cause diseases. The Polish biochemist Casimir Funk made a decisive step by linking this characteristic of beriberi with other ailments like pellagra and scurvy. In 1912 he introduced the idiom 'vitamins' – originally 'vitamines' – to label the types of nutrients that, if lacking, would cause such diseases. Still, the concept of vitamins could be applied as nothing more than a practical conceptual tool in the research of deficiency diseases. After all, it was not until 1926 that anyone identified a vitamin by isolating it from the substance it was part of.[7]

However, it became increasingly difficult to deny the existence of vitamins by the mid-1920s. To cite the title of the programmatic book by the American biochemist Elmer McCollum, these elements were at the core of a 'newer knowledge of nutrition'.[8] The traditional understanding of nutrition failed to explain the occurrence of diseases like rickets or scurvy. After all, the levels of proteins, fat and carbohydrates in the food supply of most European countries had, for the most part, remained adequate throughout the war. The newer knowledge of nutrition further stimulated the scientific search for vitamins. Academic scientists gradually identified more and more ailments as being deficiency diseases – rickets being the most notable. This was done mostly by experimenting with the addition of typical substances like milk or yeast to the *'purified'* diets – containing nothing but fats, carbohydrates and proteins – of laboratory animals. By perfecting these techniques, researchers gradually came to distinguish between the various types of vitamins that existed and to understand how they worked in the body and what the consequences of deficiencies or overdoses were.[9]

After vitamins had been discovered to be responsible for the diseases xerophtalmia, beriberi and scurvy – which had provisionally been defined as A, B and C – around 1910, the proof of rickets being caused by a different vitamin deficiency took nearly another decade.[10] Quite soon after this discovery, the relation between rickets and ultraviolet rays was established as well. Research in Germany and the US showed that irradiated rats on a rickets-producing diet seemed to remain immune to the disease. Feeding these rats with irradiated foodstuffs had the same effect. It was the German chemist Adolf Windaus from Göttingen who hit upon a fungal steroid he named ergosterol – because Windaus had isolated it from ergot – as being the sought-after active element that turned into vitamin D upon irradiation. This insight won him the 1928 Nobel Prize in Chemistry.[11] These ongoing discoveries in vitamin D research had promising consequences for industry. Companies basically needed only an ultraviolet lamp and an amount of ergosterol (or foodstuffs containing ergosterol, such as yeast) to produce a remedy against rickets – at least once they had paid the patent fee to the Wisconsin Alumni Research Foundation.[12]

Taking Vigantol, the vitamin D preparation that Merck had developed with Windaus's assistance as an example, the Dutch company Organon started producing vitamin D preparations in 1928. The producer of pharmaceuticals had itself been founded only five years earlier, among others by the pharmacologist Ernst Laqueur from Amsterdam. The owner of a butchery and meat-processing factory in the provincial town of Oss in the south of the Netherlands had asked Laqueur to help him find new uses for the animal waste he would otherwise throw away. By the 1920s, industry experimented with the medical uses of several animal glands, like the thyroid or the pituitary gland. It is likely that this inspired the factory owner to start his own pharmaceutical enterprise for processing organic waste.[13] Under Laqueur's scientific guidance, Organon started extracting insulin from cattle pancreases. It was the first continental European company to produce the life-saving drug insulin for diabetics. Laqueur soon began experimenting with sex steroids as well.[14]

Whereas Laqueur strictly supervised all hormone preparations marketed by the company, he asked his assistant Lodewijk Karel Wolff to conduct experiments on vitamin production for the company from 1927 onward.[15] An educated ophthalmologist, by the time he started working for Organon, Wolff could look back on an extensive career. Born in 1879, he had had his own practice in Amsterdam since 1909. He had also conducted research at a number of university laboratories on bacteriological and biochemical topics. In Laqueur's laboratory, Wolff had focused on bacteriological problems, but had increasingly turned his attention to the relatively new field of vitamin research.

As an advisor to Organon, Wolff started showing the company how to make a vitamin preparation of its own. Vitamin A could be extracted from cattle livers and vitamin D from fish oil. In combination, these vitamins would give the company a brand new and potentially better-tasting alternative to cod liver oil.[16] Davitamon (from D-A-vitamin) was the first vitamin product Organon launched in 1928. To this day, it is one of the most established brand names for vitamins in the Netherlands.

Wolff and Organon had good reasons for starting the production of vitamin preparations with just these two vitamins. For one, they could be produced without much difficulty. More importantly, however, of all vitamin deficiencies, shortages of vitamin A and D were by far the most widespread in the Western world at that time. Deficiency diseases like scurvy, beriberi or pellagra hardly appeared in Europe and the US any more. Rickets, on the other hand, was still very common among children in Western Europe and the US. The disease, caused by vitamin D deficiency, manifested itself most clearly in the weakening and deformation of the bones.

In 1930, the Dutch paediatrician J. J. Soer concluded that 70 per cent of the children he supervised in his clinic that had not been given extra vitamin D, had developed symptoms of rickets by the end of winter. In cooperation with the Leiden professor of pediatrics, Evert Gorter, Soer had done experiments with both ultraviolet radiation and vitamin preparations in search of a cure or as a prophylaxis against the disease. Both methods worked well and the results differed little.[17] As a consequence, vitamin D products were bound to produce large sales, especially because the most common remedy against rickets at the time, cod liver oil, was greatly disliked.

'On a Scientific Basis'

By 1930, pharmaceutical, chemical and food companies all over the Western world started focusing on the profitable production of vitamin D. In 1927 Windaus himself, in cooperation with Bayer and Merck, turned it into a commercial preparation called Vigantol. Vitamin D products like these were marketed as superior alternatives to cod liver oil. Needless to say, the fish processing industry thought little of these new competitors, although sales of cod liver oil didn't collapse after the introduction of vitamin preparations. On the contrary, cod liver oil also profited from the growing awareness amongst consumers of vitamins' benefits.[18]

Nevertheless, industrial vitamin preparations had one important trump card. Although naturally produced cod liver oil also contained vitamin D (and A), their levels fluctuated and were oftentimes unknown. The industrial preparations could boast that they delivered stable and scientifically tested vitamin levels. When Organon launched its Davitamon in 1928, it explicitly emphasized this fact. The company used the sentence 'for the production of organic preparations *on a scientific basis*' as a slogan; and these were anything but empty words. Wolff had every batch of preparations checked in the Amsterdam laboratory and later, after 1929, in his own laboratory in Utrecht, where he held a chair in public health. He personally supervised production and distribution and no batch was marketed without his consent. What for Organon was a marketing strategy, was a matter of scientific professionalism and medical responsibility for Wolff.[19]

The standard method to determine the efficacy of vitamins D preparations were in vivo tests. The Organon preparations were also analysed in this way. Wolff used the rat colony he had set up with the aid of Organon to test the quality of the biologically active substances. First, a group of young laboratory rats would be completely deprived of vitamin D until they developed symptoms of rickets. Second, the rats would be administered a product containing vitamin D. The level and speed of the rats' recovery revealed something about the vitamin level of the product. The activity of preparations was, accordingly, expressed in so-called 'curative rat units', i.e. the amount of the preparation required to cure a rat of rickets. The same method could be applied to determine the level of a product needed to keep a rat from getting rickets. This level was expressed in so-called 'prophylactic rat units'. The method dated back to the work of the London biochemist Katharine Hope Coward.[20]

A New Method

The second Dutch company to market a vitamin product domestically, Philips-Van Houten, criticized this kind of quality control – more specifically, its scientific legitimacy. This company, a subsidiary to the electro-technical company Philips, unleashed a remarkable propaganda campaign in connection with the introduction of its own vitamin preparation two years after Organon's. The central message of the campaign was that its product should be regarded as the first preparation containing a guaranteed and reliable level of vitamin D. This claim was based on a new, spectrographic calibration method that two Philips researchers had developed to determine the quantity of ergosterol in their preparations. Encouraged by executive Anton Philips, the two had joined forces with chocolate producer Van Houten to jointly produce vitamin D chocolates, labelled Dohyfral, from the autumn of 1930.[21]

The spectrographic calibration method determined the vitamin concentration in a solution by measuring the solution's absorbance of a specific wavelength of light. This technique allowed researchers to express the quantity of vitamin D in milligrams.[22] Consequently, the Philips-Van Houten researchers could express the dose of pure vitamin in their preparations using exact and comprehensible measurements, contrary to the majority of its competitors. Naturally, for companies like Organon the use of rat units was a necessary, but hardly ideal technique. Apart from the rather obscure scientific language and the inevitable association with rats, this standard did not clarify the exact amount of vitamins. It was a measurement of efficacy.

However, Philips-Van Houten's standardization method failed to do exactly this. The researchers were able to express the vitamin level of its preparations in milligrams, but these metric figures in themselves could not make any claims about efficacy. Therefore, the company still needed to establish the link between the test results and the actual effects of Dohyfral: the preparation contained vitamin D, but was it effective and was it present in sufficient quantity to actually cure rickets? To develop such a method, Philips-Van Houten approached the pharmaco-therapeutical laboratory of the University of Leiden, where two students of the pharmacologist Willem Storm van Leeuwen turned this challenge into a PhD project. At the same time, Philips had the actual efficacy of Dohyfral clinically tested. The paediatrician mentioned above, professor Evert Gorter, was asked to carry out these tests in his department of the Leiden University Hospital.[23]

Gorter and his colleagues tested the Dohyfral preparation, as well as other industrial vitamin D preparations and cod liver oil, on eighteen infants between the age of eight and twenty months. They published their results in the prominent Dutch medical journal *Nederlandsch Tijdschrift voor Geneeskunde* in August 1930. At this point Dohyfral hadn't been officially marketed yet. Moreover, the research conducted in Leiden would not be published for another six months. In spite of this, the medical researchers wrote that they had 'used a preparation in our clinics that for the first time was standardized by physical research methods'.[24] What Gorter and his colleagues tried to stress with this statement was not so much the superiority of physical calibration as opposed to less accurate techniques in vivo. Instead, they were expressing a tacit assumption that physical tests should be regarded as the one and only calibration method. The Leiden researchers stated that competing products like Davitamon and Vigantol contained 'unknown amounts' of vitamin D.[25]

Calibration, Efficacy and Standardization

The article came as a surprise to Organon, but it reacted forcefully. The company's head of scientific staff, Marius Tausk, published a firm reply to the Leiden researchers (and to a second, polemical publication on the subject that Gorter had published) in the same journal a few weeks later. Tausk not only pointed out a series of technical flaws, but also zeroed in on the weak spot in their argument: the fact that the relationship between the essentially more accurate physical calibration method and the efficacy of Dohyfral remained unclear. To make his point even more forcefully, Tausk kept stressing the international scientific communities' consensus on the central importance of biological tests.[26]

His goal was, naturally, to dispute claims about the uncertainty of Davitamon's vitamin level. Gorter in turn had raised objections to the in vivo calibration method.[27] These were widely shared, as can be concluded from Tausk's reply. He stated that in theory there were good reasons to 'fully agree with prof. Gorter that any trustworthy physical or chemical calibration method is preferable to in vivo tests'.[28] After all, the spectrographic calibration technique was quantitatively much more accurate and comprehensible than the use of rat units could ever be. Moreover, the calibration methods using laboratory rats contained some perplexing issues. Most importantly, who could guarantee that the results from one laboratory would match the results from another? Laboratories didn't necessarily use the same types of rats, the same diets and – crucially – their own method and scale of calibration.

In the spring of 1931, the two students in Leiden would address the same problem in an article based on their research about 'the standardization of vitamin D-preparations'.[29] The in vivo method would be valuable only if vitamin D preparations from different producers could be compared using the same measures. Otherwise, the 'mutual comparison' between preparations expressed in rat units would remain 'unjustified'. More than that, the rat units themselves would continue to have 'mere relative significance'.[30] To bypass this problem, the students called attention to the repeated plea of vitamin researchers for an international standard for vitamin D preparations.

However, by the time the article was published, this argument about incommensurability had effectively become outdated. The Medical Research Council (MRC) in London had just responded to this plea for an international vitamin standard. It had very recently proclaimed its vitamin D preparation as the international standard in order to resolve the problem of comparison. Tausk had already mentioned this in his reaction to Gorter in the *Nederlandsch tijdschrift voor geneeskunde*. The MRC had decided to define the common curative rat unit as the activity of one milligram of its standard preparation. As long as all vitamin researchers conformed to this standard, calibrations carried out in different laboratories would be comparable.[31]

In his letter, Tausk also emphasized the fact that Davitamon had indeed been calibrated using the MRC preparation and that its vitamin level was expressed in its internationally acknowledged standard. As long as the spectrographic technique hadn't overcome its teething problems, Tausk concluded (at great length) that it could not match the internationally accepted in vivo tests. The fact that the Permanent Commission on Biological Standardization of the League of Nations' Health Organization would adopt standard preparations like the MRC to determine official 'international vitamin units' soon thereafter, only affirmed this view. These neutral-sounding international units came to replace the provisional rat units.[32]

Wolff, as Organon's scientific advisor, also became personally engaged in the matter. In a letter he sent to the two Leiden researchers, he strongly urged his young colleagues to publicly rectify the omission of the MRC standard.[33] He had his reasons not to take the matter light-heartedly. To justify the spectrographic calibration method, the Leiden researchers had elaborated an algorithm that could link the results they physically obtained with the efficacy of the analysed preparation – i.e. quantity with quality. This was to become an important tool for biological calibration in the Netherlands. By neglecting existing practices in this field, and indeed by ignoring the fact that these practices already made use of internationally accepted standards, Wolff felt that the authors had discredited the way Organon had been evaluating its own vitamin products the past few years. Although this was undoubtedly unintentional, the two researchers essentially maintained that Organon did not posses any solid knowledge to substantiate the claims it made about vitamin levels. By clearing up this misunderstanding, the various researchers associated with both companies ended their dispute over the superior calibration method – for the time being.

Standardization and Marketing

The calibration dispute between the two main Dutch vitamin producers Organon and Philips-Van Houten shows how tightly these companies were connected to academic scientists. This scientific connection formed the hallmark of both companies. Philips-Van Houten made use of scientific publications, clinical research and the like as a means of disseminating and propagating its Dohyfral preparations. Organon mobilized its scientific potential in the same way. The 'science-industry nexus' – to quote the title of a notable conference on the topic in 2002 – of which these relations are an early illustration, has been a topical object of research in both history and science studies for many years.[34] The topics most often addressed in this field of study, like the structure, direction and confiscation of knowledge, go beyond the scope of this chapter. They can, however, offer useful ways of looking at the early forms of collaboration between science and industry. This holds, for example, for Nelly Oudshoorn's analysis of the production process of Organon's sex hormones preparations.[35] She shows how drugs were conceptualized 'in networks of different groups of actors' and can therefore be considered as 'the embodiment of interests that become mutually defined through social networks'.[36] In these networks, Oudshoorn emphasizes clinical trials as 'major devices in bringing the relevant groups of actors together'.[37] These trials played such a central role in the marketing of sex hormones, because Organon had first to create a market for these products.

In my opinion, the case of vitamins was different, in particular the case of vitamin D. After all, the larger public was already familiar with the drug, although without knowing it. Cod liver oil had been a household remedy for centuries. Clinical trials were not necessary in order for the vitamin industry to raise public awareness about the usefulness of their products. The case described in this chapter illustrates that industry couldn't do without scientists. Oudshoorn shows this as well. In the vitamin production no less than in the production of sex hormones, academic researchers provided physicians and the general public with 'tools to delimit the boundaries between quackery and scientific medicine'.[38] Above all, these tools consisted of standards and methods of standardization. In the vitamin industry, standards not only established boundaries between the growing numbers of quack products and pharmaceutical compounds on the market, but also affirmed the superiority of vitamin preparations over natural cod liver oil. Standards became the principal marketing tool for the vitamin industry.

Considering this, it should hardly be surprising that Organon and Wolff made such an issue of the rather technical judgements of Gorter and his colleagues. Organon considered the questioning of its standards by Philips-Van Houten to be a marketing ploy directed against its products. Wolff must have taken it as an attack on his professionalism and scientific authority. After all, in the standardization of industrially produced drugs, science and marketing coincided. This is why disputes like these were quite common within vitamin research and the vitamin industry during the 1920s and 1930s. In particular due to the lack of commonly acknowledged standards throughout this period, vitamin manufacturers persistently tried to push through the calibration methods from which they hoped to profit most.

To name just one instance, in 1937 Organon found itself entangled in controversy with the incomparably larger German companies Bayer and Merck. It was brought about by Wolff's discovery that the Vogan preparation of the German companies contained a considerably (fourfold) lower level of vitamin A than Bayer and Merck claimed. Apparently, the German standards were four times higher than Organon's. That is why the Organon researchers had simply opted for multiplying the level of their own vitamin A preparation by four, thereby meeting 'the new international units from Bayer', as they called them.[39] Obviously irritated by their naivety, Wolff explained to his colleagues that 'there is only one international unit ... We cannot "adapt" our calibrations to those of Bayer and still describe the outcome in terms of international units on the label'.[40] The only thing Organon could do, according to Wolff – 'though it may not be quite common'[41] – was to depict the level of vitamin A both in international units and in Vogan units on the Davitamon label.

According to Wolff, the better solution was for all three companies to agree to the Permanent Commission on Biological Standardization's official conversion factor between the biological calibration techniques Bayer and Merck used and Organon's colorimetric testing method. However, Merck bluntly stated it was not willing to accept Wolff's proposal. As far as this company was concerned, 'if a conversion factor should be established, this would have to be a great deal higher than the League of Nation's factor'.[42]

Although one has to be aware of the distinct time and setting of this particular dispute, the example illustrates that the introduction of official international standards by the League of Nations did not resolve all the standardization issues in the vitamin industry. Disputes would continue for as long as the League of Nation's authority was not recognized by all countries. More importantly, they would not stop before the complete synthetization of vitamins. This eventually made in vivo tests abundant and brought an end to the use of debatable standards.

Conclusion

The industrial production of vitamins as preparations or additives dates from the 1920s. To a large extent, this originated from academic researchers teaming up with pharmaceutical companies to convert their growing knowledge of vitamins into drugs or medicinal additives. This was the case, for example, for the Dutch companies Organon and Philips-Van Houten. Still, many pharmaceutical and foodstuff companies in Europe – including the Netherlands – and the US recognized the commercial potential of vitamins on their own as well. The promise that vitamins could be used for the prevention or treatment of certain diseases naturally sounded quite profitable. This is why the Quaker's Oats Company, for example, started adding vitamin D to its products once it had acquired the right to use the patented procedure to produce vitamin D by ultraviolet irradiation from the Wisconsin biochemist Harry Steenbock in 1927. Around the same time, the Dutch manufacturer of children's biscuits, Liga, started experimenting on its own with the addition of vitamin D taken from cod liver oil to its foodstuffs. Liga brought in an academic vitamin expert to supervise the procedure and to test the results. Such cooperative arrangements were not uncommon. Many companies that wanted to commence the production of vitamins as food supplements or medicine needed academic scientists for advice or to back up their claims. The Swiss company Cristallo S.A. from Thusis, for example, was able to introduce its vegetable 'phosphor-vitamin-complex' preparation called Eviunis onto the European market at the end of the 1920s thanks to a wide range of academic researchers who guaranteed its efficacy.[43]

At the same time, standardization in the pre-synthetics era became increasingly a matter of product marketing. Initially, Organon's scientific supervision more or less resulted from the close cooperation between the company and its academic advisors. For these advisors, it would have been inconceivable to sell products that did not meet their scientific standards. As competition in the vitamin branch grew during the 1930s, the relevance of these calibrations – and of scientific supervision in general – started to play a growing role in the advertising campaigns that were gradually appearing in newspapers and magazines. Slogans and the strategic branding of products became serious business.[44] When it came to marketing though, standardization was not only about scientific standards, but also about convincing consumers. It was only as a result of its calibration dispute with Philips-Van Houten that Organon first truly learned this lesson.

Philips-Van Houten continued advertising its Dohyfral preparations with explicit references to Gorter's critical article, even after Wolff personally had tried to convince the Philips researchers of its misleading claims. Gorter started the controversy with Organon anew with an informative brochure he had written about rickets in 1932. He again stated that Dohyfral was the only truly standardized vitamin D preparation and that 'the only thing known about Davitamon, is that it is strong enough to cure a certain number of rats of rickets'.[45] Apart from again trying to debunk Organon's internationally acknowledged type of calibration, with his statement Gorter again evoked an unseemly association between Davitamon and rats – which naturally enough did not appeal to a lay public and was not very good advertising for Organon.

For consumers, it was of little concern whether Gorter's characterization was right or not. His authority as a medical scientist was far more crucial. Rima D. Apple, the author of the acclaimed book on the history of the American pre-occupation with vitamins *Vitamania: Vitamins in American Culture*, eloquently summarizes the function of science and scientific standardization in this manner:

> Granted, little was known about their structure or about the way they worked in the body, but the science of vitamins held out the promise of great benefits. It was this promise, the aura of science, that pharmaceutical companies used to create a new market; it was the promise of science and the aura of science that convinced consumers to embrace these new products.[46]

The aura of reliable and credible standardization was increasingly regarded as an essential part of selling vitamins. This became all the more so, as vitamins were increasingly marketed as commodities promoting health and strength as opposed to treatments against particular diseases. This resulted in a practice that saw vitamin manufacturers increasingly relying on scientific standards. Scientific authorities were able to convince consumers of their trustworthiness, whether they were right or wrong, honest or not. The fact that these scientists were dealing with biologicals – as complex materials, the efficacy of which could not be expressed unambiguously – was essential. After all, this complexity gave them the flexibility to strategically mix standardization with marketing.

Illustrative in this regard is how quickly Organon learned to play this game. For Wolff's successor at the University of Utrecht and at Organon, Hendrik Willem Julius, the use of his calibrations for the company's marketing purposes was perfectly clear. In a letter to the company written in 1940, he stated that 'I want to stress that our principal of calibrating in vivo [*and not otherwise*] has to do with the aim of enhancing profits as far as the vitamin levels of our preparations are concerned. This has undoubtedly led to results'.[47]

9 THE GERMAN PHARMACEUTICAL INDUSTRY AND THE STANDARDIZATION OF INSULIN BEFORE THE SECOND WORLD WAR

Ulrike Thoms

Recent historiography has examined the invention and introduction of insulin chiefly from the perspective of medical science. Drawing on medical sources, popular histories of insulin have often concentrated on the role of the genius-inventors who philanthropically handed over the patents for the production process to the University of Toronto and the newly founded Insulin Committee, which then controlled the patent's use in other countries.[1] This interpretation implies that all of the problems were simply resolved when the Toronto Insulin Committee had developed a method of standardization and spread it through-out the world.[2] In fact, the use and production of the drug in different countries turned out to be a complex process, encountering different national health systems, therapeutic cultures and economic situations.

This essay investigates how insulin was introduced and standardized in Germany. Two years after Banting and Best had discovered insulin, German newspapers were full of articles about it. A typical article began: 'For some time, an American medication from the pancreas, insulin, has been causing the greatest interest in medical science. In certain cases of diabetes mellitus it has proved to be a real wonder drug'.[3] Another one stated: 'The discovery of insulin by the American researchers Macleod, Banting and Best and its utilization in the therapy of diabetes belongs to the major achievements of medical science'.[4] Both of these articles are part of a collection of newspaper clippings in the Bayer business archive. The fact that such clippings were collected and kept is remarkable, giving evidence of the firm's interest in public opinion on the newest medical developments as well as its own products.

When insulin was introduced into drug therapy in 1923, this was indeed breaking news, changing the treatment of diabetics in a variety of ways. Until then, therapy had relied exclusively on strict dietary measures, which meant permanent hunger, unbalanced dietary regimes with lots of meat and fat, emaciated patients and a very limited life expectancy for diabetics, particularly diabetic children. But with insulin, they could live a more satisfactory life. Thus the good and long-awaited news spread quickly from Canada to Germany, where it was not yet produced. The many letters from Germans in the correspondence of the Canadian Insulin Committee show that its advent was desperately expected.[5] In all of these cases, the secretary of the Toronto Insulin Committee usually responded that insulin was not yet available in Germany, and asked people to be patient until standardization had made it a safe cure and helped to establish larger production.

Although important progress was made, the clippings of newspaper articles from 1923 to 1925 reveal a level of disenchantment among scientists, doctors and patients.[6] Insulin was seen as a wonder drug, but not only was it very costly; it had also become obvious that it would not be enough merely to take the drug, since the entire treatment regime had to be attuned to the unique conditions of the specific patient. This included determining how much insulin was needed, how the patient reacted to it and whether the patient's metabolism was sufficiently stable, and would lead to a complicated system involving both insulin and dietary measures, which was worked out and had to be closely adhered to. The patient's entire lifestyle had to be disciplined, with permanent controls implemented to monitor the sugar content of urine and eventually blood.[7] Moreover, it became clear that the standardization and stabilization of German insulin would take time, while foreign insulin was neither available in large amounts nor affordable for most of the patients.

Despite the complications, standardization of the biological drug was seen as the basic precondition for changing the situation for diabetic patients. The Canadian inventors of insulin had laid the foundation for boosting production in order to secure provision for everyone in need. In fact, the Toronto Insulin Committee took care to globalize insulin by establishing national insulin committees all over the world, attempting to make its production and use known everywhere as soon as possible. In the case of Germany, achieving this goal was difficult under the economic and social circumstances of the 1920s. The deep economic problems included inflation and then runaway inflation, as well as very limited international trade due to import barriers. Moreover, the Franco-Belgian occupation of the Ruhr area in 1923 made the situation even worse, as it isolated Farbwerke Hoechst: the German pharmaceutical company with the most experience, knowledge and contacts in this field. In comparison to other countries, the German meat trade was much more decentralized and relied on smaller slaughterhouses. Consequently, pancreases were much harder to obtain and under the given economic conditions their quality worsened even further.

On the other hand, much of the founding work on metabolism and diabetes had come from Germany. In fact, lively research was already being undertaken at Farbwerke Hoechst, and the company was very close to the solution of the problem at the point when Banting and Best announced their sensational findings. Based on archival sources from industrial and state archives, as well as articles from the popular press and from medical journals, this essay searches out the contributions of different actors, which ended up with the regulation of the drug, thus securing its safety and its affordability for the patient, and finally allowing the companies to make some profit.

The chapter follows the path of insulin from the Canadian research laboratory to the German pharmacy, examining the different phases in the standardization and later life of standardized insulin. It aims to show that in this case regulation was by no means driven forward by the German State and its institutions. In fact, it was based on a well-established system of drug research and drug marketing, which relied on the collaboration of firms, industrial scientists and physicians. Within this system, researchers, doctors and pharmaceutical companies had different motives to strive for the standardization of insulin. In the laboratory, standardization was an indispensable tool of research, since only the standardization of a drug can lead to reproducible test results that will allow investigation of the effects of certain substances. Physicians need to be able to predict drug effects and fix the necessary doses in order to cure rather than kill their patients. Of course, the pharmaceutical industry shares this interest, for the obvious reason that only a safe and efficacious drug with no or only a few side effects will create trust. And it is only trust in drugs that will make doctors prescribe and patients buy and use the products. In addition to these motives, standardization is a precondition for setting up mass production and reducing production cost. As will be shown, German pharmaceutical companies were very well aware of this fact, and were confident that they would be able to realize this aim soon. As the introduction to this book has pointed out, drug research as well as production, regulation and sales of biological drugs were situated in different national contexts. Therefore, I will briefly recall the development of the physiological and clinical insulin that began in Canada, where insulin was founded in 1921, in order better to characterize German developments. In contrast to the situation in the US, Canada and Great Britain,[8] the German case was marked by the complete absence of any state institution to examine or authorize insulin preparations.

The Discovery of Insulin, the Insulin Committee and the Physiological Insulin Standard

German researchers had been experimenting with pancreas extracts since the late nineteenth century, which had seen the introduction of some oral preparations. German pharmaceutical firms were very interested in this problem and kept in close contact with several researchers. Among them was Georg Zuelzer (1870–1940), who had already taken out a patent for his 'Acomatol', as well as Josef Blum from Frankfurt and Ernst Vahlen, who had his 'Metabolin' patented.

All of these early efforts were unsuccessful, either because the side effects were deemed too severe or because it was not possible to stabilize the effect of the drug. Nevertheless, Hoechst did not give up. In 1921 it renewed its attempts to isolate the active agent using veal and cattle pancreases.[9] In the same year, Frederick Grant Banting (1891–1941) and Charles H. Best (1899–1978), managed to isolate a substance from canine pancreases, through the relatively simple and cheap method of extraction by alcohol. As they showed, the injection of this extract caused a reasonable drop in the blood-glucose level of dogs.

John R. MacLeod (1876–1965) became interested in the problem and provided Banting and Best with more funds and the technical assistance of the biochemist James Collip (1892–1965), who worked on the purity of the extract. By late 1921, Collip's insulin was pure enough to begin clinical tests, first in animals and later in humans.[10] In January 1922 the substance was administered to Alexander Thompson, a 14-year-old who was near to death, but then quickly recovered after the injection.

In May 1922 they published their discovery in the *Journal of the Canadian Medical Association*,[11] and handed production over to the Connaught Laboratories at the University of Toronto, which had been originally created to produce antitoxins. But the relatively small laboratory was neither able to increase insulin production to the amount needed, nor to maintain and stabilize the quality of the extract. Following a proposal of Eli Lilly's research director, George Clowes (1877–1958), Eli Lilly was included in the enterprise in May 1922. The university then decided to hand over the entire production process to the large, well-established pharmaceutical firm, thus benefiting from its experience in the standardization of glandular extracts.

It is well known that Banting and Best refused any financial gain from their finding, handing over the patent rights to the University of Toronto and asking the dean of the university to speed up the process of patenting. Following their wish to make good quality insulin available to all patients who needed it, and at a reasonable price, the dean established the so-called 'Insulin Committee'. This consisted of three members of the Board of Governors of the University of Toronto. Attached was an advisory committee including Banting, Best, MacLeod, Collip and Clowes. The committee's task was to supervise insulin production and, more importantly, to manage patents and finances.[12] The university agreed with Eli Lilly that the firm should have the exclusive right to market insulin, but only for one year. In return Eli Lilly agreed to deliver insulin samples to a specific group of researchers for clinical trials, to test all batches of insulin in the laboratory of the Insulin Committee at Toronto, to give 12 per cent of the insulin production to Connaught Laboratories for free, and to inform the committee of all improvements in production methods. Last but not least, all rights derived from patents on improvements were to be assigned to the University of Toronto.[13]

Although this was a long list of expensive concessions, the offer seemed promising for Eli Lilly since it allowed the firm to present itself as a modern, research-driven scientific enterprise.[14] For its part, the Insulin Committee acquired enormous moral authority, thanks to its abjuring conduct and strong connection with the state, which seemed to guarantee its material disinterestedness. And Banting and Best so enhanced their scientific and ethical reputations that by 1923 they were awarded the Nobel Prize for Medicine.[15]

The researchers were highly aware of diabetics' need for a cure, and indeed, once public knowledge of the discovery of insulin spread through the popular press, demand for the new substance increased rapidly, forcing production to be ramped up as quickly as possible. This was despite the conditions of growing mistrust in pharmaceutical companies.[16]

The major problem was a uniform standard, which would ensure stable and reproducible results in treatment. In this regard, the character of insulin as a biological posed a special problem, because it was clear that chemical analysis would not suffice in determining the product's physiological properties. Collip had discovered that rabbits would develop identical clinical signs to humans, these signs (i.e. hypoglycaemia and its expression in cramps and faintings) and their physiological reactions to the injected biological substance would be used to measure and standardize the strength of the insulin, to evaluate and to calibrate the batches.

There was nothing entirely new about this method; it had been used in the production of sera according to the standards set down by the League of Nations. But this method also relied on the standardization of the animals themselves. Collip decided to use only rabbits that weighed 2 kg and that had been fasting for twenty-four hours. Blood samples of the rabbits were taken every one-and-a-half, three and five hours after the insulin injection. The amount of insulin needed to cure the animals from hypoglycaemia and to bring their blood-glucose levels back to normal was then defined as the 'Insulin Unit'. The animals played more than a simple or transient role in the discovery phase, since such tests became standard procedure within the industry; every single production batch came to be tested in this way before it was sent out to clinics and pharmacies, to determine the physiological value of the insulin and to measure its effects in medical practice.

The Development of the Clinical Standard in Canada and the US

From early on, different standards were used by different firms and institutions. Lilly, for example, used different standards for the rabbits compared to Banting and Best, while other researchers used different animals to define a physiological standard, achieving nearly identical results.[17] Clowes went so far to ask whether the convulsions would not be more useful than the measurement of blood sugar levels. Over time, it became clear that defining the physiological standard was one thing, whereas defining the clinical standard was quite another. This had a lot to do with the special character of insulin as a biological substance, and the biological diversity of different diabetics. More than other drugs, insulin needed to be attuned to the specific conditions of every single diabetic body, and its action needed to be observed continuously. In this sense, insulin relied very much on a holistic view, as it was pursued by the alternative medical systems such as the German 'biological medicine', although diabetes specialists most often did not adhere to biological medicine. Furthermore, although insulin was a natural substance extracted from organisms, it was dangerous if overdosed. And yet it was not possible to define the level of overdose or to put an exact figure on it. Insulin, it turned out, was a special case.

Insulin levels had to be adjusted according to food intake and bodily activity day by day and against the background of a thorough understanding of the underlying cybernetic regulation cycle. Being able to find out how this cycle functioned and to generalize how insulin injections would steer its functioning, relied on the collection of as much clinical data as possible, from as many patients as possible. In principle, diabetes specialists were well prepared to do this, since different kinds of tests and the application of standards had already become part of the diagnostic and surveillance procedures applied to diabetic patients. In particular, urine tests together with several quantifying procedures had already become part of the daily work routines in clinics, and were ready to be applied in the testing of insulin. Tables and records documenting patients' food intake and excretions formed the basis on which so-called carbohydrate tolerance was calculated. Using such patient data, Elliot Joslin had developed a dietary regime that reduced food intake to a minimum. Though influential in America, his standard diet had not been introduced in Germany, where treatment depended on doctors' respective scientific opinions.[18]

Collecting such large volumes of data about patients' treatment surpassed the narrower, more technically orientated aims of the Insulin Committee, and therefore another, less formal committee was established, which was also called the 'Insulin Committee'. Comprising such well-known diabetes specialists as Elliot Joslin (1869–1962), Frederick Allen (1878–1964) and Rollin Woodyatt (1878–1953),[19] it was designed to establish a network of hospitals that would gather data and develop practical clinical methods of insulin application. Its responsibilities were not extended to legal issues, which were instead addressed by the administration of the University of Toronto. The Insulin Committee was instead concerned with quality control. Moreover, it was charged with publishing the diabetes research in the medical press and promoting the standardization of treatment by practitioners.

One of the first findings of this clinical committee was that the original Toronto standard unit was useful for the production of insulin, but ill-suited for clinical practice. Therefore, the committee decided in December 1922 to divide the physiological unit by four, in order to be better able to calibrate the dosage for the individual patient's needs.[20]

Insulin goes International: The German Insulin Committee 1923–4

The Canadian Committee tried to deploy knowledge about insulin and to collect and evaluate the practical experiences derived from its use. In so doing, it decided to approach the League of Nations and Henry Dale. In May of 1923, Dale then convened a meeting of the Standardizing Committee of the League of Nations,[21] in which the standard clinical unit was fixed at one-third of the original Toronto unit and the standard powder preparation was designated to contain eight units per mg.[22] At this point, insulin as such was already known to the German scientific and lay public.[23] Some physicians had read about it in the English press in late 1922,[24] and reports on the miraculous substance and articles about the Canadian, American and English findings had reached the German press by January of 1923. Very often with strong nationalist undertones, publications stressed the immense role of German research in laying the foundation for this important new drug. From March 1923 reports could be found in German chemical journals,[25] and by April the news had spread to the popular press, where it was carefully monitored by the pharmaceutical industry.[26] The clinicians disliked such reports about new therapies, fearing they would 'raise hope in the patients and force doctors to try out such novelties in their patients', before sufficient experience had been made, or in other words, before the treatment had been standardized.[27] Instead, the clinicians asked for careful tests and warned against the dangers of the new treatment,[28] as well as against the products of unreliable companies, which would throw unsafe preparations on the market and sell them for high prices.[29]

In the spring of 1923, the Toronto Committee contacted medical organizations and experts abroad to expand the use of the drug for the benefit of mankind. The experts were encouraged to convene national insulin committees, whose members were chosen on the basis of their scientific reputation and experience. How they built and organized their respective national committees, however, was left solely to the experts' discretion. Just how different these national organizations became can be surmised from the fact that although Albert Calmette initially offered the Institut Pasteur's services for the control of insulin, there are no traces of any activity related to insulin in the Institut Pasteur archives.[30] In fact, no such committee was established in France, where insulin was predominantly marketed by smaller firms. In Germany no state institution was involved. This fits well into established patterns that, until the second half of the twentieth century, saw German governmental institutions playing only a marginal role in the control of drugs. Instead, professional bodies decided on the value of new therapies.[31] Although, as we will see, the Imperial Health Office (*Reichsgesundheitsamt*) was responsible for the regulation of the drug market, its activities were later limited to the designation of dangerous substances, which required a prescription. In general, however, German health officials left the development of insulin to market forces.

The first contacts between German scientists and the Insulin Committee were established by Ernst Fuld, a professor for internal medicine at the University of Berlin. On 28 November 1922, Fuld wrote to the University of Toronto in order to learn more about insulin, about which he had read in the Manchester Guardian, but had not been able to find further information.[32] Oskar Minkowski must have heard about insulin only shortly after Fuld. He sent some reprints to the committee in January 1923, and received back the latest reprints on insulin together with some admiring remarks about his 'monumental work'.[33] On 6 April 1923, MacLeod wrote identical letters to Ernst Fuld, the diabetes specialist Carl von Noorden (1859–1944) and Oskar Minkowski. They were informed that the University of Toronto 'has been trying to exercise some control' over the manufacture and distribution of insulin 'by taking out patents in various countries'. Minkowski, von Noorden and Fuld were asked to communicate with Ludolf von Krehl (1881–1938) from Heidelberg, the physiologist Friedrich von Müller (1858–1941) from Munich and the clinicians Fritz Umber (1891–1946) and Hermann Strauss (1868–1944) from Berlin, 'with regard to what steps might be taken to supply manufacturers with the necessary information for the manufacture of insulin'.[34] Three weeks later, Minkowski wrote to MacLeod that he had 'entered into correspondence with the confreres you mentioned', while Fuld was already told to enter a second motion at the *Reichspatentamt* (Imperial Patent Office) in order to take out a patent, after the first motion had failed.[35] In his eyes it was necessary to produce insulin in Germany because foreign preparations were too expensive, and the place to do so was Hamburg or Berlin because only these two towns had 'great and well organised abbatoires' to deliver enough pancreases of good quality.[36]

Interestingly enough, German firms reacted in a somewhat reluctant manner to the insulin question.[37] Even in April 1923, when German doctors tried to obtain insulin from the Toronto Committee, Hoechst's representatives thought that it was quite unclear whether insulin was at all useful.[38] Only when the foundation of the German Insulin Committee was officially announced in July 1923 did the firm realize how far things had been pushed in Toronto;[39] they then tried everything to catch up and to secure their share of the market.

Unlike the governmental character of the French and British committees, the German one more closely resembled the American Clinical Committee, which was likewise only informally organized.[40] It was independent of the state and relied exclusively on the clinical work of physicians, while the standardization of insulin was left to industry. This goes back to Minkowski, who never intended to establish a formal institution for checking insulin, but thought 'that the best course to pursue in the interest of the matter would be to entrust the manufacture to a reputable chemical firm (Merck or Höchst)'.[41]

On 5 July 1923, Minkowski informed industrial firms of the committee's existence and queried them about their progress in the production of insulin. He underscored the committee's intention to avoid the centralization of production or the exclusion of certain firms. If the committee had contacted only some firms, it did so because it was already aware that they produced good products. Due to the high price of insulin, he did not expect firms to distribute production samples to practitioners, but he definitively stated the importance of the committee as well as the firms' need to collaborate:

> If you attach any importance to the recommendations of the German Insulin Committee, then it will be necessary for you make available a certain amount [of insulin] to all the members of the Insulin Committee, either free of charge or at substantially reduced prices.[42]

With that, the members of the committee would be first in line to test the insulin and publish the results of their trials.[43] Ultimately, the firms agreed to supply each member of the German Committee with 500 units of insulin for initial tests. Depending on the amount of insulin that their patients needed, this amount would barely suffice to treat a single person on a continuous basis. More insulin was forthcoming only to test its quality. According to the testing system agreed to by industry and the committee, two committee members would test the product of a given firm, and each member would test two products. This agreement was obviously meant to establish a certain neutrality, but the firms seem to have engaged in preferential treatment of those physicians deemed important, from time to time arbitrarily providing them with extra insulin.[44] The committee members were then required to report the results of their clinical experiences directly to the companies and garner information about improvements and changes in the production process.

The firms were very well aware of the fact that, for the sake of their prestige, they needed to outperform their competitors by providing the first, purest and cheapest insulin on the market, and they did not expect standardization to be too difficult. A Bayer employee, for example, remarked that: 'The work cannot be too difficult. [The Norwegian insulin specialist] Krogh came back [from Toronto] on 12 December and on 21 December he had self-made insulin for trials in rabbits'.[45] Specialized in chemistry and not in the extraction of organic substances, however, the firms clearly underestimated the problems associated with the supply of good quality pancreases, extraction and biological standardization. Moreover, they saw the biological nature of the drug as being 'naturally only temporary'.[46] Like Fuld, firms such as Hoechst simply expected that its chemists would soon be able to synthesize the active principle, as they had been able to do in the case of other biological substances like adrenaline and thyroxine.[47] They did not expect to make high profits at the very start of this business, but they did see their engagement as an investment in the future. And apart from that, they had their reputations to protect. One Hoechst employee stressed that insulin would once again provide the firm with the 'opportunity to leave its scientific calling card at the doctor's office'.[48] Subsequent developments proved that they had overestimated this opportunity. Even a firm like Merck, which in principle had extensive experience with organic materials, abandoned production after their first attempts failed both to extract insulin of stable quality and to acquire the dried extract from other firms.[49] A basic problem of these post-war years of scarcity and need lay in the low number of well-nourished animals in Germany, and hence in the dearth and low quality of the harvested pancreases.

The companies, however, were very well aware of the fact that doctors and firms depended on each other. As a local representative of Bayer put it in October 1923, their policy explicitly followed the rule that 'one hand washes the other',[50] and representatives did everything to maintain and cultivate these contacts to clinicians, hoping for positive evaluations that would substantiate the efficacy of their product and underline the firm's competence.[51] The firms regarded authorization by the committee to be of the utmost importance and in their correspondence they spoke directly of 'official approval' by the committee.[52] Therefore, they did everything they could to acknowledge the committee's authority and retain close contact using their pharmaceutical salesmen, who acted as the firm's local representative, something that was rarely mentioned or discussed in the medical press. In any case, Bayer appealed to the Insulin Committee's authority in refusing to grant the wishes of many doctors, who wanted to purchase insulin to treat their patients. The firm pointed to the agreements with the Insulin Committee and insisted on the necessity of getting the quality of insulin officially approved before they brought it onto the market. Although this implied waiting for approval, and thus losing some profits, in the long run this practice helped to underscore the respectability and reliability of the firm and its refusal to exploit the needs of seriously ill people.

In return, the firms somehow expected that *their* examiner would use their products in clinical practice. Failure to do so provoked angry reactions, as in the case of Fritz Umber, who was responsible for testing Hoechst's insulin. Queried as to the reasons why Umber didn't use Hoechst's product, the local Hoechst salesman assured his superiors that he had made the firm's expectations clear to Umber: 'We have stressed that it would be very disadvantageous for us if the clinic that tests our insulin does not subsequently use it'.[53]

In general, the German Insulin Committee protected the firms by not extending the list of firms subject to regular scrutiny.[54] This aroused suspicion that firms and committee members were conspiring to keep prices high and exclude competitors. Moreover, from the outset these competitors could not earn the important designation 'tested by the Insulin Committee'. Responding to these accusations, the committee declared that it had been authorized by the Canadians, and suggested that they had already preselected the firms designated to produce insulin.[55] The committee argued that, given the high expenditures involved in starting production, it was for the time being only fair to protect the chosen firms. Later, in the 1940s, the committee stated that its members were simply unable to expand the number of firms, because of their limited capacity to carry out testing.[56] However, the entire biotechnological task of standardizing insulin as a substance was left to industry, while physicians were responsible only for a final quality check. Physicians' assessments of single batches of insulin were based on observation of the amount needed to keep the blood-glucose levels of their patients stable, as well as on the side effects provoked by the samples.[57]

The Imperial Health Office did nothing either to evaluate the quality of insulin or to further encourage its use. Very much in line with its general policy of refusing any requests to test drugs or to provide producers with seals of approval, it left the task of assessing the usefulness of new drugs to medical experts and the scientific public.[58] The case of insulin was seen as somehow particular, but it was still only briefly discussed. Overall, it took until October 1923 for the Imperial Health Office to issue any official statement on insulin. The short statement, which was published in the office's official journal, mentioned the International Standardization Conference and the International Congress of Physiologists, which had taken place in Edinburgh on 19–21 July 1923, and described the standardization as having been agreed upon there.[59] Apart from that, it referred to the report of the Canadian Insulin Committee, which had been published in the Journal of the American Medical Association in July, and mentioned the translation of McLeod's presentation, published in the German medical journal *Therapie der Gegenwart* in August.[60] In general, the statement echoed the views of the first publications by German physicians and in popular journals,[61] which warned readers not to expect too much from insulin.[62] Although the employees of the Imperial Health Office clearly recognized the hazards of insulin, especially the danger of severe and possibly life-threatening hypoglycaemia,[63] they were quite sure that the misuse of insulin would be prevented simply by the fact that it had not yet been produced in Germany[64] and furthermore that imported insulin was extremely expensive. The fact that insulin was only used in hospitals, where patients were under the constant scrutiny of doctors, also reassured officials that its risks were limited.[65] In other words, they recognized the risks, but at this point they left the developments to market forces, which they believed would limit any dangerous effects. This laissez-faire attitude shifted only after rapid improvements in the production process, which made larger amounts of insulin available on the market and helped to lower the prices.

Although the Imperial Health Office was hardly interested in the insulin question, the committee obviously felt obliged to deliver reports on its activities and at least on one of its (rare) meetings. The files of the Imperial Health Office contain one single report on a meeting of the German Insulin Committee. In May 1924 president Minkowski reported to the Imperial Health Office on the activities of the Insulin Committee. His report devoted considerable space to the use of the trademark 'Insulin' by a German factory owner. Overall, the report clearly shows that the committee viewed the sera as a model case for the standardization and licensing of insulin.[66] Aside from its request to have insulin made a prescription drug, the committee demanded that apothecaries' profit margin be reduced, as in the case of Salvarsan and other sera. The last sentence of his long report alludes specifically to future policies of insulin surveillance, suggesting that 'steps be taken as soon as possible to organize the state's oversight in a manner similar to that governing other sera'.[67]

The committee clearly expected more from this state institution, and when the first application for an insulin patent failed, it expected that an *arbitrium* from the Imperial Health Office would make a successful second motion.[68] Fuld and the German Committee's patent attorney, Armand Mestern, were sure to get such a document on insulin's quality,[69] after they had made contacts with the office's key employee, Eugen Rost. But as Fuld reported to Toronto on 7 January 1925, the Imperial Health Office changed their mind. They declared that they were unable to give their *arbitrium* in a cast of contestation according to one part's wish. They were willing to answer a query of the Imperial Patent Office, but 'declared themselves opposite in general to any trademark'.[70] According to Fuld, this did not result from Rost's opposition. In fact, Rost supported the Insulin Committee's approach; at his suggestion a declaration signed by prominent colleagues was handed in. But since his standpoint was opposed by the president and the attorney of the Imperial Health Office, it failed.

The last and final attempt to install some kind of state-authorized insulin regulation and control was made in November 1925. In order to obtain some of the standard preparation of insulin, Hoechst had written to the British Medical Research Council, which kept these samples. The council, though, refused to send any, and argued that it would hand in 'the preparation only to a national testing institution or similar organization, which would on its part provide for the manufacture of a national standard preparation and the distribution thereof to the various firms'.[71] It is unclear whether this meeting was provoked by a concerted action of the Toronto Committee, Fuld and Hoechst, but it seems likely, since Fuld strongly advocated a double check of insulin. The National Health Office should keep a small quantity of the insulin standard and was responsible for testing the insulin preparation with respect to its pharmacological quality, while the Insulin Committee was in charge of distributing samples of the standards to the producers and was also responsible for clinical tests by the committee members. This double testing should be noted on the label.[72] Although he might once have agreed with the Canadian Insulin Committee on this position, Fuld was opposed by the other members of the German Insulin Committee. Minkowski frankly declared that he 'considered an international standard preparation for pharmacological assay superfluous' because the insulin unit was – unlike the diphtheria serum – fixed absolutely and defined so exactly, that the strength of the preparation could be easily determined. Fritz Umber considered the standard preparation superfluous for clinical testing, which was done against diet and sugar excretion on an individual basis. In his eyes, the development was not yet completed and so he feared that 'a state assay might have a rather arresting effect on account of the relatively strict conditions'.

As might be expected, industry looked at this problem from the perspective of cost. So did Eichholtz from E. Merck, while Weyl, who represented the company C. A. F. Kahlbaum from Berlin, and Linder, as a representative of Hoechst and Bayer alike, shared Minkowski's view. But they underlined 'that the use of the Toronto Standard preparation for testing and a corresponding reference were certainly important for advertising and especially for export'.[73] As Fuld reported in frustration to Toronto,

> everything would stay as it is: no central instance for animal experiments, no ingerence of the *Reichsgesundheitsamt*, the manufacturers would continue to do experimental work on rabbits (or would perhaps not) and the insulin committee would examine the single preparation on patients.[74]

In fact, it took until 1928 for the Imperial Health Office finally to acknowledge some need for action and add insulin to the list of organic extracts generally classed as strongly acting drugs.[75] From 30 April 1928 onwards, patients therefore needed a doctor's prescription to obtain insulin from pharmacies.

This hardly bothered the pharmaceutical companies. Although they may have been somewhat slow off the mark, after the German Insulin Committee had been established in July 1923, German firms did their utmost to quickly produce and market sufficient quantities of their own high-quality insulin. Bayer was able to send out its first insulin samples to the members of the committee in July of 1923. But the fact that the first reports on clinical trials appeared in the medical press in mid-July 1923 makes it highly probable that the initial trials were conducted using imported insulin.[76] These imported products were extremely expensive, as were the first German products. Firms like Bayer would thus not provide complimentary samples to doctors, but instead sold the insulin to them directly and insisted on immediate payment.[77] For many patients it was almost impossible to afford the recommended dosage. Firms continued to complain about poor profits and low profit margins.

In spite of its high price, however, insulin still held out the prospect of high profit margins and thus drove firms to expand sales, establish their priority and corner their share of German markets by all possible means. Bayer, for example, was unable to obtain enough pancreases of acceptable quality to decisively expand production. Therefore the company decided to buy insulin from Organon's overproduction, which they then simply checked, cleaned and – if necessary – titrated, before bottling and packing it.[78] This shows that at least some firms were able to install a production system quickly and indeed so successfully, that they had ample insulin and could sell it in bulk.

Bayer began marketing their products in October of 1923. The firm's pharmaceutical salesmen were informed on 4 and 5 October, and were instructed to keep in close personal contact with the members of the Insulin Committee. On the very same day, Hoechst began sending out its first batches to regional offices and to some clinicians not on the Insulin Committee.[79] The clinicians were eager to receive samples and to begin trials and treatments. The firm anticipated that doctors would expect to receive free samples before regular sales began, but at this point insulin was simply too expensive to distribute free of charge. In order not to disappoint the doctors, the firm proceeded very cautiously.[80] On 17 November, Bayer informed Minkowski about the different package sizes and prices, assuring him that the prices had been set as low as possible.[81] The company emphasized that it would do its utmost to expand production as soon as possible. To encourage the use of insulin, Minkowski accepted these claims and officially allowed Hoechst to describe its product as 'checked by the German Insulin Committee'.[82] Such labelling was not necessary in order to market insulin, but it was necessary to sell the product under the protected trade mark 'Insulin'. As such, the Insulin Committee served as a professional board, which supervised and thus assured the standard quality of all preparations that were marketed under this name, thus protecting patients from both ineffective drugs and exploitative sales practices.[83]

Such protection had been a major goal of Banting and Best, who wanted to improve and speed up the circulation of the knowledge of insulin between industry, researchers and physicians. This in turn would help to reduce the price of insulin. In order to do so, the Canadians wanted to protect their patent rights, allowing them to control the licensing of production. They expected the German Insulin Committee to respect the patents held by the Connaught Laboratories in Toronto, which had acquired the rights from the inventors on the condition that they would be granted free of charge to other companies.[84] The committee was supposed to obtain a German patent for the Connaught Laboratory. This was the job of Insulin Committee member, Heinz Fuld.

On behalf of the Connaught Laboratories, Fuld therefore applied for a patent at the Imperial Patent Office.[85] But the Patent Office refused to issue the patent, echoing arguments put forward today in discussions about patenting certain biological products, species or genes.[86] In the eyes of the patent office, *insulin* was the scientific name for the active principle of the pancreatic gland, which was no invention, but had simply evolved into a free brand name. According to German law, it was not possible to register such products as brands on the Brand Name Role (*Warenzeichenrolle*). Thus, at first *insulin* was only enrolled as a free trade sign (*Freizeichen*), which was less well protected. The committee made a second, successful attempt to acquire a patent, pointing to the unique method of extraction, which was finally acknowledged as an intellectual property right. The Patent Office now accepted the argument that, as a biological substance, insulin was indeed produced by the pancreas, but as a marketable substance it was a product of the applicant, Connaught Laboratories.

Yet a lawsuit was brought against the approval of the patent, the suitor arguing that insulin was indeed produced in at least thirteen different ways, so that the Canadian method was not unique at all.[87] He claimed that it was not Connaught Laboratories, but the two Canadian scientists, Best and Banting, who were to be regarded as the real inventors of the production.[88] Moreover, he claimed that Banting and Best had called their product 'Iletin', not 'Insulin'. In fact, J. de Meyer had already coined the name *insulin* in 1909.[89] Nevertheless, the lawsuit was unsuccessful. In 1932 the Patent Office reiterated its decision to approve *insulin* as a brand name. It argued that the owner of the brand had been the first to launch a marketable product. Moreover, the professional literature had always acknowledged the scientific priority of the Connaught Laboratories and seen their product as the accepted standard. Consequently, insulin was judged to be a special case, in so far as the scientific name used to describe a substance had now become a brand name used by the patent applicants. Similar preparations were not forbidden, but they were marketed under names like 'seaxulin', 'cholosulin' and 'paninsulin'.[90] The only difference was that they had not received the certification 'tested by the Insulin Committee'. As a consequence, they lacked an important seal of quality and were therefore hampered in the marketing of their product.

All these activities were ultimately designed to reduce the price of insulin by mass-producing it, and indeed price was a major point of contention. The German problems with insulin production were not so much rooted in the inability of German researchers or pharmaceutical firms quickly to develop safe and stable production procedures, as historians have maintained time and again. Instead, it was more a problem of producing insulin at a low cost and selling it at a low price.[91] In the spirit of the Toronto Committee, and very much contradicting established practice in the German pharmaceutical industry, information about the preparation process was freely distributed. This prevented the development of a knowledge monopoly, which in turn would have allowed companies to dictate prices. In fact, the prices of insulin were very high in 1923 and remained so throughout 1924. The first batches of 'Insulin Bayer' were marketed for the incredible sum of seventeen Goldmark for 100 units.[92] But already in November 1923 a Bayer representative remarked that the competition from so many firms lowered prices, so that insulin 'obviously becomes even less profitable'.[93]

In principle, this result corresponded with the Canadian policy and the intentions of the German Insulin Committee, but even the German firms believed it was important to reduce the price. This was not based on the humanitarian grounds envisioned by the Insulin Committee, but rather on their recognition that high prices would clearly reduce their sales figures. As early as October 1923, Bayer therefore discussed the possibility of cutting prices by circumventing pharmacies and wholesalers, and selling directly to hospitals. They did so mainly out of concern that the price of imported *American* and *English Insulin* would undercut *German Insulin*.[94] At this point, the cost of insulin treatment was not yet covered by national health insurance, making individual consumer choice key to marketing strategy. It seems that Bayer attempted to work through regional governmental boards, leading to the District President approaching the Prussian Welfare Ministry to secure approval for Bayer's strategy.[95] But these efforts were blocked by the state boards, which cited the dire economic situation of German pharmacists, who would lose an important source of income, and did not allow Bayer to sell directly to hospitals and clinics.[96]

Insulin in Germany after 1923: Shifting from the Standardization of Drugs to the Rationalization of Treatment

It soon became clear that the standard was in fact not as uniform as one might have expected. Given the elaborate techniques of standardization and their international communication, one might have expected the insulin standard to be uniform. But this turned out not to be the case. The first reports had stated that Hoechst had a preparation at hand in spring 1923, which was produced by a process similar to the Canadian one, but was very effective and seemed to give better treatment results.[97] Clinical experience showed that American and Canadian insulin was much stronger than German insulin. This fed suspicion that German insulin was of inferior quality, the reasons for which puzzled German firms. It is possible that this was due at least in part to the general effect that products of companies that first move into new markets are often trusted more with regard to the quality than products of the latecomers, which may be regarded as mere *imitators*.[98] Nevertheless, experienced, ethical companies like Schering, Bayer and Hoechst struggled to ensure the quality of their products, even though they had been given the original preparation rules by the Canadian Insulin Committee. Time and again, German clinicians observed 'that the Americans can do with much smaller doses'.[99] The German Insulin Committee carefully examined all available products and finally, at the end of 1923, had to admit that all German products were indeed less strong than American ones. As late as 1925, such renowned diabetes specialists as Georg Klemperer saw the need to write articles on the question: 'Is German insulin full-fledged?'[100] Such publications were a major blow to German insulin's image and trustworthiness, which formed the basis of the business.

The reactions towards these findings differed, but in general nourished suspicions of unfair competition. One member of the committee, Ludolf von Krehl, went so far as to insinuate that 'the Americans make their insulin stronger in order to keep down German production and to seize the whole business for themselves'.[101] It seems more likely, however, that German firms used the smaller units introduced at the conference in Edinburgh, whereas the American firms stuck to the older, far stronger standard. A member of the committee found this stronger effect even in English insulin. Finally it turned out that Canadian as well as American firms (including Eli Lilly) had indeed increased the concentration of the insulin by 40 per cent – without notification.[102]

In November 1928, Schering's scientists turned to Minkowski in despair. They admitted that the difference in efficacy was largely a problem of durability, since the quality of the Schering insulin degraded when kept in storage. But although the scientists had tried hard, following and improving the production instructions, they had not managed to produce a solution as durable as the American one.[103] They turned to the Canadian Insulin Committee in order to have their insulin judged in Canada, but received no reply; even though Minkowski forwarded their letter to the secretary of the Canadian Insulin Committee, the files contain no response.

In other words, establishing a standard for the product as such was one problem, while the stabilization and maintenance of quality was another. The standard itself, as set by Banting and Best, also began to present new challenges. It was based on the evaluation in living animals, which differed more than had first been assumed. Over time, it appeared that the animals' feed could influence the test results, that white rabbits gave unreliable results and that animals (as well as humans) showed inexplicable variations in their reactions to insulin. As a consequence, researchers drove the standardization of both the rabbits and the tests even further. The original standard rabbit unit of Banting and Best had been defined as the amount of insulin that lowered the blood sugar of a rabbit by 50 per cent during the initial one to three hours after injection.[104] The Toronto unit of 1923 then took the rabbits' weight and diet into account. It defined the insulin unit as the amount of insulin needed to lower the blood sugar to 45 mg per cent in three to four hours in rabbits that had been fasting for twenty-four hours. But on a practical level, the blood-glucose levels had not been measured in every rabbit. Instead, the cramps that normally occurred at this blood-glucose level were taken as signs that the level had been reached, even though cramps may occur at very different individual blood-glucose levels. Finally, industry grudgingly turned to regular blood sugar measurements at one-and-a-half, three and five hours after the injection.[105] In addition, numerical calculations of the units were made in order to fine-tune the doses.[106]

All in all, three international conferences were dedicated to the further standardization of insulin. The first one, in Edinburgh in 1923, has already been mentioned. A second followed in 1926, organized by the Health Organization of the League of Nations. Its participants agreed to continue working with an insulin standard product that had been produced by the International Institute for Medical Research.[107] Thereafter, every batch of insulin had to be tested against the international standard, which contained 8.4–8.8 E. per mg of insulin. In order to facilitate the calculation, one mg of the English standard was equated with eight units, or in other words: 1 international unit was equivalent to 0.125 mg of the standard product. Small amounts of these standard products were sent out to the national insulin committees, which in turn were responsible for ensuring that firms produced their own standard products by comparing them with the international one.

When in 1935 only small amounts of the standards remained, a second conference of the League of Nations was convened. It introduced a new standard which relied on the crystallization of insulin, as had been introduced in 1935.[108]

Nevertheless, there were various different opinions about the mg content of the standard unit. After long discussions with different laboratories, the views of Henry Dale (1875–1968) prevailed.[109] Shortly thereafter, however, in October 1940 the standardization of the so-called *old* insulin was abandoned entirely. The reasons for this were twofold. First of all, in recent years the committee members had found little reason to complain about the old insulin, especially since the crystallized insulin was of generally high purity. Second, after 1934, depot insulins had been gradually introduced. Because they promised to save up to 20 per cent of insulin, they became the drugs of choice in the treatment of diabetics under Nazi rule, including the compulsory treatment of *normal* patients in the national health insurance system. Patients treated with depot insulins showed different blood sugar curves and had to follow a different diet scheme, so that it was not possible to test the old insulin on them without returning to the old model and thus prolonging their stay in hospital. Health insurance providers rejected this as an undue burden on their budgets.[110]

Nine years after its foundation, the German Insulin Committee was reorganized. Several members had already left the committee: Carl von Noorden had returned to Vienna in 1930 and Oskar Minkowski had died the following year. Succeeding him as president of the committee was Friedrich Umber, who had been very active in the field of diabetes during the preceding years. His relationship to the pharmaceutical firms was different from Minkowski's, as we have already glimpsed with his unwillingness to adopt more widely the insulin he tested in his clinic. In 1932 he reintroduced the revamped Insulin Committee to the public in an article in the *Deutsche Medizinische Wochenschrift*.[111] Neither he nor the committee worked silently as it had before; nor was their relationship to industry based on gentlemen's agreements. The more the political climate changed after the National Socialists seized power in 1933, the more the committee cooperated with governmental and health care institutions.

The direct impact of Nazi rule manifested itself in the person of Umber, who became a member of the Nazi Party and who, during the war, was responsible for the rationing of food and insulin.[112] Umber in his publication did not even mention Ernst Fuld and his merits, most probably because he rejected his pacifist and international attitude.[113] A Jewish member of the committee, Hermann Strauss, was expelled and dismissed from his position as professor at the Charité in 1933. Eleven years later, Strauss died in the concentration camp Theresienstadt.[114] It's unclear why another member, Friedrich von Müller, left the ranks of the committee, but his advanced age may have played a role; he died in 1941. Another more marginal figure, who had served on the German Committee from its inception, Hermann Fuld, was not included in the new committee and went unmentioned in Umber's article.

After its reconfiguration the new committee was comprised of Max Bürger (1885–1966) from Leipzig, Gerhardt Katsch (1887–1961) from Greifswald, Erich Grafe (b. 1881) from Würzburg, Karl Gutzeit (1903–57) from Breslau, Wilhelm Stepp (1882–1963) from Munich and Wilhelm Falta (1875–1950) from Vienna. Although the structure of the Insulin Committee's work remained largely unchanged, a new standardization process was introduced. The focus of this new process had clearly shifted, although the insulin unit as such remained the same. Unlike in the US, where Elliot Joslin had established a rigid dietary system and had systematically collected treatment data from his patients, the original German Insulin Committee had shown little interest in diet. German diabetes diets differed from doctor to doctor and were based on widely varying amounts of carbohydrates, fats and proteins. The new committee set out to change this by standardizing the diet in order to get the most out of each standard unit.[115]

The new system of diabetes treatment, as developed mainly by Gerhardt Katsch, was a lifestyle system, including not only insulin and food, but also physical exercise. This change reflected the impact of a holistic body image, based on the understanding of it as a cybernetic system of regulation. As the introduction to this book set out, this model formed part of the biopolitical agenda of the National Socialists and their notion that diabetics were people of lesser value. Deemed to be only 'conditionally healthy' (*'bedingt gesund'*), they were urged to follow rational and disciplined lifestyles.[116] Only if they managed to adhere to a strict dietary and lifestyle regime would they prove their mental and physical strength, be able to reduce their insulin requirements to a minimum, and be accepted as 'conditionally healthy', but fully useful members of society. This argument was further buttressed by the German war economy, in which many drugs were rationed and production was limited to domestic sources.[117]

Conclusion: The Role of Industrial Standards in the German History of Insulin

Standards have multiple forms and origins, but industrialization certainly played a very important role in the history of standardization.[118] The German pharmaceutical industry, which was used to build monopolies and cartels in order to maximize profits and protect business from competitors, struggled mightily in developing the production of insulin under the conditions set down by the Toronto Insulin Committee. Industry was accustomed to working together with university scientists as well as with clinicians, and knew quite well how to establish and maintain contacts. Against the backdrop of the Insulin Committee's reputation and the acknowledged standing of German doctors, industry was not inclined to question the corporatist governance of the German Insulin Committee. But industry did not need simply to submit itself to the committee's rule. Instead, it drove the process forward for its own sake.

It was the stable and secure action of the new drug that engendered the trust of doctors and patients in certain brands. But this trust did not exist from the outset; it had to be created, not least because the use of insulin had to be carefully calibrated on a daily basis. In other words, insulin's *wildness*, its character as a natural substance of varying quality, had to be tamed by standardization. Moreover, chemical synthesis remained the ultimate goal, because it promised to solve the problems and complications that arose in the standardization of a highly variable biological substance. The production of trust remained a central problem of the early history of German insulin and the modern techniques used to market it. Even before the thalidomide scandal of the second half of the twentieth century, industry recognized that mistrust could and would destroy their entire business. The history of American insulin in Germany and the long-lasting mistrust in German brands illustrates this quite nicely.

There is also a second aspect that needs to be taken into consideration. Standardization is a basic element of the industrial production of goods. From a historical viewpoint, standardization was the very basis for the enormous development of industry since the nineteenth century, for the maximization of output, and for the tight control of costs once the production of insulin had begun. On the one hand, more comprehensive monitoring complicated the production process and thus increased costs. But on the other hand, it increased efficiency by reducing the need for raw materials and avoiding product degradation. Just how important this could be was demonstrated, for example, when in 1938 Schering had to recall 10 million units (the equivalent of one year's production) because they were ineffective.[119] Following procedures that secured a certain level of quality could protect firms from such disasters. Strict surveillance of the production process not only helped to make insulin treatments medically safe; it also helped to make insulin a rewarding business.

As mentioned above, some firms initially took up the production only to enhance their image and not to make a profit. Only by cutting costs was it possible, in the long run, to generate real profits. This ability to cut costs was based on growing experience with the production process and was bound to the ever greater exactness of the production rules. In the case of Schering, the description of the production process expanded from only three pages in 1924 to fifteen pages in 1946, including a description of the production process, five pages on the production line and eight pages on the standardization of insulin.[120] While developing its own rules of standardization came at a cost, it resulted in an enormous reduction in production cost. The price of insulin was reduced in the initial phase of production in 1923 and 1924, but later on it remained stable and revenues grew. Even in the early years of the war, when transportation of the pancreases was difficult, and when meat and pancreas prices rose as their quality declined, the cost of insulin from cow pancreases fell by half from thirty-four *Pfennig* per 100 units to seventeen *Pfennig* per 100 units, and the price of insulin made from calf pancreases fell from sixty to ten *Pfennig*.[121] Two articles from 1929 and 1932 best illustrate just how important the standardization really was, especially as a marketing tool. Both were published in Schering's *Medizinische Mitteilungen,* a journal that was distributed free of charge to doctors.[122] Above all, the second article from 1932 describes the standardization process in minute detail. Its layout, rich illustrations and excellent photos document the enormous importance of standardization for the company; it had become an integral and indispensable part of the firm's self-fashioning and, as such, it was an element of the marketing efforts of an industry that used standardization as a tool for the production of trust.

10 'THERE IS A FROG IN SOUTH AMERICA / WHOSE VENOM IS A CURE': POISON ALKALOIDS AND DRUG DISCOVERY1

Klaus Angerer

Whereas there are many known cases of bioactive compounds obtained from medicinal plants and used in drug discovery, substances isolated from animal sources are less frequently utilized in pharmaceutical research and rarely the subject of historiographical analysis. The present essay focuses on the trajectory of epibatidine, an alkaloid isolated from poison frog skin secretions that turned out to be a decisive contribution to research on analgesic substances binding to nicotinic receptors and, thus, 'a possible first step toward producing a long-sought drug: a powerful non-sedating, non-opioid painkiller'.[2]

In the 1970s, the National Institutes of Health (NIH) chemist and pharmacologist John Daly and his colleagues undertook several field trips to Ecuador and collected a large number of skins taken from tiny poison frogs belonging to *Epipedobates anthonyi*, a species endemic to southern Ecuador and a small part of northern Peru.[3] Back in their laboratories at the NIH, they investigated the properties of the frog skin extracts and, among many other alkaloids hitherto unknown to science, also managed to isolate a small sample of a highly toxic alkaloid that, much later, was named 'epibatidine'. Quite soon they realized the alkaloid's enormous potential for analgesic drug discovery, but only in the 1990s, after many delays, dead ends and confusing results were they finally able to determine its molecular structure and mechanism of action, thus rendering it suitable for further research and development.

Following the rather broad concept of biologics proposed in the introduction to this volume, epibatidine can certainly be considered a biologic, not just because of its biological source material, but also because it was considered to be a substance with a specific natural origin that would soon become contested amongst environmentalists. Nevertheless, after being made available as a structurally defined, patented and synthesized compound, its biological origin became – or rather, was rendered – irrelevant for many actors, particularly for researchers in drug discovery and development working with synthetic compounds derived from the originally isolated molecule. However, more than twenty years after the first Ecuadorian poison frogs were collected by Daly and his colleagues, the biological origin of epibatidine regained enormous importance because of controversies about access to biological materials and the sharing of benefits arising from those materials' utilization after the adoption of the Convention on Biological Diversity (CBD) in 1992. Thus, rather than addressing the general question of what a biologic might be, this essay analyses in which settings and by which means the biological origin of a substance is taken into account or made negligible in natural product research and drug discovery.

It should be noted that contemporary actors draw a clear distinction between 'natural products' (secondary metabolites isolated from biological materials, usually small molecules) and 'biologicals' (larger peptides or proteins isolated from organisms or cell lines or produced by biotechnological means).[4] The present essay adopts the categories proposed in the introduction to this volume and uses 'biologics' as a generic term that includes 'natural products'. This essay is based on a review of published literature (mainly in natural product and drug discovery journals) and on the results of fieldwork undertaken in Ecuador and Germany.

'The Indiana Jones of the NIH' – Collecting Frogs and Screening their Skin Extracts

John Daly had not yet focused his research on amphibian alkaloids when he joined the NIH in 1958 as a postdoc in the Laboratory of Chemistry at the National Institute of Arthritis and Metabolic Diseases (NIAMD). He became interested in frog toxins in 1963 when Bernhard Witkop, then his laboratory chief, asked him to undertake a field trip to western Colombia to collect additional skins of *Phyllobates aurotaenia*, a poisonous frog from which Witkop and his colleagues had previously isolated the highly toxic alkaloid batrachotoxin.[5] A few years later, Daly and his colleagues also published the structure and a thorough characterization of this alkaloid,[6] thus initiating an unprecedented chemical, biological and pharmacological research programme on amphibian alkaloids and a series of field trips from the 1960s and still continuing in the present day to collect amphibian specimens in Panama, Colombia, Ecuador, Peru, Venezuela, Brazil, Argentina, Madagascar, Australia and Thailand.[7] It was likely crucial to the further development of this research endeavour beyond the initial trips to Colombia that, by chance, the herpetologist Charles Myers noticed an article published in 1966 in *Medical World News* about the properties of batrachotoxin and Daly's field trip in 1963. At the time, Myers was a graduate student in Panama and would later become the curator in vertebrate zoology (herpetology) at the American Museum of Natural History in New York. Myers contacted

Daly and proposed that they collaborate on poisonous frogs from Panama in order to investigate whether the frogs' coloration was linked to their toxicity.[8]

Even though this initial hypothesis proved incorrect, it marked the beginning of an interdisciplinary collaboration between the chemist and pharmacologist Daly and the taxonomist Myers – a collaboration that ultimately extended to more than sixty species of poisonous frogs of the neotropical *Dentrobatidae* family and their skin toxins.[9] A homage to the 'frog man' John Daly published after his death in 2008 suggested that his research on amphibian alkaloids would have been unlikely 'outside the unique intramural research structure of the NIH and would have been given short shrift in a more applied environment'.[10] Daly's forty-year-long collaboration with Myers illustrates that he was able to conduct basic research not only free of any directly foreseeable application but also in a truly interdisciplinary manner alongside other pharmacologists, chemists and biologists from inside and outside the NIH. In hindsight, Daly himself maintained that 'Without Chuck Myers, this program would never have happened. He came up with a great deal of the money for the field work, planned the logistics and worked on requisite permits'.[11] Obviously, the role of chance and serendipity in the encounter between Daly and Myers turned out to be decisive in the discovery of epibatidine and to a whole research programme on amphibian toxins. But it was only the 'unique environment at NIH'[12] that seems to have been able to provide the necessary long-term funding and infrastructure to pursue such an interdisciplinary research agenda (involving chemistry, biology and pharmacology) without too much pressure to produce immediately applicable results or to justify every detail of work in progress. Presumably, Daly's approach was quite unorthodox in the 1960s because its usefulness had yet to be established. Daly readily recognized the critical role of the NIH in allowing him to proceed with his rather serendipitous approach to research:

> [the] NIH has been a blessing to me. I don't think I would have prospered in an academic world where I'd have to defend my research and lie about where it was going, because, in many cases, I didn't know where it was going to go.[13]

In the field, Daly and Myers often employed – quite literally – a trial-and-error method in order to discern which frogs to collect:

> Once in the field, the two had a simple test to decide whether to take a particular frog. 'It involved touching the frog, then sampling it on the tongue. If you got a burning sensation, then you knew this was a frog you ought to collect', says Daly.[14]

This general screening of extracts obtained from frogs based on their colour or the burning sensation caused by touching them finally led to the discovery of epibatidine. It was part of an approach to finding interesting amphibian alkaloids that involved 'searching for the always interesting unknown', as some of

Daly's colleagues aptly recalled in hindsight.[15] On other occasions, however, their collections did not rely on trial-and-error-methods, but rather on what they retrospectively described as the 'classical paradigm of targeting'. This approach relied on so-called traditional knowledge of the local population, for example on reports about the indigenous use of frog skin secretions to poison blowgun darts.[16] It was used during their early field trips to Colombia which led to the discovery of batrachotoxin alkaloids from the golden frog *Phyllobates terribilis*, the most toxic vertebrate species worldwide. Applying these strategies on their early field trips, Daly and Myers were able to obtain an enormous number of poison frog skins in several tropical countries between the 1960s and the early 1980s: seven field trips to Colombia between 1964 and 1977 yielded more than 10,000 frogs (mostly from one single site) belonging to different *Phyllobates* species; and four trips to Ecuador between 1974 and 1982 produced approximately 2,000 skins of *E. anthonyi* (likewise from a single site or nearby sites).[17] The large number of specimens gathered by Daly and his colleagues in various countries and the key role of collecting for their research clearly demonstrates that bioprospecting is not only 'an activity dedicated to exploration and discovery' but also, 'fundamentally, about the practice of collecting, that is, removing material from one location and concentrating it in another' and as such subject to changing conditions of access to biological materials.[18]

The arduous research justifying his nickname 'Frog Man'[19] and the frequent description of Daly as the 'Indiana Jones of the NIH'[20] evoke images of heroic explorers in search of unknown treasures in the most exotic regions of the planet. And those images were further reinforced by numerous accounts of 'the personal risks associated with acquiring and handling' poison frogs.[21] Skinning frogs in the field was extremely demanding and risky, so much so that one of Daly's colleagues suffered a year-long partial paralysis of one of her hands.[22] Presumably, skill needed to deal safely with poison frogs could only be achieved through many years of experience in the field; in Daly's case, this amounted to no less than forty-four years of collecting and analysing hundreds of different frog skin extracts.[23]

'Like Captain Ahab' – Precarious Substances and Contested Collecting Practices

Around 1970, Daly and his co-workers already enjoyed a degree of success with their work on amphibian alkaloids thanks to having isolated batrachotoxin from frogs obtained in Colombia and having resolved the structure of this alkaloid. After their work in Colombia, Daly and his colleagues continued their research on poison frogs in 1974 with an exploratory field trip to south-western Ecuador, where they gathered a large number of skins of *E. anthonyi*, a species they presumably selected using the trial-and-error-method mentioned above. After returning from this first trip to Ecuador, Daly routinely assessed the in vivo effects of the frog skin extracts by injecting them subcutaneously in mice and 'serendipitously stumbled upon' a totally unexpected effect which he had hitherto never observed'.[24] The mice arched their tails over their backs, an effect known as 'Straub-tail reaction' and typical of opioid alkaloids. In his notebook, Daly recorded his observations of a typical injection as follows: 'agitation, labored breathing, pronounced S-T, running convulsions, 3 min on side twitching, still pronounced S-T, rolling convulsions, arching back, extends hind feet ... cannot locomote, still rights itself readily'.[25] This phenomenon had not been seen before in any frog alkaloid and aroused enormous interest in the compound responsible for this reaction. That interest grew even more once the extract was shown to have powerful analgesic properties in hotplate tests with mice: a common way of testing pain response in animals that involves placing them on a heated surface and that is often used to assess the efficacy of analgesics. In fact, the compound proved to be 200-fold more potent than morphine in eliciting Straub-tail reactions and in hotplate assays, a feature often quoted as one of its key traits.

After further investigations had exhausted their initial supply of extracts, Daly and Myers returned to Ecuador in 1976 for more skins, hoping to detect a novel, very potent opioid structure in the frog poison. However, the frogs at one of the previous lowland collection sites had disappeared and the skin secretions of a population from nearby banana plantations contained no alkaloids. At a highland collection site, Daly and Myers were able to obtain skins from approximately 800 frogs, yielding 60 mg of a mixture of alkaloids. From this alkaloid cocktail they obtained no more than 500 µg of relatively pure so-called 'Straub-tail alkaloid'. Nevertheless, it was this very sample, collected in 1976, that was ultimately used to determine the compound's molecular structure sixteen years later.

In 1978, Daly was able to show that, surprisingly, the opioid receptor antagonist naloxone did not block the alkaloids' effects; in other words, only then did they realize what they had found: a non-opioid analgesic, much more powerful than morphine, which potentially eliminated the risk of dependency that characterizes opioid analgesics.[26] However, the exact mechanism of action could not be established at that time since the sensitivity of nuclear magnetic resonance (NMR) spectrometers did not suffice to allow structure elucidation using the available trace sample. Thus, Daly and Myers had to return again and again to Ecuador for more frog skin extracts. Yet on subsequent field trips in 1979 and 1982, they were not as lucky as before and only found frogs with insignificant amounts of alkaloids in their secretions. Worse still, frogs raised in captivity were completely alkaloid-free. Given the lack of sufficient and adequate source material, structure determination remained impossible with the available instruments.[27]

Even without knowledge of the compound's molecular structure, the investigation of the pharmacological, toxicological and biochemical properties of the sample isolated from extracts from the collection of 1976 continued. The compound appeared to be the first alkaloid that contained chlorine found among the approximately 200 amphibian alkaloids known at that time, hence the 'impurity possibility was entertained for years, mainly because of the capricious appearance of the S-T effect'.[28] Only in 1984 did Daly overcome his initial scepticism and convince himself that the alkaloid had been originally present in the frog skin and was not just an impurity or artefact of isolation.[29] This sceptical attitude, however, seems to be quite normal in natural product research, which is prone to impurities, particularly when working with small trace samples that are not synthetically available.[30] Daly's former colleagues stress that at the time, 'every cutting edge or routine MS instrument available had been tried but often ambiguous data resulted'.[31] So in the mid-1980s, the sample of Daly's research group was as interesting as it was irreplaceable, albeit ill-suited for further research until structure elucidation could be accomplished or more frog skins obtained.

To make things worse for Daly and his colleagues, further collection became much more burdensome in 1987, shortly after a last collection of specimens in Ecuador.[32] The conditions governing access to frog specimens changed dramatically with the protection of the *Dendrobatidae* family (to which *E. anthonyi* belongs) under Appendix 2 of the Convention on International Trade in Endangered Species (CITES) in 1987 (not in 1984, as Daly states).[33] CITES, an international convention between states aiming 'to ensure that international trade in specimens of wild animals and plants does not threaten their survival' had been discussed since the 1960s and was finally agreed upon in 1973 at a meeting in Washington, DC (hence, it is also known as the Washington Convention) and came into effect in 1975.[34] With currently 178 signatories, CITES ranks among those conservation organizations with the largest membership.[35]

In any case, the inclusion of the *Dendrobatidae* family in Appendix 2 of CITES in 1987 meant that, from then on, the frogs were subject to strict regulations that involved authorization and a non-detriment finding by the exporting country.[36] Although permits under CITES are obtainable and even routinely granted by exporting countries, according to Daly it had become nearly impossible 'to obtain permits to collect the requisite hundred or more specimens required for structure elucidation of minor and trace components found in dendrobatid frogs'.[37] Apparently, the problem was not access *per se*, but rather obtaining an adequate amount of specimens.

Thus, for Daly and his group, the conditions for accessing and removing biological materials in foreign, mainly tropical, countries had changed significantly in the wake of international measures designed to protect species. During the 1960s and 1970s, they had been able to collect huge numbers of frogs and to skin them in the field with few restrictions placed on their work. In most of their earlier papers, they mentioned no permits whatsoever in the acknowledgements section and expressed no complaints about the difficulty of obtaining permits. In later articles, however, they listed the collection of permits as a standard feature and frequently stressed regulatory burdens. Of course, this does not necessarily imply that there were no permits solicited for the earlier collections, but it does suggest that obtaining permits was not considered problematic.

In hindsight, Daly also lamented the restrictions imposed on access to tropical poison frogs and suggested a rather more pragmatic than political way of dealing with this obstacle, namely collecting different species or doing so in countries with less cumbersome regulatory systems:

> The research has been hindered by difficulties in obtaining permits to collect any amphibians for scientific investigation, especially in neotropical countries of Central and South America, where the alkaloid-containing dendrobatid frogs are found. For this reason, in the past decade our research has shifted to bufonid frogs of Argentina and to mantellid frogs of Madagascar.[38]

Whereas it seems that Daly's collecting practices were not politically contested or subject to major public debate, they were nonetheless affected by species conservation measures which made the collection of sufficient amounts of specimens much more cumbersome. Hence, in the mid-1980s, lacking further access to a sufficient amount of frog skins from *E. anthonyi*, and after the original poison samples had been 'partially consumed in fruitless chemical reactions' designed to explore the compound's molecular structure and properties, Daly had no other choice but to temporarily 'lock away' the alkaloid sample. He decided to wait for improved technologies instead of putting the remaining sample at risk in further chemical experiments. Accordingly, he interrupted his group's work with the trace alkaloid and 'adopted a moratorium on further bioassays, purification or chemical characterization work', out of 'fear of losing the world's last supply' of this promising but elusive alkaloid.[39]

Finally, in 1991, technological developments again changed the conditions of Daly's research programme. Thanks to an alternative method of detecting NMR signals, the sensitivity of the new 500 MHz-NMR spectrometers increased up to a hundredfold;[40] that is, it had evolved to such an extent that a return to the source of the alkaloid was rendered unnecessary. Daly and his colleagues dared to lift their self-imposed moratorium and to subject their unique sample to NMR analysis; a rather basic 1D ^{1}H-NMR analysis allowed them to reveal the molecular structure of the alkaloid, and the structure elucidation of the compound was reported in 1992.[41]

Only now did they name the compound 'epibatidine', inspired by the name of the species from which the alkaloid had been originally obtained. Earlier designations of the compound had either referred to its molecular weight as 'alkaloid 208/210' or to its effects as 'Straub-tail alkaloid'. After having waited for 'eighteen tortuous, patient years ... for the right technology'[42] the immediate possibility of structure determination represented for Daly a 'striking example of how technical advances in instrumentation have made possible what was impossible 15 years ago'.[43] In order to highlight the 'stubborn tenacity'[44] needed by Daly and his colleagues to bridge the time gap between the first isolation of the frog skin alkaloid in 1974 and the identification of its structure in 1992, Daly's endeavour has even been compared to fictional icons of perseverance and obsessive behaviour:

> John, like Captain Ahab obsessed with Moby Dick, continued to invest time, manpower and instrument dollars into solving the structure of the elusive m/z 208/210 substance whose presence in *P. anthonyi* (*D. tricolor*) skins was erratic and whose amounts were frustratingly variable.[45]

The degree of tenacity and patience that was necessary for determining the structure of epibatidine, however, is not entirely unusual for biologics, which often tend to be precarious substances, as stressed in the introduction to this volume.[46] Epibatidine was precarious in various senses, not just in terms of its toxicity. On the one hand, the alkaloid was extremely rare, it exhibited erratic effects and was secreted in highly varying concentrations by frogs of restricted availability due to CITES. On the other hand, the decisive factor that ultimately enabled a determination of the compound's molecular structure was that 'the partially purified extract containing minor amounts of the m/z 208/210 substance that remained, had been shown to be stable in long-term storage at -5°C'.[47]

Indeed, the history of epibatidine was 'less a linear accumulation of data but was, over the period 1974 to the early 1990s, more of an up and down journey with frequently confusing results, false premises, many detours and dead ends'.[48] Epibatidine's development was characterized by unpredictable and 'suspended transactions', a concept Parry introduces in her analysis of the trade in bio-information and biological materials.[49] In this case, the delays and breakthroughs in investigating biologics seem to have depended as much on the availability of sufficient amounts of adequate raw material as on serendipity, on the elusive traits of isolated natural products, on their stability in storage and on advances in instrumentation.

Epibatidine: Drug Lead Trajectories and Derivatives

The trajectories of drug lead compounds like epibatidine – bioactive compounds with structures that serve as starting points for further chemical modifications in drug development –tend to be anything but linear or straightforward. Instead, they unfold in complex and entangled networks, just like the trajectories of drugs once they reach the market.[50] Transactions and trajectories can be suspended not only because of delays in the time between access to biological materials and the use of isolated compounds, but also because their utilization often meanders over several years due to a variety of factors, decisions and coincidences, instead of transpiring all at once at a single and precise moment in time. Epibatidine's fate as a lead compound illustrates this point because after many years of waiting for its structure to be determined, it was hyped twice, once after the publication of its structure and again after news broke about a derivative. And yet, it remains difficult to assess its impact nowadays, since there is no derivative on the market.

The publication of epibatidine's molecular structure in 1992 had an almost immediate impact, with more than 300 papers and an entire issue of *Medicinal Chemistry Research* having been published about it by 2003.[51] Public interest in epibatidine further increased after it was popularized in a report in *Science* as nothing less than 'a possible first step toward producing a long-sought drug: a powerful non-sedating, non-opioid painkiller'.[52] Soon afterwards, following 'a furious race to synthesize the chemical',[53] several syntheses of the alkaloid were reported and its mechanism of action was determined – the analgetic activity is blocked by mecamylamine, a nicotinic antagonist.[54] Furthermore, epibatidine could be purchased in standardized quality as early as 1993 or 1994 from companies that produced research chemicals, so it had become generally available, in stark contrast to its extreme scarcity up until 1992.[55] Notwithstanding the considerable impact of the publications on epibatidine, it seems never to have been in development as an analgesic because it possesses a poor therapeutic window, that is to say, its analgesic effects 'are accompanied by adverse effects (for example, hypertension, neuromuscular paralysis, and seizures) at or near the doses required for antinociceptive efficacy'.[56] Hence, epibatidine's influence in drug discovery derived mainly from its impact on the development of synthetic derivatives and as a research tool.

By the early 1990s, Abbott Laboratories had already conducted several years of research on nicotinic cholinergic receptor (nAChR) agonists – the substance class that epibatidine also belongs to – as drug leads for cognitive disorders like Alzheimer's. This drug discovery programme was a rather risky endeavour and was viewed with considerable scepticism within the company, with one member of the scientific advisory board even wondering: '[I]f it's so good, why isn't Merck working on it?'[57] The programme led to one clinical candidate, but apparently Abbott made real progress in this area only once they heard about epibatidine. Due to their previous research on nAChR agonists, presumably they were more than ready to realize the alkaloid's potential and to work on related substances. One of Abbott's scientists, who was interviewed for a press release on an epibatidine derivative, recognized this 'head start' for his group as follows: 'Chance favors the prepared mind ... We had a slew of compounds that we knew interacted (with the nicotine receptors). We then looked through them for some that had analgesic potential'.[58]

Actually, it was not even someone from the group working on nAChR ligands but rather a chemist from Abbott's inflammation research programme who incidentally noted the report on epibatidine in *Science* and 'immediately recognized that NCEs [new chemical entities] with similar structural motifs were being made at Abbott as part of its exploratory effort in nAChR-based analgesics'.[59] Michael Williams, a chemist from the nAChR group,

> then immediately contacted Daly to see whether the MoA [mechanism of action] of epibatidine was known. John [Daly], in his usual gracious manner, indicated that a paper was in press on this topic and after being asked whether it was nicotinic receptor-mediated, agreed.[60]

Since the mechanism of action of epibatidine was published the following year anyway and its structure had already been disclosed, arguably Daly's sharing of information prior to publication did not reveal any details completely beyond the reach of Abbott's scientists. Nevertheless, it probably helped the company speed up the development of derivatives. Furthermore, it might have been instrumental in reassuring Abbott that further research on nAChR-based analgesics was worth the effort since, until 'the discovery of epibatidine, it appeared that there existed an affinity barrier or ceiling beyond which it was almost impossible to venture'.[61]

In the following years, Abbott used the knowledge of the mechanism of action in an undisclosed way to design a library of more than 500 optimized compounds. The screening of this library finally led to the identification of ABT-594, a compound as potent as epibatidine but lacking its severe side effects.[62] The article on this new drug lead 'was published in *Science* in the first week of January 1998, a "quiet news week" because of the New Year holiday season that resulted in full media coverage, print, radio and cable TV'.[63] In the midst of this considerable hype, TV crews even wanted to shoot videos of the frogs at Abbott and were disappointed to learn that the company did not have a frog colony and no one there had ever seen the frogs except in photographs.[64] The hope for a frog-derived magic bullet against pain was even hailed in a song by Paul Simon:

> Nothing but good news
> There is a frog in South America
> Whose venom is a cure
> For all the suffering
> That mankind must endure
> More powerful than morphine
> And soothing as the rain
> A frog in South America
> Has the antidote for pain
> That's the way it's always been
> And that's the way I like it.[65]

Notwithstanding the hype around the drug lead derived from frog poison, Abbott had never developed epibatidine as a drug candidate. Rather, the company explored its pharmacological profile in vitro and in vivo and published a thorough characterization of the compound.[66] Thus, the knowledge of the properties, structure and mechanism of action of the alkaloid served as an inspiration for the design of compound libraries. It seems that the precise relation between epibatidine and its derivatives is as difficult to assess as that between the research undertaken by Daly's group at the NIH and the screening and development at Abbott. The initial contact with Daly and his sharing of information was rather informal, with no agreements mentioned in published sources and no disclosed transfer of materials. While there was no collaboration taking place and Abbott's research was not directly based on Daly's previous work, in hindsight scientists involved in the development of ABT-594 readily admit that 'Abbott researchers along with others in both academia and industry benefited significantly from the basic research efforts funded by the NIH'.[67]

But if Abbott never worked on the development of epibatidine as a drug candidate, can ABT-594 and other related compounds still be considered derivatives of a biologic substance? In their article on ABT-594 in *Science*, Bannon et al. compare the efficacy and side-effect profile of the compound to nicotine, morphine and epibatidine, so some connection to the frog alkaloid exists. But it's hard to say whether this reference implies that it had been instrumental in library design or rather employed as a rhetorical device for the sake of enhanced credibility. Furthermore, in this case the exact degree of derivation is particularly hard to measure, since the alkaloid turned out to be a surprisingly adaptable molecule with a striking 'amount of structural change that is tolerated by epibatidine without loss of affinity': some derivatives are quite similar to the parent compound while others are only remotely related.[68] However, this chemical adaptability, while being a key feature of the usefulness of any lead compound in drug discovery, exemplifies that 'derivative' is a very loosely defined category that encompasses many different modes of designing substances. Compounds can be imitated, copied, 'turned around' to produce a differently 'handed' enantiomer, and certain molecular fragments can be added or removed (usually as a first, rather routine step in creating a library of derived compounds). And all of this might be accomplished via total synthesis from scratch or by semi-synthesis with some initial biological material.[69]

Epibatidine apparently served Abbott mainly as a source of inspiration in library design and reassured the company that targeted research on nAChR ligands was worthwhile, particularly in the area of analgesics. But what, if anything, might we consider to be the core of epibatidine as a substance isolated from frog poison and its derivatives? Some pattern in a structural formula of a natural product that chemists might recognize as a so-called 'core-structure'?

After all, it remains an open question whether the frog skin extract can, in any meaningful sense, be seen as the source of epibatidine derivatives like ABT-594 and, if so, how these derivatives are related to their rather remote biological origin.

'The Invasion of the Frog-Snatchers' – Contested Biologics, Serendipity and Derivatives

While the biological source of the alkaloid – as well as most details about the frogs – had been rendered rather irrelevant for most pharmaceutical researchers, the hype around ABT-594 also led to new kinds of claims that tried firmly to reattach epibatidine and its derivatives to their material or inspirational source in living beings from concrete geographical locations. This occurred against the backdrop of controversies over access to biological materials and the sharing of benefits derived from their utilization between the providers and the users of specimens following the adoption of the CBD in 1992.

The CBD had been discussed and prepared in several working groups within the United Nations Environment Programme (UNEP) since the late 1980s before it was opened for signature in 1992 at the United Nations Conference on Environment and Development in Rio de Janeiro, the so-called 'Earth Summit'.[70] Currently it has 193 signatories, that is, all UN member states except Andorra, the Vatican, South Sudan and, more significantly, the US. The convention's text was a rather vague compromise that ensued from long-standing north–south conflicts over the control of natural resources, particularly the so-called 'seed wars' of the 1980s, which centred on the question of whether germplasm should continue to be treated as a common heritage of mankind – with more or less free access to biological specimens abroad – or instead reconfigured as the sovereign property of nation states.[71] Frequently, concerns were voiced that

> Third World nations have little to gain from the quixotic pursuit of common heritage in plant genetic resources. But they have a great deal to gain through international acceptance of the principle that plant genetic resources constitute a form of national property. Establishment of this principle would provide the basis for an international framework through which Third World nations would be compensated for the appropriation and use of their plant genetic information.[72]

Finally, the CBD formally stated the sovereign right of member states to determine the conditions under which access to their so-called genetic resources is granted and called for the sharing of the benefits arising from their utilization under mutually agreed terms; in a kind of bargain, it 'also *requires* that these resources be made available to outside parties (that is, that access not be "unreasonably" restricted)'.[73] Although the CBD is only 'soft law', i.e. a mere framework agreement that has to be implemented in national law in order to be enforceable, it contributed to the designation of 'resources once (not unproblematically) characterized as part of the *international* commons – such as wild plants, microbes, and cultural knowledge – as *national* sovereignty' and thus widely affected the conditions under which biological materials were collected abroad.[74] Thus, whereas so far CITES had imposed restrictions only on the trade in certain endangered species, the CBD aimed at facilitating the conservation of biodiversity at large through the sustainable use of any species in a move sometimes called 'green developmentalism', and was either hailed or criticized as a way of 'selling nature to save it'.[75] The CBD proclaimed a positive correlation between the sustainable use of biodiversity, its conservation and the equitable sharing of the ensuing benefits, thus also reinforcing the relationship between the so-called 'genetic resources' and the benefits generated, for example, through bioprospecting.

At the same time, the discussions which flourished in the context of the CBD provided new ways of contesting the legitimacy of the use of biological materials collected abroad, often in tropical countries. That legitimacy could no longer be questioned – chiefly by scientists concerned about conservation, taxonomy and natural products – if the protection of a certain species, for example through CITES, was scientifically sound or environment-friendly. Instead, researchers and companies faced scrutiny within a political and socio-economic arena as to whether the commercial exploitation of genetic resources was equitable and in compliance with relevant legislation.

Thus, not only the legitimacy of collecting biological materials could be contested but also the perceived or actual failure to share benefits arising from the sustained use of substances somehow derived from living beings a long time ago, for example in drug discovery programmes with natural products. This quickly led to new sorts of claims being 'attached' to biological materials, as Hayden shows in her study of bioprospecting in Mexico:

> Most significant ... is the way in which the CBD has provided an institutional focal point for a new articulation of biological resources: not just as productive, but as a resource that comes with (new kinds of) potential claimants attached.[76]

McAfee also highlights the new kind of local–transnational alliances that started to articulate their claims in the political space provided by the convention:

> [T]he CBD has become a gathering ground for transnational coalitions of indigenous, peasant, and NGO opponents of 'biopiracy' and the patenting of living things, and advocates of international environmental justice. They have begun to put forward counter-discourses and alternative practices to those of green developmentalism.[77]

In the case of epibatidine, these new claimants made themselves heard once the hype around ABT-594 had been noticed in Ecuador. This soon led to fierce debates as to whether the collection of the frogs more than twenty years ago had been in compliance with the regulations for accessing biological materials in force at that time. Daly and his co-workers retrospectively insist that in the mid-1970s there was no competent regulatory agency in Ecuador and thus the collected samples were legally exported with the required US Fish and Wildlife import documentation.[78] However, other sources assume that in 1976 there was an Ecuadorian regulatory agency and an applicable law in force (*ley de protección de la fauna silvestre y de los recursos ictiológicos* of November 1970), but admit there are no archival records from the *Ministerio de la Producción*, which at the time was responsible for enforcing the law.[79] Ultimately, the delay of almost twenty years between the collection of the frog specimens and the use of substances isolated from their skin extracts in drug discovery has rendered any proof of the legitimacy or illegitimacy of the original access to the frog skins impossible, since nowadays it is not feasible to document how the collection permits were granted or rejected.

Other claims focused on Daly's alleged use of traditional knowledge about the frogs' local utilization without already having obtained the necessary informed consent to do so and without benefit-sharing agreements. Actually, it is quite frequently stated that the frogs from which epibatidine was isolated were traditionally used in dart poisoning and that – beyond mere serendipity in choosing adequate frogs – the knowledge of this usage guided Daly's endeavour in the field, even in Bradley's report on the newly described alkaloid in *Science*.[80] These claims gave rise to accusations of biopiracy, but they are probably inaccurate, since apparently there was no local use of *E. anthonyi*.[81] On other occasions, however, as stated above, Daly and Myers relied heavily on information from locals and extensively recorded their knowledge and practices, for example during field trips in the early 1970s to the Emberá indigenous people in the Colombian Chocó region which led to the isolation of batrachotoxin from *P. terribilis*.[82] And yet, this does not tell us much about the case of epibatidine – beyond the fact that Daly and Myers sometimes did use traditional knowledge – since on another field trip epibatidine was obtained from a different species in another country.

Nevertheless, in 1998 the *Instituto Ecuatoriano Forestal y de Áreas Naturales y Vida Silvestre* (INEFAN, now part of the Ecuadorian Ministry of the Environment) filed an official claim that Abbott Laboratories should share any benefits generated by its epibatidine derivatives with the Ecuadorian state. In order to support this claim, the INEFAN alleged that indigenous knowledge had been instrumental in the development of epibatidine and that any potential benefits were derived from this knowledge. Beyond the fact that the frog species *E. anthonyi* was probably not used in traditional dart poisoning, in a strictly legal sense there was not very much that Ecuador could do, since the collection of the frogs had taken place a long time before the CBD was ratified and the convention does not apply retroactively to resources obtained pre-CBD. Hence, in this case, one cannot *de jure* insist upon compliance with the framework for accessing biological materials and sharing the benefits arising from their utilization established by the CBD. Furthermore, even today there is no readily enforceable international agreement on access and benefit sharing under the CBD in force.[83] Given the lack of legal instruments to enforce the benefit sharing, it is hardly surprising that the official Ecuadorian claim failed.[84] Furthermore, 'Abbott Laboratories said that it owes nothing to Ecuador because it merely got the inspiration for its drug by reading a scientific paper about the frog chemical', presumably referring to the papers by Daly's group or the report on epibatidine in *Science*.[85]

Alongside the unsuccessful official claim, Ecuadorian NGOs started a campaign accusing Abbott and Daly of biopiracy and insisting on the purported traditional use of the frog poison and its importance for Daly's collecting activities. The campaign soon led to international media echoing allegations of an '[i]nvasion of the frog-snatchers'.[86] In some of these publications, quite colourful details were added to the accusations, for example the frequently cited claim that the frogs must have left Ecuador by diplomatic pouch because there was no proof that an export permit had been granted.[87] While almost certainly inaccurate, these accusations may well have clouded the legal issues involved, such as the lack of any retroactive enforcement of conventions like CITES or the CBD and the territorial jurisdiction of the Ecuadorian legislation. Be that as it may, the accusations are part of an 'idiom of expectation and ... accountability that has made some powerful marks on the shape of academic and industrial resource collection worldwide' against the background of the CBD.[88]

From this vantage point there seems to exist among many scientists who depend on access to biological specimens a kind of generalized sentiment that regulations governing specimen collection in the wild are too restrictive. There are plenty of sources in which scientists' concerns are voiced as expressions of a retrospective nostalgia for an age of free collecting, undisturbed by public scrutiny, media attention, NGO campaigns and regulatory burdens, 'in the days when the world was a kinder and gentler place', as one senior researcher at Merck interviewed by Parry states.[89]

Countering the charges of biopiracy raised against them, in retrospective accounts Daly and his co-workers deny explicitly the existence of any local traditions concerning the use of the poison frogs from which they isolated epibatidine.[90] Instead, they claim that their work illustrates the importance of serendipitous findings and curiosity-driven research which they contrast with hypothesis-driven ways of practising science.[91] Arguably, serendipity and chance lay at the very heart of their endeavour because they did not find a species that always secretes bioactive alkaloids; the frogs they collected happened to belong to a population of *E. anthonyi* which is able to secrete toxins accumulated from a dietary source of uncertain origin (probably an arthropod species like ants or mites), leading to highly variable alkaloid profiles in different populations belonging to the same species.[92] This means that highly contingent local ecological conditions and the possibility of long-term storage of the unique trace sample resulting from only one of their various collections of the *E. anthonyi* skins were crucial in the discovery of epibatidine. Thus, at least in the case of epibatidine, Daly and his colleagues are probably right in highlighting the role of serendipity in their research trajectory more so than the importance of traditional knowledge. But, at the same time, this recurrent and insistent retrospective emphasis on serendipity also serves to justify their collecting activities from earlier decades and to invalidate accusations of biopiracy based on their purported illegitimate use of traditional knowledge.

But there is also another lesson that can be drawn from the history of epibatidine and its contested use. Even if Daly's field work in Ecuador were to take place today and the collected resources not brought to the US – a country that has signed but never ratified the CBD and is therefore not obliged to share benefits under the CBD – a more fundamental question remains: have there been any benefits generated by epibatidine – beyond the general advancement of biological, pharmaceutical and chemical knowledge – that could be shared?

Epibatidine has helped to open up the entirely new area of research on nicotinic analgesics that had been relatively unexplored before and inspired work on a novel class of drug leads for various targets. And so its indirect impact in drug discovery and development can hardly be overestimated. However, today it is mainly used as a standardized research tool for diverse purposes and sold in bulk as a chemical compound, so the direct monetary benefits obtained from epibatidine are very low. And if there are revenues from derived compounds, how are these related to the frog alkaloid and to what degree of modification do substances still count as derivatives? While precisely identifying the derivatives of a compound like epibatidine may be almost irrelevant for many actors, including the scientists conducting research on such compounds (not to mention the difficulties it poses for historians), it might amount to a key issue in regulatory deliberations about whether the revenues generated by a certain drug must be shared with the provider of the biological source material from which its active principal has somehow been 'derived'.

In the context of the CBD, the role of derivatives and whether these are covered by the provisions for access and benefit sharing established under the convention has been one of the issues most fiercely debated. In the Nagoya Protocol, which constitutes a mandatory albeit rather vague framework for the regulation of access and benefit sharing under the CBD, a derivative is defined as 'a naturally occurring biochemical compound resulting from the genetic expression or metabolism of biological or genetic resources, even if it does not contain functional units of heredity'[93] and as such does not literally cover isolated biochemicals subject to posterior modifications. Furthermore, the derivatives defined in art. 2 (e) are not explicitly included in art. 3 which delimits the scope of the protocol. Nevertheless, as Vogel et al. highlight,

> many delegates and scholars are not disheartened. They have inferred 'derivative' in the phrase 'utilisation of such sources' [in art. 3]. Unfortunately for the advocates, such an inference is not obvious and would morph 'utilisation of such sources' into a 'panchrestron', Garrett Hardin's neologism for something that signifies everything and therefore means nothing.[94]

Regardless of these legal issues, the 'utilisation of' biological materials in research and development seems to be as difficult to circumscribe as the relation between isolated compounds and their derivatives. If anything, the controversies around the notion of derivation and the adequate scope of benefit sharing, as well as the accusations of biopiracy that attempt to reconnect the epibatidine derivatives to Ecuadorian poison frogs, clearly show that, as Gaudillière stresses, the notion of biologics 'is less a problem of natural versus artificial ontology, than of socio-technical order'.[95]

Conclusions: Contested Ways of Taking Nature out of Biologics (and Reattaching it)

The current situation of epibatidine derivatives illustrates the high failure rates even with promising lead compounds, as well as the insecure prospects and long delays that characterize drug development in general and natural product research in particular. So far, no product based on the epibatidine pharmaco-phore is known to have reached the market. Notwithstanding the hype that surrounded ABT-594 some fifteen years ago, the clinical trials of the compound as an analgesic were discontinued after phase 2 due to gastrointestinal side effects like nausea and vomiting. However, further research based on ABT-594 continues at Abbott with the aim of retaining its desired analgesic activities while reducing its side effects.[96] Some other related substances are still being investigated, among them ABT-894, a compound with an as yet undisclosed structure that, after disappointing phase 2 trial results for neuropathic pain, is currently being developed by Abbott and NeuroSearch for ADHD.[97]

Furthermore, the discovery of epibatidine has not only been a key inspiration to drug discovery in the area of nicotinic analgesics. It has also contributed to new forms of basic biological and biochemical research in the field and in the laboratory. For example, the study of alkaloids from animal sources has expanded enormously and nowadays tries to account for the original dietary sources that provide amphibians with alkaloids or their precursors, particularly ants and mite that sequester toxins. Thus, vast and complex chemical ecologies are sketched out and often visualized in tables comprising a high numbers of amphibian and arthropod species, as well as the alkaloids shared by both, in an effort known as 'combinatorial bioprospecting'.[98]

In general, the history of epibatidine shows some typical features of biologics in drug discovery and development. Since the work with substances obtained from living beings is often a risky endeavour with uncertain prospects of success, the role of publicly funded research institutions – in this case, the NIH – in collecting materials, isolating compounds and testing for bioactivity can hardly be overestimated. Today, research in this area is undertaken mainly by university organic chemistry groups, after several large pharmaceutical companies shut down their natural product departments in the 1990s.[99] One reason why many companies tend to avoid the risks involved in doing research on substances derived directly from natural resources is due to the frequently insecure supply and resupply of adequate amounts of raw or processed material, a condition that is further exacerbated by variations in the quantity and quality of compounds from different batches of material extracted from the same species. In this regard, epibatidine might represent an extreme case of severely restricted availability and highly varying alkaloid profiles, but is not totally atypical for the role of natural products in drug discovery, as Pauli et al. highlight in a recent review of natural product research:

> The majority of pure NPs [natural products] represent rare chemicals of extremely limited supply. Frequently, particularly in the case of newly reported structures, such compounds are also unique commodities and are only immediately available from a single source, namely, the original investigators, or by re-isolation.[100]

In the case of epibatidine, the supply issue could only be solved once the compound was synthesized and, after many detours and delays, transformed from an irreplaceable trace sample confined to Daly's laboratory into a synthetically available and highly adaptable chemical molecule. And yet, the synthesis of natural products isn't always possible, at least not on an economically viable scale – as in the case of Taxol. Furthermore, even synthesized biologics may still exhibit the typical traits of precarious substances. For this reason, medicinal chemists often view them as 'too "dirty", too difficult to assay or too time-consuming to be competitive with companies' chemical collections', in other words, 'as "ugly ducklings"', possessing undesirable features such as structural complexity, multiple hydroxyl moieties, ketones and chiral centers'.[101] As the history of epibatidine illustrates, even after the synthesis of natural products it tends to require a lot of effort to remove undesired properties and reduce side effects.

After all, 'taking the nature out of NP [natural products]'[102] is hard and expensive work, does not always succeed and is in no way accomplished by merely synthesizing a compound originally obtained from a biological source. Instead, it involves getting rid of certain traits while retaining the desired activities of biologics or their derivatives, as well as enhancing the compatibility with high-throughput screening and other drug-like properties for the sake of increased 'drugability'. Finally, a structurally optimized natural product derivative ought to fit in the library of a pharmaceutical company like any other chemical compound, as disentangled and decontextualized as possible from its original material or inspirational source in a living being. Thus, while natural products are touted as providing drug discovery with a degree of 'chemical diversity unmatched by any synthetic chemical collection or combinatorial chemistry approach',[103] most companies seek to render the sources of compounds irrelevant for their further work on derivatives.

Ultimately, the relevance of the biological origin of substances in the research and development of pharmaceuticals is hard to grasp, depends on the specificities of each case and changes over time. However, these changes are not necessarily unidirectional: in addition to being taken out of natural products, nature might also be reattached to compounds derived from living beings by various sorts of claims and regulatory measures. Whereas epibatidine, for example, was treated as a chemical substance with interesting bioactivity in drug discovery, the NGO campaigns accusing Daly and Abbott Laboratories of biopiracy, as well as the official claims for benefit sharing, insisted on its character as a biologic that had been isolated from the secretions of Ecuadorian poison frogs. Some of the proposed regulatory measures currently being debated among policymakers with regard to the implementation of access and benefit sharing under the CBD also aim at reinforcing the relationship of chemical compounds to their source organisms, for example via certificates of origin for biological materials or mandatory disclosure of origin when filing patents. And yet, the history of epibatidine shows that it is rather improbable that these measures – if they are implemented – will allow one to definitively trace the entangled trajectories of biologics and to fix their role in drug discovery as long as there is no clear answer to the question of what it means for a compound to be 'derived from' a biological source.

COMMENTARY: BIOLOGICS, MEDICINE AND THE THERAPEUTIC REVOLUTION: TOWARDS UNDERSTANDING THE HISTORY OF TWENTIETH-CENTURY MEDICINE[1]

Christoph Gradmann

One of the peculiarities of the historiography of twentieth-century medicine is that it has so far delivered little in the way of grand narratives on the period as a whole. While grand narratives such as the 'birth of the clinic' or the 'laboratory revolution' have done their part in furthering our understanding of earlier periods, the larger picture of twentieth-century medicine has remained somewhat fragmented.[2] There is, of course, no shortage of historical monographs, yet reflection on how such works figure in larger historical processes falls short of the level of reflection that has been achieved elsewhere. By comparison, general history has been engaged in debates about comprehensive twentieth-century narratives since the mid-1990s. The lesson to be drawn is not that historians of medicine should adopt these narratives, for example the notion of a short twentieth century (1914–90), which seems to be the dominant framework of interpretation in general history. Historians of medicine have long been aware that their histories follow different trajectories and there is no reason to assume that what holds for earlier periods should not apply to the recent past.[3] But there are a number of candidates from which grand narratives could be developed. One such candidate comes into view if we relate the essays in this volume on biologics to a historical phenomenon that is usually described as the therapeutic revolution that transpired, roughly speaking, between 1930 and 1970.[4] Its most conspicuous feature was the invention and application of several classes of potent drugs over a relatively short period: insulin, beta blockers, hormones, psychoactive drugs and antibiotics. While these medicines differed in many respects, they shared some common features and in their entirety they transformed clinical medicine, pharmacology and public health. Their efficacy gave drugs a pivotal position in clinical medicine. As standardized industrial products, they became part and parcel of the standardizations of clinical protocols and they paved the way for the widespread use of statistical evaluations. For example, the introduction of streptomycin in the therapy of tuberculosis not only replaced a formerly drawn out process of therapy with a short and rather uniform therapeutic protocol, it also facilitated the application of methods of evaluation such as the randomized controlled trial.[5]

Assessing the twentieth century in terms of the therapeutic revolution, one must be aware that that *revolution* is but a slogan for a host of interrelated processes culminating in the twentieth century, but originating at different points in time and in different disciplines such as chemistry, medicine and pharmacology: the industrialization of pharmaceutical production gained momentum in the late nineteenth century; modern antihypertensive drugs didn't emerge until the 1950s; and the fungal antibiotics developed in the 1940s were actually preceded by so-called rational case management in the treatment of infectious disease and the sulphates in the 1930s.[6] The example of anti-infective medicines can also serve to highlight traditions of a more cultural and far-reaching sort that were related to the therapeutic revolution: the anti-infective medicines of the 1930s and 1940s seemed to fulfil the promise of remedies associated with the work of Robert Koch and Louis Pasteur two generations earlier.[7] Generally, the late nineteenth century's enthusiasm for interventions targeting clearly identifiable causes remained a driving force in twentieth-century medical science. The time lag between the establishment of a causal mode of explanation and the development of an intervention based on such an explanation, as was the case in anti-infective chemotherapy, seems to be the rule rather than the exception.[8]

Rather than delving into the essays of this volume in detail, my commentary attempts to further explore the suitability of the therapeutic revolution as a grand narrative for the history of twentieth-century medicine. Studying how biologics were made and employed over time can crucially deepen our understanding of what the therapeutic revolution entailed in at least three respects. First, since many of the drugs in question were in fact processed biologic substances, studying biologics arguably provides insight into an object that cuts across those classes of drugs. Second, although the use of biologic substances in pharmacology and medicine was hardly new in itself, we face challenges in reflecting on the uses to which natural substances were put and how those uses differed in comparison with preceding or subsequent periods. Finally, we must also reflect on the dynamics that evolved between medicine, pharmacology, biology and chemistry. Unsurprisingly, a term such as biologics, although frequently used, is employed in a variety of ways to denote a multitude of different objects. Whatever the theoretical challenges lurking within this multitude, I would prefer to use the wealth of historical data contained in the contributions to this volume and in the history of the term biologics as presented in the introduction as a background and point of departure in addressing these challenges. I will try to sketch out what can be called a historical phenomenology of biologics. Studying the shifting uses of those terms helps us accomplish the historian's task of distancing us from an object of study, the twentieth century, which lies in the very recent past – a terrain that is notoriously difficult for historians.[9]

Understanding Biologics

When it comes to biologics, the term's variety of meanings reflect, as the editors have emphasized in their introduction, different trajectories in the production, regulation, application and marketing of biologic drugs. Moreover, the term was used to describe both an actor-centred and an analytical category. The analytical category predominated and those adopting an actor-centred category did so in relation either to very recent histories or to US drug regulation where the semantic field seems to have originated. Furthermore, the terms were used in reference to different substances with different properties. To grasp the potential scope of the history of biologics, we can discern five such variations. They are listed below in a loose chronological order, the intricacies of which will be discussed later. In so far as they relate to essays in the volume, I have pointed this out. Yet, the nature of the task at hand requires that I address some themes not covered in the essays.

First, biologics are things that are collected from and originate in nature. Think of plant extracts, cola and coca, hormones, sperm, organs. This seems to be a rather traditional practice of relating to biologics and it reminds us of eighteenth-century naturalists and collectors, in other words of a world of taxonomy and proto-industry. Jean-Paul Gaudillière's chapter on kola, its refinement and entry into the French pharmacopeia is a fine illustration of this. There is a longe durée that connects pre-modern and often colonial exploration and appropriation with modern bioprospecting and it is very relevant to our story.[10] Sophie Chauveau's chapter on the commodification of human tissue or Sven Bergmann's investigation of the political economy of sperm and egg donation tell us that, while such a practice may seem traditional, it is nonetheless an important trait of what biologics became in the twentieth century.

Second, biologics are things that result from industrial processing of biologic substances. Unlike our first group of biologics, we are talking about industry proper in this case. The classical example is provided in Jonathan Simon's chapter on the diphtheria antitoxin. As Simon's analysis makes clear, this way of making biologics has three interconnected origins: (1) the industrialization and standardization of biologic phenomena, such as when antitoxins or vaccines are produced from blood serum or bacterial cultures; (2) such medicines were conceived as applications of the germ theory of diseases by contemporaries and indeed also in subsequent historiography; and (3) the industrial mode of production and the strong effects of such drugs led to innovations in the regulation and standardization of biologic drugs that involved testing their efficacy.[11] The interwar years were the heyday of such medicines. If we consider substances like vaccines, plant extracts or hormone extracts, we realize that their origin in complex and sometimes even physiologically active molecules acted as another strong incentive to standardize them by testing their efficacy rather than by chemical analysis. Again, more recent examples fall into that same category: first-generation antibiotics were clearly a product of that type. Likewise, it is not limited to medicines and indeed the industrial production of food such as yoghurt seems to fall into the same family of phenomena.[12]

Third, biologics are substances that imitate variations one and two by synthesis on an industrial scale. It is Pim Huijnen's chapter on vitamin C that gives the most obvious example of this case. Note that over time many biologics move from groups 1 or 2 into 3, as in fact vitamins themselves did. Historically, synthesis was a later addition to the existing approaches of collection/refinement or industrial processing. Although in evidence earlier, industrial synthesis seems to have become the dominant framework after the Second World War. In pharmaceutical industries this entailed a shift in the strategy used to discover new active substances from collecting or bioprospecting to large-scale screening. Lea Haller's chapter on cortisone presents the history of a hormone as it evolved from early twentieth-century gland extracts to chemically defined and synthesizable medicines after the Second World War. Similarly, insulin was transformed from an organic to a synthetic substance in the 1980s – a transition that, however, lies beyond the framework of Ulrike Thom's chapter in this volume. The list of examples of such histories is surprisingly long and includes, for example, second-generation semi-synthetic antibiotics[13] or steroids that have become so central to the development of modern contraceptives.

Fourth, biologics are abstractions of life. This variant is not covered in the contributions to the volume and indeed the term biologics is usually not even employed in relation to it. It can be best explained in relation to laboratory animals. Studies of their selection, production and use convey to us the insight that a biologic is as much an abstraction from the chemical as it is from the social. The social dynamics between laboratory animals and scientists are notorious and the technologies employed in breeding varied widely across time – from selection and cross-breeding via in-line breeding, all the way to biotechnological manipulation.[14] In most of these applications, the use of animals (e.g. as experimental organisms) required certain changes to be made, whereby animals' sociality was brought in line with the ways in which researchers thought about and used them as biologics. The character of such an endeavour is inherently limited and a comparable phenomenon in relation to humans is highlighted in Ulrike Thoms's chapter: the limits that patients impose on standardization in clinical practice.

Finally, hybridization or biologics are conventions. I was inspired to think of this variant by the recent career of the term biosimilars that the editors explore in the introduction. Here the term biologics would be used to describe complex molecules that may resist chemical analysis. We can also think of the plethora of products that biotechnological industries usually derive from controlled manipulations of biologic substances such as microbes. Interestingly, it would very often be an actor-centred category employed in the late twentieth century. A good example is the way the WHO's Committee on Biological Standardization handled the distinction between biologicals and chemicals. In a paper by a WHO official, biologicals are simply substances that have to be defined through an assay of their potency because their complexity or impurity does not permit analysis. Once this can be done, they are dropped from the agenda: 'These substances cannot be assayed by simple physic-chemical means' he explains, and continues 'whenever the structure and the chemical composition of a chemical substance becomes known … the corresponding international reference materials are discontinued'.[15] In other words, the same substance would now be a chemical and we learn that such a framing cuts across the traditional biologic/synthetic distinction and is mostly conventional: protein synthesis as an experimental practice and somatic gene therapy using viruses as an example of a medical technology clearly fall into that category. It seems that the distinction between biologics and syntheticals that seemed fairly straightforward for a long time is becoming less and less applicable to objects related to recent biotechnology. At least it seems somewhat outdated when, for example, applied to an understanding of PCR-technology.[16]

Summing this up, it seems that our small historical phenomenology of biologics can help organize a history of biologics, as well as their definition and uses in modernity (from the nineteenth century onward). Two characteristic features meet here: first, the object of our curiosity, the therapeutic revolution, takes up a central position. It appears as a point of culmination of several interrelated processes that cover a much longer period. Second, this history is not one of a succession of phases, but of added layers under which previous practices remain prevalent. Their succession would be: collecting/refining – industrial processing – synthesis – abstractions of life – hybridization. Summing up this point, we can now qualify the usefulness of *biologics* as a category of historical analysis: it seems to work well as an analytical category for a process from the late eighteenth to the mid-twentieth century, but functions somewhat less impressively in describing present practices. Ironically, this coincides with its increasing use as an actor-centred category.

Conclusions

What does this tell us about the suitability of the therapeutic revolution as a narrative for the history of twentieth-century medicine and pharmacology? While confirming its centrality, it appears that, taken on its own, its focus is too narrow. Given that the essential trajectories of what surfaced in the period from 1930 to 1970 originated in the late nineteenth century, it seems attractive to argue for a longer and somewhat transposed twentieth century: historically the therapeutic revolution of the twentieth century appears as an echo or answer to the laboratory revolution of the previous century.

Putting it that way, we can draw parallels with other historical processes. Think of the history of diseases, where the period in question saw two major epidemiologic shifts that are likely to be intimately connected to our story. The first shift from infectious diseases to chronic conditions, cancers and coronary heart diseases transpired in the early decades of the twentieth century. This shift was the outcome of what is known as the demographic transition.[17] The second shift relates to post-Second World War medicine and the rise of lifestyle medicine and what is known as the pharmacopeia of risk. Clearly, this fits very nicely with that model: early examples of biologic medicines – just think of vaccines – were often related to infectious disease and developed in an historical period in which new medicines appeared to be targeting an established panorama of conditions such as common infectious disease. Later on, over the course of the twentieth century, the relationship between disease and cure became one of mutual definition. The example in this volume is of vitamin deficit disorders and other such mutual definitions – think of the example of hypertension – that have been highlighted in recent historiography.[18] Finally, the era of commodification and hybridization corresponds to an increasing interest in body design, including its normal and pathological states. Think of patents on body parts, somatic gene therapy or cell cultures.

Another aspect that becomes transparent is the centrality of industrial standardization to the history of biologics and of the therapeutic revolution. It is not the use of biologic substances as such, but rather their industrial processing, that defines our period. In that sense, the history presented here is, by and large, a post-1850 history. Industrial standardization differed from earlier practices like collecting, labelling or refining. However, these were not so much abolished as incorporated into a larger framework of technological standardization. A quick comparison between the smallpox vaccine and the diphtheria antitoxin serves to explain what changed over the course of the nineteenth century: while the first was calibrated in its application, the later was intimately connected to the technological standardization that drove the nascent pharmaceutical industries of the late nineteenth century.[19] By this interpretation, the standardization of biologics in the modern era would be a specific trait of the industrialization of natural products and processes and, in that sense, be confined to a specific period of history.

The history of biologics that I have drafted spans the era from the laboratory revolution to the therapeutic revolution. Unsurprisingly, it is intimately connected to the history of technological modernity, to which it adds a specific pharmacological and medical dimension. Biologics figure prominently in that history. Given that it entails not just industrial production, but also clinical protocols, tools of evaluation and even animal or human behaviour, it may well be paraphrased as a history of industrialization that went far beyond industries. We can assume that such a spirit characterized medicine to some degree from about 1850, but it was only after 1930 that it came to be dominant. There is some indication that such an innovative spirit has faded recently. From the 1990s, we find complaints about the declining nexus of industrial innovation and medical intervention. And the definition of what a biologic is seems to have become blurred. Yet, to come to grips with this is a task that for the time being we can leave to future historians.

NOTES

Von Schwerin, Stoff and Wahrig, 'Biologics: An Introduction'

1. W.-H. Boehncke and H. H. Radeke, 'Introduction: Definition and Classification of Biologics', in W.-H. Boehncke and H. H. Radeke (eds), *Biologics in General Medicine* (Berlin, Heidelberg: Springer, 2007), p. 1.
2. See J.-P. Gaudillière's contribution to this volume, specifically p. 62.
3. On the 'therapeutic revolution', see C. Rosenberg, 'The Therapeutic Revolution: Medicine, Meaning and Social Change in Nineteenth-Century America', *Perspectives in Biology and Medicine*, 20 (1977), pp. 485–506; L. Engelmann, 'Workshop Report: Is This the End? The Eclipse of the Therapeutic Revolution. 04.10.2012–06.10.2012, Zürich', *H-Soz-u-Kult*, 27 November 2012, at http://hsozkult.geschichte.hu-berlin.de/tagungsberichte/id=4488 [accessed 28 May 2013]; see also C. Gradmann's contribution to this volume on p. 194; for the impact of standardization, see C. Bonah, C. Masutti, A. Rasmussen and J. Simon (eds), *Harmonizing Drugs: Standards in 20th-Century Pharmaceutical History* (Paris: Editions Glyphe, 2009); for regulation, see J.-P. Gaudillière and V. Hess (eds), *Ways of Regulating: Therapeutic Agents between Plants, Shops, and Consulting Rooms*, Preprint series 363 (Berlin: Max-Planck-Institut für Wissenschaftsgeschichte, 2008).
4. Compare I. Hacking, *Representing and Intervening: Introductory Topics in the Philosophy of Natural Science* (Cambridge: Cambridge University Press, 1983).
5. On the DRUGS network sponsored by the European Science Foundation (ESF), see http://drugshistory.eu./?Activities [accessed 1 February 2013].
6. Korwek provides a thorough comparative analysis of the history of biological product definitions in human and veterinary biologics legislation. We concentrate here on the use of the terms themselves. Also, we will not delve into the important aspect of veterinary medicine. E. L. Korwek, 'What Are Biologics? A Comparative Legislative, Regulatory and Scientific Analysis', *Food and Drug Law Journal*, 62 (2007), pp. 257–304.
7. R. A. Kondratas, 'Biologics Control Act of 1902', in J. H. Young (ed.), *The Early Years of Federal Food and Drug Control* (Madison, WI: American Institute of the History of Pharmacy, 1982), pp. 8–27, on p. 17.
8. P. M. Banta, 'Federal Regulation of Biologicals Applicable to the Diseases of Man', *Food, Drug, Cosmetic Law Journal*, 13 (1958), pp. 215–21, on p. 216; Kondratas, 'Biologics Control Act', pp. 15–16; J. Parascandola, 'The Public Health Service and the Control of Biologics', *Public Health Reports*, 110 (1995), pp. 774–5; Anon., '100 Years of Biologics Regulation', *FDA Consumer*, 36:4 (2000), pp. 8–10.

9. *The Pharmacopoeia of the United States of America, Eighth Decennial Revision, by Authority of the United States Pharmacopoeial Convention held at Washington, A.D. 1900, revised by the Committee of Revision and published by the Board of Trustees, 1 September, 1905* (Philadelphia: P. Blakiston's Son & Company, 1905), p. xliii. In 1900, the National Convention for Revising the Pharmacopoeia had voted against the introduction of sera in the 8th revision of the United States Pharmacopoeia because these preparations did not seem to have much in common with others made from medicinal plants or chemical substances.

10. D. P. Carpenter, *Reputation and Power: Organizational Image and Pharmaceutical Regulation at the FDA* (Princeton, NJ: Princeton University Press, 2010), p. 137.

11. Young (ed.), *The Early Years*. In 1980, Merill and Hutt stated that the 1902 act was commonly called the Biologics Act. R. A. Merrill and P. B. Hutt, *Food and Drug Law: Cases and Materials* (New York: The Foundation Press, 1991), p. 661.

12. The original text is cited in Kondratas, 'Biologics Control Act', on p. 21. The first documented use of the expression 'Biologics Act' is in a report of the Public Health Service in 1927. Ralph C. Williams, Assistant Surgeon General, also used it in his large history of the United States Public Health Service. In 1958, the General Counsel of the Department of Health, Education and Welfare, P. M. Banta, wrote a short account of the law's denotation. Anon., 'Some Special Features of the Work of the Public Health Service', *Public Health Reports*, 42 (1927), pp. 287–324, 375, on pp. 319, 395; R. C. Williams, *The United States Public Health Service, 1798–1950* (Washington, DC: Commissioned Officers Association of the United States Public Health Service, 1951), pp. 182–3; Banta, 'Federal Regulation'.

13. Kondratas, 'Biologics Control Act', p. 8. In 1914, Congress enacted a separate Animal Virus, Serum, and Toxin Act to regulate veterinary biological products as part of the appropriations legislation for the US Department of Agriculture Bureau of Animal Industry. Merill and Hutt, *Food and Drug Law*, p. 664. On the contemporary language, see for instance W. Wyman, 'The Present Organization and Work for the Protection of Health in the United States', *Public Health Reports*, 25 (1910), pp. 1303–13, esp. p. 1308; F. Lackenbach, 'Pharmacy in its Higher Development', *Journal of Pharmaceutical Sciences*, 1 (1912), pp. 959–67, on p. 967.

14. Cited in Kondratas, 'Biologics Control Act', p. 21.

15. Korwek, 'Biologics', p. 258.

16. For an analysis of the shifting definition of this expression see Korwek, 'Biologics'.

17. Lackenbach, 'Pharmacy', p. 960.

18. L. F. Schmeckebier, *The Public Health Service: Its History, Activities and Organization* (Baltimore, MD: The Johns Hopkins University Press, 1923), pp. 26–7; V. A. Harden, *Inventing the NIH: Federal Biomedical Research Policy, 1887–1937* (Baltimore, MD: The Johns Hopkins University Press, 1986), pp. 18–21. In subsequent years, a number of regulations were promulgated in support of the 1902 Law. For details, see E. A. Timm, '75 Years Compliance with Biological Product Regulations', *Food, Drug, Cosmetic Law Journal*, 33 (1978), pp. 225–30.

19. Banta, 'Federal Regulation', pp. 217–8; Center for Biologics Evaluation and Research (US) and United States Public Health Service, *Science and the Regulation of Biological Products: From a Rich History to a Challenging Future* (Rockville: Center for Biologics Evaluation and Research, 2002), p. 1.

20. Surgeon General of the Public Health Service of the United States, *Annual Report for the Fiscal Year 1908: Operations of the United States Public Health and Marine-Hospital Service, 1908* (Washington, DC: Government Printing Office, 1909), p. 44.

21. Surgeon General of the Public Health Service of the United States, *Annual Report for the Fiscal Year 1910: Operations of the United States Public Health and Marine-Hospital Service, 1910* (Washington, DC: Government Printing Office, 1911), pp. 67, 74.

22. Lackenbach, 'Pharmacy'.

23. W. M. Bowman, 'The Sale of Biologicals', *Journal of Pharmaceutical Sciences*, 4 (1915), pp. 298–302.

24. Eli Lilly and Company, Biologic Department, *The Elements of Biologics: Recurrent Questions and Answers* (Indianapolis, IN: Eli Lilly and Company, 1917), p. 4.

25. Of these establishments, thirty-two were located in the US, one in Canada, one in England, three in France, one in Italy, two in Switzerland and one in Germany. Schmeckebier, *Public Health Service*, p. 130.

26. Anon., 'State and Insular Health Authorities, 1923', *Public Health Reports*, 38 (1923), pp. 2256–76. On the structure of the health organization, see also Wyman, 'Present Organization', p. 1308. When an official of the Rockefeller Foundation reported on the work of the League of Nations in 1926, he referred to 'vaccines and serums commonly known as "the biologicals"'. V. G. Heiser, 'The Health Work of the League of Nations', *Proceedings of the American Philosophical Society*, 65 Supplement (1926), pp. 1–9, on p. 4.

27. A. G. DuMez, 'Committee Reports', *Journal of Pharmaceutical Sciences*, 12 (1923), pp. 1132–5, on p. 1134. The US Pharmacopoeia included 'serums and other biological products' from the ninth revision onward. *The Pharmacopoeia of the United States of America, Eighth Decennial Revision, by Authority of the United States Pharmacopoeia Convention held at Washington, May 10, 1910, prepared by the Committee of Revision and published by the Board of Trustees, September 1st, 1916* (Philadelphia, PA: P. Blakiston's Son & Company, 1916), p. xxxiii.

28. Lackenbach, 'Pharmacy', p. 962.

29. For the impact of the First World War, see P. M. H. Mazumdar, 'Antitoxin and *Anatoxine*: The League of Nations and the Institut Pasteur, 1920–1939', in K. Kroker, P. M. H. Mazumdar and J. E. Keelan (eds), *Crafting Immunity: Working Histories of Clinical Immunology* (Aldershot, Burlington: Ashgate, 2008), pp. 177–97, on pp. 178–9; for strong links to European bacteriological tradition, see D. M. Morens, V. A. Harden, J. K. Houts and A. S. Fauci, *The Indispensable Forgotten Man Joseph James Kinyoun and the Founding of the National Institutes of Health* (National Institute of Allergy and Infectious Diseases, 2012), p. 21, at www.niaid.nih.gov. [accessed 1 February 2013].

30. Wyman, 'Present Organization', p. 1309. For details on the laboratory's work on biologics, see Schmeckebier, *Public Health Service*, pp. 129–33 and Harden, *Inventing*, pp. 19–30.

31. Surgeon General of the Public Health Service of the United States, *Annual Report for the Fiscal Year 1920* (Washington, DC: Government Printing Office, 1920), p. 75; Harden, *Inventing*, p. 19.

32. Schmeckebier, *Public Health Service*, p. 160.

33. Williams, *United States Public Health Service*, pp. 169–70. For a full account of this transformation, see Harden, *Inventing*, pp. 109–75. The institute was later renamed National Institutes of Health (NIH).

34. Center for Biologics, *Science and the Regulation of Biological Products*.

35. Surgeon General of the Public Health Service of the United States, *Annual Report for the Fiscal Year 1918* (Washington, DC: Government Printing Office, 1918), pp. 59, 66.

36. Parascandola, 'The Public Health Service', pp. 774–5. See also Surgeon General, *Annual Report 1920*, p. 85.

37. Surgeon General, *Annual Report 1920*, p. 75.

38. Center for Biologics, *Science and the Regulation of Biological Products*, p. 15.

39. For example, several blood fractionation products, including albumin, globulins useful for blood grouping, immune globulins, fibrin foam and thrombin (clotting agents used to control bleeding during surgery). Center for Biologics, *Science and the Regulation of Biological Products*, p. 17.

40. Korwek, 'Biologics', p. 271.

41. For a full account of this tragedy and its role in passing the FD&C Act, see Carpenter, *Reputation and Power*, pp. 73–117.

42. Merill and Hutt, *Food and Drug Law*, p. 987.

43. Ibid, cited on p. 663; L. B. Leveton, H. C. Sox and M. A. Stoto, *HIV and the Blood Supply: An Analysis of Crisis Decisionmaking* (Washington, DC: National Academy Press, 1995), p. 43.

44. E. P. Hennock, 'Vaccination Policy against Smallpox, 1835–1914: A Comparison of England with Prussia and Imperial Germany', *Social History of Medicine*, 2 (1998), pp. 49–71.

45. See the laws and regulations reproduced in M. Pistor, *Das Gesundheitswesen in Preussen nach deutschem Reichs- und preußischem Landesrecht*, vol. 2 (Berlin: Ric. Schoetz, 1989), pp. 499–560.

46. A. C. Hüntelmann, 'Diphtheria Serum and Serotherapy: Development, Production and Regulation in *fin de siècle* Germany', *Dynamis*, 27 (2007), pp. 107–33, on pp. 123–5; C. Gradmann, *Krankheit im Labor: Robert Koch und die medizinische Bakteriologie* (Göttingen: Wallstein, 2005), pp. 105–70. For a history of sera in relation to valuation and standardization, see C. Gradmann and J. Simon (eds), *Evaluating and Standardizing Therapeutic Agents, 1890–1950* (Basingstoke: Palgrave Macmillan, 2010).

47. J. Simon, 'French Serum Regulation in 1895: The Necessary Minimum or the Maximum Possible?', in Gaudillière and Hess (eds), *Ways of Regulating*, pp. 95–104, on pp. 98–100, 103 and V. Hess, 'The Administrative Stabilization of Vaccines: Regulating the Diphtheria Antitoxin in France and Germany, 1894–1900', *Science in Context*, 21 (2008), pp. 201–27.

48. N. Pemberton and M. Worboys, *Mad Dogs and Englishmen: Rabies in Britain, 1830–2000* (Basingstoke: Palgrave Macmillan, 2006), pp. 102–32; Hennock, *Vaccination Policy*, pp. 54–6; B. Latour, *The Pasteurization of France* (Harvard, MA: Harvard University Press, 1988), pp. 106, 116.

49. Simon, 'French Serum Regulation in 1895', pp. 98–100, 103 and Hess, 'The Administrative Stabilization of Vaccines'.

50. G. Canguilhem, *A Vital Rationalist: Selected Writings* (New York: Zone Books, 1994), p. 146.

51. Hüntelmann, 'Diphtheria Serum', p. 110.

52. Compare L. Haller, *Cortison. Geschichte eines Hormons, 1900–1955* (Zürich: Chronos, 2012), pp. 41–6.

53. W.-D. Müller-Jahncke, C. Friedrich and U. Meyer, *Arzneimittelgeschichte*, 2nd edn (Stuttgart: Wissenschaftliche Verlagsgesellschaft, 2005), pp. 35–44.

54. E. Hickel, *Die Arzneimittel in der Geschichte. Trost und Täuschung – Heil und Handelsware* (Nordhausen: Bautz, 2008), p. 439.

55. H. Boehnke-Reich, *Die Arzneistoffe aus dem Thier- und Pflanzenreich in systematischer, pharmakognostischer und chemischer Beziehung zusammengestellt* (Göttingen: Vandenhoeck & Ruprecht, 1864).

56. Hickel, *Die Arzneimittel*, pp. 356–7.

57. Ibid., pp. 352, 438. The word 'protein' was first used in 1839 by Johannes Mulder, following the suggestion of J. J. Berzelius.

58. J.-P. Gaudillière, 'The Pharmaceutical Industry in the Biotech Century: Toward a History of Science, Technology and Business?', *Studies in History and Philosophy of Biological and Biomedical Sciences*, 32 (2001), pp. 191–201, on pp. 194–6.

59. Ibid., pp. 192–3.

60. M. Foucault, *The Order of Things: An Archaeology of the Human Sciences* (London: Tavistock, 1970), p. 265.

61. K. T. Kanz, '" ... die Biologie als die Krone oder der höchste Strebepunct aller Wissenschaften." Zur Rezeption des Biologiebegriffs in der romantischen Naturforschung (Lorenz Oken, Ernst Bartels, Carl Gustav Carus)', *NTM Zeitschrift für Geschichte der Wissenschaften, Technik und Medizin*, 14 (2006), pp. 77–92.

62. T. Lemke, *Biopolitics: An Advanced Introduction* (New York: New York University Press, 2011), pp. 9–21.

63. U. Heyll, *Wasser, Fasten, Luft und Licht: Die Geschichte der Naturheilkunde in Deutschland* (Frankfurt/Main: Campus, 2006), pp. 201–28 and M. H. Kater, 'Die Medizin im nationalsozialistischen Deutschland und Erwin Liek', *Geschichte und Gesellschaft*, 16 (1990), pp. 440–63.

64. W. T. Reich, 'The Care-Based Ethic of Nazi Medicine and the Moral Importance of What We Care About', *American Journal of Bioethics*, 1 (2001), pp. 64–74, on p. 65.

65. H. Meng, *Das ärztliche Volksbuc. Gemeinverständliche Darstellung der Gesundheitspflege und Heilkunde*, 3 vols (Stuttgart: Hippokrates, 1924–1930); G. Madaus, *Lehrbuch der biologischen Heilmittel*, 3 vols (Leipzig: Thieme, 1938), p. 8; Heyll, *Wasser*, pp. 201–28; C. Timmermann, 'Rationalizing Folk Medicine in Interwar Germany: Faith, Business, and Science at Dr. Madaus & Co', *Social History of Medicine*, 14 (2001), pp. 459–82.

66. J.-P. Gaudillière, 'Professional and Industrial Drug Regulation in France and Germany: The Trajectories of Plant and Gland Extracts before 1945', in Gaudillière and Hess (eds), *Ways of Regulating*, pp. 37–64.

67. C. Sengoopta, *The Most Secret Quintessence of Life: Sex, Glands, and Hormones, 1850–1950* (Chicago, IL, and London: University of Chicago Press, 2006); V. C. Medvei, *The History of Clinical Endocrinology: A Comprehensive Account of Endocrinology from Earliest Times to the Present Day* (Casterton Hall: Taylor & Francis, 1993), pp. 159–94; H. H. Simmer, 'Organotherapie mit Ovarialpräparaten in der Mitte der neunziger Jahre des 19. Jahrhunderts – Medizinische und pharmazeutische Probleme', in E. Hickel and G. Schröder (eds), *Neue Beiträge zur Arzneimittelgeschichte – Festschrift für Wolfgang Schneider zum 70. Geburtstag* (Stuttgart: WVG, 1991), pp. 229–65; M. Borell, 'Organotherapy, British Physiology and the Discovery of Internal Secretions', *Journal of the History of Biology*, 9 (1976), pp. 235–68.

68. E. H. Starling, 'The Croonian Lectures on the Chemical Correlations of the Body', *Lancet*, 166:4278 (1905), pp. 339–41, on p. 340.

69. D. Hawhee, *Moving Bodies: Kenneth Burke at the Edges of Language* (Columbia, SC: University of South Carolina Press, 2009), p. 80.

70. R. Smith, 'The Emergence of Vitamins as Bio-Political Objects during World War I', *Studies in History and Philosophy of Biological and Biomedical Sciences*, 40:3 (2009), pp. 179–89; H. Kamminga, 'Vitamins and the Dynamics of Molecularization: Biochemistry, Policy and Industry in Britain, 1914–1939', in S. Chadarevian and H. Kamminga (eds), *Molecularizing Biology and Medicine: New Practices and Alliances 1910s–1970s* (Amsterdam: Taylor & Francis, 1998), pp. 83–105.

71. Haller, *Cortison*; P. Huijnen, *De belofte van vitamins. Voedingsonderzoek tussen universiteit, industrie en overhead, 1918–1945* (Hilversum: Uitgeverij Verloren, 2011); C. Ratmoko, *Damit die Chemie stimmt. Die Anfänge der industriellen Herstellung von weiblichen und männlichen Sexualhormonen 1914–1938* (Zürich: Chronos, 2010); B. Bächi, *Vitamin C für alle! Pharmazeutische Produktion, Vermarktung und Gesundheitspolitik (1933–1953)* (Zürich: Chronos, 2009); J.-P. Gaudillière, 'Professional or Industrial Order? Patents, Biological Drugs, and Pharmaceutical Capitalism in Early Twentieth Century Germany', *History and Technology*, 24 (2008), pp. 107–33; W. Wimmer, *'Wir haben fast immer was Neues': Gesundheitswesen und Innovationen der Pharma-Industrie in Deutschland, 1880–1935* (Berlin: Duncker & Humblot 1994).

72. H. Stoff, *Ewige Jugend. Konzepte der Verjüngung vom späten 19. Jahrhundert bis ins Dritte Reich* (Cologne, Weimar: Böhlau, 2004); R. D. Apple, *Vitamania: Vitamins in American Culture* (New Brunswick, NJ: Rutgers University Press, 1996).

73. H. Stoff, *Wirkstoffe. Eine Wissenschaftsgeschichte der Hormone, Vitamine und Enzyme, 1920–1970* (Stuttgart: Franz Steiner Verlag, 2012), pp. 232–77.

74. Heyll, *Wasser*, pp. 233–42; A. Harrington, *Reenchanted Science: Holism in German Culture from Wilhelm II to Hitler* (Princeton, NJ: Princeton University Press, 1999), pp. 186–7.

75. Gaudillière, 'Pharmaceutical Industry', pp. 191–2.

76. On antibiotics, see R. Bud, *Penicillin: Triumph and Tragedy* (Oxford: Oxford University Press; 2007); C. Gradmann, 'Magic Bullets and Moving Targets: Antibiotic Resistance and Experimental Chemotherapy 1900–1940', *Dynamis*, 31 (2011), pp. 305–21.

77. Haller, *Cortison*, pp. 187–230.

78. Center for Biologics, *Science and the Regulation of Biological Products*, p. 19.

79. Ibid.

80. A. Hecht, 'Making Sure Biologicals are Safe', *FDA Consumer* (July–August 1977), pp. 21–6, on p. 26.

81. R. Bud, *The Uses of Life: A History of Biotechnology* (Cambridge, New York, Port Chester, Melbourne, Sydney: Cambridge University Press, 1993), p. 147. Marschall attributes this revival more to the 1970s. L. Marschall, *Im Schatten der chemischen Synthese: Industrielle Biotechnologie in Deutschland (1900–1970)* (Frankfurt/Main: Campus, 2000), pp. 295–7.

82. DFG-Archive, Bonn, Az 60324, Fremdstoff-Kommission, 1969–70, vol. 7: Joint FAO/WHO Food Standards Programme. Codex Komitee für Lebensmittelzusatzstoffe. Entwurf eines Allgemeinen Standards für Enzympräparate. Beitrag der Delegation der Bundesrepublik Deutschland.

83. U. Thoms, 'Between Promise and Threat: Antibiotics in Food in Germany 1950–1980', *NTM Zeitschrift für Geschichte der Wissenschaften, Technik und Medizin*, 20 (2012), pp. 187–8.

84. Parascandola, 'The Public Health Service', p. 775. In 1944, the former Division of Biologics Control was renamed Laboratory of Biologics Control. In 1948, the testing of

biological products was incorporated into the NIH's National Microbiological Institute. Center for Biologics, *Science and the Regulation of Biological Products*, p. 22.

85. Leveton, Sox and Stoto, *HIV*, p. 44.

86. Ibid.

87. Hecht, 'Making Sure Biologicals are Safe', p. 23.

88. K. Reid, 'CBER and CDER Have a Long History of Being Lumped Together and Split Up', *Bioresearch Monitoring Alert* (September 2002), p. 4.

89. An influential contemporary definition of biotechnology was formulated in 1974 by DECHEMA, a West German chemical society with close ties to the chemical and pharmaceutical industry: The meaning that is most widely accepted is that it is the industrial processing of materials by micro-organisms and other *biological agents* to provide desirable products and services. It incorporates fermentation and enzyme technology, water and waste treatment, and some aspects of food technology. Its scope and potential therefore are enormous and like microelectronics before it, novel ideas and tangible benefits are being reported at an ever-increasing rate. Cited in Bud, *Uses*, p. 151 (emphasis by the authors). This definition became the basis of the widely known OECD report on biotechnology published in 1979. Ibid., p. 161.

90. Ibid., p. 177.

91. For summaries, see ibid., pp. 177–82; P. Rabinow, *French DNA: A Story of Biotechnology* (Chicago, IL: The University of Chicago Press, 1996); M. Morange, *A History of Molecular Biology* (Cambridge, MA, and London: Harvard University Press, 1998), pp. 184–203; E. J. Vettel, *Biotec: The Contercultural Origins of an Industry* (Philadelphia, PA: University of Philadelphia Press, 2006). Korwek provides a detailed overview on the key developments with respect to regulation. See Korwek, 'Biologics', pp. 276–88.

92. For the interferon story, see T. Pieters, *Interferon: The Science and Selling of a Miracle Drug* (London, New York: Routledge, 2005).

93. I. Löwy, *Between Bench and Bedside: Science, Healing, and Interleukin-2 in a Cancer Ward* (Cambridge, MA: Harvard University Press, 1996).

94. Ibid., p. 5.

95. For an overview, see J.-P. Gaudillière, 'New Wine in Old Bottles? The Biotechnology Problem in the History of Molecular Biology', *Studies in History and Philosophy of Biological and Biomedical Sciences*, 40 (2009), pp. 20–8.

96. See the Reports of the WHO Expert Committee on Biological Standardization; WHO Expert Committee on Biological Standardization, 'Thirty-Fifth Report', *WHO Technical Report Series*, 725 (1985), p. 10; WHO Expert Committee on Biological Standardization, 'Thirty-Six Report', *WHO Technical Report Series*, 745 (1987), p. 8.

97. Carpenter, *Reputation and Power*, p. 30.

98. Pieters, *Interferon*, pp. 5, 60.

99. Of fourteen new biological remedies approved by the FDA two years later, only one was genetically engineered. See Bud, *Uses*, p. 193.

100. For instance, the Biological Research Subcommittee was established within the US government's Office of Science and Technology Policy. Its purpose was not to regulate, but to explore new strategies of biotechnology research. See ibid., pp. 212–4.

101. Ibid, cited on p. 192.

102. By 1983, the NCDB had established nine 'offices' dedicated to different products. A decade later, there were sixteen such offices. In 1983, the biologics component of the NCDB was renamed Office of Biologics Research and Review (OBRR) within the Center for Drugs and Biologics (COB). In 1988, the COB was divided into two centres: the Center

for Biologics and Research (formerly OBRR) and the Center for Drug and Research (COER). In 1993, the Center for Biologics and Review was renamed the Center for Biologics Evaluation and Research (CBER). See Center for Biologics, *History*, p. 22; Leveton, Sox and Stoto, *HIV*, pp. 44–5; Carpenter, *Reputation and Power*, pp. 6, 446, 483.

103. Reid, 'CBER and CDER'. For details see www.biopharma.com/CBERtoCDER.html [accessed 22 May 2012].

104. Today, CBER's jurisdiction includes a wide range of products: vaccines; allergenic extracts; blood for transfusion and as a raw material for drug products; reagents used for blood typing and other related activities; plasma derivatives, including immunoglobulins; hyperimmune products and antitoxins; human cell tissue, as well as cellular and tissue-based products (HCT/P) such as bone, skin, corneas, ligaments, tendons, stem cells, heart valves, hematopoietic stem/progenitor and cord blood, oocytes and semen; some medical devices, specifically test kits for HIV, tests used to screen blood donations, blood bank collection machines and equipment and blood bank computer software; xenotransplantation; gene therapy and human cloning. CDER regulates biological products mostly produced by biotechnology methods, including: monoclonal antibodies designed as targeted therapies in cancer and other diseases; cytokines (types of proteins involved in immune response; growth factors (proteins that affect the growth of a cell); enzymes (types of proteins that speed up biochemical reactions), such as thrombolytics (used to dissolve blood clots) and immunomodulators (agents that affect immune response). For CBER, see www.fda.gov/BiologicsBloodVaccines/default.htm [accessed 11 March 2012]; for CDER, see FDA, *FDA Consumer Health Information*, 101 (25 July 2008, at www.fda.gov/ForConsumers/ConsumerUpdates/ucm048341.htm#Whatbiol ogicalproductsdoesFDAregulate [accessed 25 March 2013]; see also S. R. Scott, R. P. Brady and E. Y. Chung, 'What is a Biologic?', in M. P. Mathieu (ed.), *Biologics Development: A Regulatory Overview*, 3nd edn (Waltham, MA: PAREXEL International Corp., 2004), pp. 1–16, on p. 12.

105. The biological products included four categories: '– human, e.g. human blood and human blood products, animal, e.g. micro-organisms – whole animals, parts of organs, animal secretions, toxins, extracts, blood products – vegetable, e.g. micro-organisms, plants, parts of plants, vegetable secretions, extracts – chemical, e.g. elements, naturally occurring chemical materials and chemical products obtained by chemical change or synthesis. *Directive 2001/83/EC of the European Parliament and of the Council of 6 November 2001 on the Community Code Relating to Medicinal Products for Human Use*, at eur-lex.europa.eu/en/index.htm [accessed 11 March 2012], p. 9.

106. Compare www.ema.europa.eu/ [accessed 11 March 2012; emphasis by the authors]. Also, the terms 'biologics' and 'biologicals' are used extensively by the EMA. Keyword search on the webpage of the EMA (www.ema.europa.eu/), responsible for the authorization and supervision of medicinal products for human and veterinary use [accessed 22 May 2012].

107. The first approval procedure that describes the standard procedures for medicinal products comprises '*biological medicines* such as recombinant proteins'. The second approval procedure involves '*similar biological medicines*', that is, generics of 'biological medicines', also known as biosimilars. The third application procedure encompasses substances from which biologics have originated, including plasma-derived medical products such as albumin, coagulating factors and immunoglobulins of human origin, as well as vaccines, toxins, sera and allergen products, now referred to as '*biological medicinal products*'.

'Herbal medicinal products' are also included here. Finally, the fourth category of the EU drugs approval requirements includes '*gene therapy and somatic cell therapy*'. *Directive 2001/83/EC*, p. 72 (emphasis by the authors).

108. A similar difference between regulation and legislation can be attributed to the US context as well. Compare Korwek, 'Biologicals', pp. 295–302.

109. For example, German regulatory bodies today use different terms. The Federal Institute for Vaccines and Biomedicines – better known as the Paul Ehrlich Institute (PEI) – is (mainly) responsible for the regulation of 'biomedicines' ('*biomedizinische Arzneimittel*'), including vaccines, antibodies, allergens, blood and blood products, tissue products, gene therapy, somatic cell therapy and xenogenic cell therapy. The institute was established in 2009 when German law renamed the PEI. *Gesetz zur Änderung arzneimittelrechtlicher und anderer Vorschriften* (AMGuaÄndG) v. 17.7.2009, at www.buzer.de/gesetz/8873/a162161.htm [accessed 20 June 2011]. However, 'biomedicines' do not include all 'biological products' as defined in the German Drug Law or the European Medicinal Products Directive. Hence, the German Federal Institute of Drugs and Medicinal Devices (*Bundesinstitut für Arzneimittel und Medizinprodukte*, BfArM) is responsible for the regulation of recombinant proteins with the exception of blood products and monoclonal antibodies, i.e. hormones, immune modulators and enzymes (para. 77 of the German Medicinal Product Law (*Arzneimittelgesetz*) in the version published 2005, last amended May 2011). Some experts prefer the term '*Biologika*' to describe this group of biotechnologically produced substances or products using recombinant organisms. Most of these 'biomedicines' (e.g. gene therapeutics, industrially processed tissue products) are licensed and monitored by the EMA, but both the BfArM and the PEI are substantially responsible for surveillance and coordination of producers, consumers and various European and national bodies. The division of labour between the BfArM and the PEI began in 1996 when the German Federal Health Office (*Bundesgesundheitsamt*) was dissolved as a consequence of the HIV contamination of blood supplies.

110. Internationally, the use of 'biologicals' by the World Health Organization (WHO) had long covered immunological substances as well as antibiotics, hormones and enzymes.

111. Korwek, 'Biologics', pp. 269–70. The status of homoeopathic and herbal medicinal products remains confusing. One reason for this may be that regulatory measures for herbal medicines usually differ substantially from established medical standards. For instance, their compliance with quality standards must be documented, but not their efficacy in the sense of established medical standards.

112. Korwek, 'Biologics', p. 266.

113. 'For biological medicinal products, starting materials shall mean any substance of biological origin such as micro-organisms, organs and tissues of either plant or animal origin, cells or fluids (including blood or plasma) of human or animal origin, and biotechnological cell constructs (cell substrates, whether they are recombinant or not, including primary cells)'. *Directive 2001/83/EC*, p. 84 (Amendment to Directive 2001/83/EC by Commission Directive 2003/63/EC of 25 June 2003).

114. FDA, *FDA Consumer*.

115. For this characterization, see also J.-P. Gaudillière, 'Introduction: Drug Trajectories', *Studies in History and Philosophy of Biological and Biomedical Sciences*, 36:4 (2005), pp. 603–11, on p. 606.

116. For West Germany, see Stoff, *Wirkstoffe*, pp. 302–5; for the US, see N. Langston, *Toxic Bodies: Hormone Disruptors and the Legacy of DES* (New Haven, CT: Yale University Press, 2010), pp. 61–82.

117. For a thorough analysis, see Langston, *Toxic Bodies*.

118. For an example taken from hormone research, see Haller, *Cortison*, p. 116.

119. E. Hickel, *Arzneimittel-Standardisierung im 19. Jahrhundert in den Pharmakopöen Deutschlands, Frankreichs, Großbritanniens und der Vereinigten Staaten von Amerika* (Stuttgart: Wissenschaftliche Verlagsgesellschaft 1973); C. Bonah, J.-P. Gaudillière, C. Gradmann and V. Hess, 'Standard Drugs and Drug Standards: A Comparative Historical Study of Pharmaceuticals in the 20th century', in Bonah, Masutti, Rasmussen and Simon (eds), *Harmonizing Drugs*, pp. 17–27.

120. See the literature in the second section of this introduction, and also Pieters, *Interferon*. See also the contributions in J.-P. Gaudillière (ed.), *Drug Trajectories*, special issue of *Studies in History and Philosophy of Biological and Biomedical Sciences*, 36:4 (2005); Mazumdar, 'Antitoxin and *Anatoxine*'; C. J. Rutty, 'Canadian Vaccine Research, Production and International Regulation: Connaught Laboratories and Smallpox Vaccines, 1962–1980', in Kroker, Mazumdar and Keelan (eds), *Crafting Immunity*, pp. 273–300.

121. M. Grmek, *Raisonnement expérimental et recherches toxicologiques chez Claude Bernard* (Geneva, Paris: Librairie Droz, 1973).

122. H. Dale, 'Biological Standardization', *Analyst*, 64 (1939), pp. 554–67, on p. 554; compare Haller, *Cortison*, pp. 100–7.

123. A. Helmstädter, 'Antidiabetic Medicinal Plants between Phytotherapy and Lead Structure Research', *Pharmacy in History*, 55 (2013), in print.

124. Gaudillière, 'Drug Trajectories', p. 606.

125. Anonymous, 'Some Special Features', pp. 397–8 (emphasis by the authors).

126. See also K. Angerer's contribution to this volume on p. 195.

127. See J.-P. Gaudillière's contribution to this volume on p. 48.

128. Merill and Hutt, *Food and Drug Law*, pp. 664–5.

129. CBER, 'What are Biologics Questions and Answers', at www.fda.gov/AboutFDA/CentersOffices/OfficeofMedicalProductsandTobacco/CBER/ucm133077.htm [accessed 22 May 2012].

130. K. C. Zoon, 'Well-Characterized Biotechnology Products: Evolving to Meet the Needs of the 21st Century', in F. Brown, A. Lubiniecki and G. Murano (eds), *Characterization of Biotechnology Pharmaceutical Products, Washington D.C., USA, December 11–13, 1995* (Basel: Karger, 1998), pp. 3–8, on p. 4.

131. Schmeckebier, *Public Health Service*, p. 143.

132. P. Sizaret, 'Evolution of Activities in International Biological Standardization since the Early Days of the Health Organisation of the League of Nations', *Bulletin of the World Health Organization*, 66 (1988), pp. 1–6, on p. 2.

133. W. A. Timmerman, 'International Biological Standardisation', *Journal of Pharmacy and Pharmacology*, 3 (1951), pp. 65–77; Dale, 'Biological Standardisation', pp. 558–60; Mazumdar, 'Antitoxin and *Anatoxine*'.

134. For more details, see P. M. H. Mazumdar, '"In the Silence of the Laboratory": The League of Nations Standardizes Syphilis Tests', *Social History of Medicine*, 16 (2003), pp. 437–59.

135. Mazumdar advances this argument. Mazumdar, 'Antitoxin and *Anatoxine*', p. 189.

136. Pieters, *Interferon*, pp. 68–9, 107.

137. Haller, *Cortison*.

138. Ibid.

139. On the battle metaphor, see E. Martin, *Flexible Bodies: Tracking Immunity in American Culture – from the Days of Polio to the Age of Aids* (Boston, MA: Beacon Press Books, 1994), pp. 23–44.

140. P. Sarasin, *Reizbare Maschinen. Eine Geschichte des Körpers 1765–1914* (Frankfurt/ Main: Suhrkamp, 2001); P. Sarasin, S. Berger, M. Hänseler and M. Spörri (eds), *Bakteriologie und Moderne: Studien Zur Biopolitik des Unsichtbaren, 1870–1920* (Frankfurt/ Main: Suhrkamp, 2007); S. Berger, *Bakterien in Krieg und Frieden. Eine Geschichte der medizinischen Bakteriologie in Deutschland, 1890–1933* (Göttingen: Wallstein, 2009).

141. A. Labisch, *Homo Hygienicus. Gesundheit und Medizin in der Neuzeit* (Frankfurt/Main, New York: Campus, 1992), p. 255 (trans. AvS, HS and BW).

142. Stoff, *Ewige Jugend*.

143. Stoff, *Wirkstoffe*, pp. 64–82, 232–79.

144. For these aspects, see J.-P. Gaudillière, 'Biochemie und Industrie. Der "Arbeitskreis Butenandt-Schering" im Nationalsozialismus', in W. Schieder and A. Trunk (eds), *Adolf Butenandt und die Kaiser-Wilhelm-Gesellschaft. Wissenschaft, Industrie und Politik im 'Dritten Reich'* (Göttingen: Wallstein, 2004), pp. 198–246; Bächi, *Vitamin C für Alle!*; Stoff, *Wirkstoffe*.

145. Pieters, *Interferon*, pp. 163, 168–75.

146. E. Hickel, '"Bei Risiken und Nebenwirkungen fragen Sie" ... die Wissenschaft? Nebenwirkungen: das paradigmatische Problem der Arzneimittelforschung', *Mitteilungen der TU Braunschweig*, 29 (1994), pp. 50–7.

147. Pieters, *Interferon*, pp. 60–1.

148. H.-J. Rheinberger, 'Precarious Substances: A Brief Commentary', in V. Balz, A. von Schwerin, H. Stoff and B. Wahrig (eds), *Precarious Matters/Prekäre Stoffe: The History of Dangerous and Endangered Substances in the 19th and 20th Centuries*, Preprint series 356 (Berlin: Max Planck Institute for the History of Science, 2008), pp. 181–2, on p. 182.

149. B. Wahrig, H. Stoff, A. von Schwerin and V. Balz, 'Precarious Matters: An Introduction', in Balz, von Schwerin, Stoff and Wahrig, *Precarious Matters*, pp. 5–13, on p. 12.

150. A. von Schwerin, *Strahlen. Biologie und Politik staatswichtiger Dinge. Eine Geschichte der Deutschen Forschungsgemeinschaft 1920–1970* (Stuttgart: Franz Steiner Verlag, 2014), pp. 27–33.

151. See U. Thoms's contribution to this volume on p. 161.

152. Pieters, *Interferon*, p. 61.

153. In Germany, animal lymph was declared the standard lymph in 1897. Pistor, *Gesundheitswesen*, p. 54.

154. Hennock, *Vaccination Policy*, pp. 58, 60–5; D. Porter and R. Porter, 'The Politics of Prevention: Anti-Vaccination and Public Health in Nineteenth-Century England', *Medical History*, 32 (1988), pp. 231–52 and E. Wolff, 'Medizinkritik der Impfgegner im Spannungsfeld zwischen Lebenswelt und Wissenschaftsorientierung', in M. Dinges (ed.), *Medizinkritische Bewegungen im Deutschen Reich* (Stuttgart: Steiner, 1996), pp. 79–108.

155. C. Bonah, 'Le drame de Lübeck: la vaccination BCG, le 'procès Calmette' et les Richtlinien de 1931', in C. Bonah, E. Lepicard and V. Roelcke (eds), *La Médecine expérimentale au tribunal: Implications éthiques de quelques procès médicaux du XXe siècle européen* (Paris: Editions des Archives Contemporaines, 2003), pp. 65–94.

156. J.-P. Gaudillière, 'Hormones at Risk: Cancer and the Medical Uses of Industrially-Produced Sex Steroids in Germany, 1930–1960', in T. Schlich and U. Tröhler (eds), *The Risks of Medical Innovation: Risk Perception and Assessment in Historical Context* (London and New York: Routledge, 2006), pp. 148–69.

157. D. Cantor, 'Cortisone and the Politics of Drama, 1949–55', in J. V. Pickstone (ed.), *Medical Innovations in Historical Perspective* (Basingstoke, London: Macmillian, 1992), pp. 165–84; D. Cantor, 'Cortisone and the Politics of Empire: Imperialism and British Medicine, 1918–1955', *Bulletin of the History of Medicine*, 67 (1993), pp. 463–93; Haller, *Cortison*, pp. 187–230. See also J.-P. Gaudillière's contribution to this volume on pp. 47–63.

158. For a selection, see K. Philip, 'Imperial Science Rescues a Tree: Global Botanic Networks, Local Knowledge and the Transcontinental Transplantation of Cinchona', *Environment and History*, 1 (1995), pp. 173–200; St J. Harris, 'Long-Distance Corporations, Big Sciences, and the Geography of Knowledge', *Configurations*, 6 (1998), pp. 269–304; M. R. Dove, 'The Life-Cicle of Indigenous Knowledge, and the Case of Natural Rubber Production', in R. Ellen, P. Parks and A. Bicker (eds), *Indigenous Environmental Knowledge and its Transformations: Critical Anthropological Perspectives* (Amsterdam: Harwood Academic Publishers, 2000), pp. 213–51; A. Barrera, 'Local Herbs, Global Medicines: Commerce, Knowledge, and Commodities in Spanish America', in P. H. Smith and P. Findlen (eds), *Merchants and Marvels: Commerce, Science, and Art in Early Modern Europe* (New York: Routledge, 2002), pp. 163–81; W. Beinart and K. Middleton, 'Plant Transfers in Historical Perspective: A Review Article', *Environment and History*, 10 (2004), pp. 3–29; L. Schiebinger, *Plants and Empire: Colonial Bioprospecting in the Atlantic World* (Cambridge, MA, and London: Harvard University Press, 2004); M. Flitner, *Sammler, Räuber und Gelehrte: Die politischen Interessen an pflanzengenetischen Ressourcen 1895–1995* (Frankfurt/Main and New York: Campus, 2005). Many thanks to Klaus Angerer who introduced us to recent debates on bioprospecting.

159. L. Schiebinger and C. Swan, 'Introduction', in L. Schiebinger and C. Swan (eds), *Colonial Botany: Science, Commerce, and Politics in the Early Modern World* (Philadelphia, PA: University of Pennsylvania Press, 2005), pp. 1–16, on pp. 2–3.

160. M. Frein and H. Meyer, *Die Biopiraten. Milliardengeschäfte der Pharmaindustrie mit dem Bauplan der Natur* (Berlin: Econ Verlag, 2008), pp. 164–5.

1 Simon, 'Standardization and Clinical Use: The Introduction of the Anti-Diphtheria Serum in Lyon'

1. This essay is a follow-up to the DFG project HE 2220/4–1 and 2, 'The Industrialisation of Experimental Knowledge' on the development and production of anti-diphtheria serum in France and Germany at the end of the nineteenth century, carried out in collaboration with Axel Hüntelmann and Ulrike Klöppel under the direction of Volker Hess at the Charité in Berlin.

2. Vaccines were used prophylactically, except for the vaccine treatment for rabies developed by Louis Pasteur. Rabies was not, however, a very widespread disease.

3. A. I. Hardy, 'From Diphtheria to Tetanus: The Development of Evaluation Methods for Sera in Imperial Germany', in C. Gradmann and J. Simon (eds) *Evaluating and Standardizing Therapeutic Agents, 1890–1950* (Basingstoke: Palgrave Macmillan, 2010), pp. 52–70; A. Hüntelmann, 'Evaluation as a Practical Technique of Administration: The Regulation and Standardisation of Diphtheria Serum', ibid., pp. 31–51 and for the French side, see J. Simon, 'Quality Control and the Politics of Serum Production in France', ibid., pp. 89–104.

4. Annex 1 of EC/1084/2003, at http://eur-lex.europa.eu/, p. L159/7 [accessed 20 July 2010]. I have quoted the second sentence accurately, but, as if to exemplify how the meaning of this text is largely implicit for those working in the field, I believe that certain crucial words would need to be added for it to make literal sense.

5. For a more complete discussion of this tradition of *Wertbestimmung* and its influence, see Gradmann and Simon (eds), *Evaluating and Standardizing*.

6. For more details, see C. R. Prüll, 'Paul Ehrlich's Standardization of Serum: Wertbestimmung and its Meaning for Twentieth-Century Biomedicine', in Gradmann and Simon (eds), *Evaluating and Standardizing*, pp. 13–30.

7. E. Roux and L. Martin, 'Contribution à l'étude de la diphtérie (Sérum-thérapie) (3e Mémoire)', *Annales de l'Institut Pasteur*, 8:9 (1894), p. 621; for the logic of remaining loyal to this form of evaluation, see Simon, 'Quality Control', p. 98.

8. S. Timmermans and M. Berg, *The Gold Standard: The Challenge of Evidence-Based Medicine and Standardization in Health Care* (Philadelphia, PA: Temple University Press, 2003), p. 24.

9. Hüntelmann, 'Evaluation as a Practical Technique', p. 42.

10. J. Simon, 'French Serum Regulation in 1895: The Necessary Minimum or the Maximum Possible?', in J.-P. Gaudillière and V. Hess (eds), *Ways of Regulating: Therapeutic Agents between Plants, Shops and Consulting Rooms*, Preprint series 363 (Berlin: Max Planck Institute for the History of Science, 2008), pp. 95–104.

11. L. Bard, 'Des conditions de propagation de la diphtérie. Relation de l'épidémie d'Oullins', *Lyon Médical*, 60 (1889), pp. 199–209.

12. Ibid.

13. Several authors have argued for the role of new diagnostic and therapeutic technologies in the rise in the status of hospitals at the turn of the nineteenth and twentieth centuries. For an argument around the place of X-rays and other diagnostic techniques in Philadelphia, see J. D. Howell, *Technology in the Hospital: Transforming Patient Care in the Early Twentieth Century* (Baltimore, MD: The Johns Hopkins University Press, 1996). Paul Weindling has also suggested that serotherapy contributed significantly to the acceptability of hospital care for bourgeois families, see P. Weindling, 'From Medical Research to Clinical Practice: Serum Therapy for Diphtheria in the 1890s', in J. Pickstone (ed.), *Medical Innovations in Historical Perspective* (New York: St Martin's Press, 1992), pp. 72–83.

14. B. Latour, *Microbes: Guerre et Paix* (Paris: Métailié, 1991), a theme also picked up by David Barnes in the characterization of his 'sanitary bacteriological synthesis'. D. S. Barnes, *The Great Stink of Paris and the Nineteenth-Century Struggle against Filth and Germs* (Baltimore, MD: The Johns Hopkins University Press, 2007).

15. Bard, 'Des conditions de propagation', p. 206.

16. Ibid., p. 259.

17. E. Aschkinazi, *Le Stérésol (vernis antiseptique) et ses applications spécialement dans la diphtérie* (MD thesis, Paris Faculty of Medicine, 1893).

18. For a full report of Roux's announcement of these results in Budapest, see J. Sacaze, 'Huitième congrès international d'hygiène et de démographie tenu à Budapest du 2 au 8 septembre 1894', *La Semaine Médicale*, 14 (1894), pp. 405–10.

19. *Salut Public*, 7 September 1894, p. 1 (trans. JS).

20. F. Rabot, 'Prélude à la sérothérapie', *Lyon Médical*, 77 (1894), pp. 527–43, on p. 538 (trans. JS).

21. Ibid., p. 539.

22. Ibid., p. 540.
23. Ibid., p. 540.
24. P. Patet, *La sérothérapie à Lyon* (Lyon: MD thesis, Lyon Faculty of Medicine, 1895).
25. *Nouveau Montpellier médical*, 1894.
26. Archives Municipales de Lyon, 1125 WP 023.
27. It seems that Pasteur's treatment for rabies escaped this type of criticism, despite the dangers associated with using an attenuated virus. G. L. Geison, *The Private Science of Louis Pasteur* (Princeton, NJ: Princeton University Press, 1995).
28. Zolot-Nisky, 'Revers de la médaille', *Lyon Médical*, 79 (1895), pp. 94–8, 162–5, 194–201.
29. Ibid., p. 94.
30. S. Arloing, 'Sur quelques effets non mentionnés par Roux des injections de toxines diphtériques sur le cheval', *Lyon Médical*, 79 (1895), pp. 82–3, see the footnote on p. 82.
31. See the chapters on serotherapy in Gradmann and Simon (eds), *Evaluating and Standardizing.*

2 Gaudillière, 'Biologics in the Colonies: Emile Perrot, Kola Nuts and the Industrial Reordering of Pharmacy'

1. This essay is dedicated to the memory of Nina Inckes-Schultze who introduced me to the trajectory of kola.
2. See, for example, the papers assembled in J.-P. Gaudillière (ed.), *Drug Trajectories*, special issue of *Studies in History and Philosophy of Biological and Biomedical Sciences*, 36:4 (2005), pp. 603–780; V. Balz, A. von Schwerin, H. Stoff and B. Wahrig (eds), *Precarious Matters/Prekäre Stoffe: The History of Dangerous and Endangered Substances in the 19th and 20th Centuries*, Preprint series 356 (Berlin: Max Planck Institute for the History of Science, 2008).
3. J.-P. Gaudillière, 'Professional and Industrial Drug Regulation in France and Germany: The Trajectories of Plant Extracts', in J.-P. Gaudillière and V. Hess (eds) *Ways of Regulating Drugs in the 19th and 20th centuries* (Basingstoke: Palgrave, 2012), pp. 66–96.
4. J.-P. Gaudillière, 'Une marchandise scientifique? Savoirs, industrie et régulation du médicament en Allemagne', *Annales*, 65 (2010), pp. 89–120.
5. On Heckel, see G. Aillaud, 'Edouard Heckel, un savant organisateur. De la botanique appliquée à l'Exposition Coloniale de 1906', *Province historique*, 43 (1993), pp. 153–65, on p. 153. M. A. Osborne, 'Edouard-Marie Heckel', in N. Koertge (ed.), *New Dictionary of Scientific Biography* vol. 21 (Farmington Hills: Charles Scribner's Sons, 2008), p. 272.
6. E. Heckel and F. Schlagdenhauffen, 'Du kola au point de vue botanique, chimique et thérapeutique', *Journal de Pharmacie et de Chimie*, 7–8 (1883), p. 556.
7. M. Osborne, 'The Emergence of Tropical Medicine in Marseille', forthcoming.
8. On these developments, see ibid.
9. E. Heckel, *Les végétaux utiles de l'Afrique. Les kolas africains. Monographie botanique, chimique, thérapeutique, pharmacologique* (Paris: Société des Editions Scientifiques, 1893).
10. Ibid., p. 127 (trans. J-PG).
11. E. Knebel, 'Zur chemischen Kentniss der Kolanuss', *Apotheker Zeitung*, 7 (1892), p. 112.

12. On the uses of the graphic method in late nineteenth-century physiology, see R. M. Brain, *The Graphic Method: Inscription, Visualization and Measurement in Nineteenth-Century Science and Culture* (PhD thesis, University of California Los Angeles, 1996).

13. The firm was called the *Compagnie Francaise de Spécialités Pharmaceutiques au Kola*. Little is known about its origins and operations. For evidence of its existence, see J. B. Jacob, *Spécialités pharmaceutiques anciennes à base de caféine ou des drogues à caféine* (Thèse Faculté de Pharmacie, Paris V, 1992).

14. Faculté de Pharmacie de Paris, 'Dossier biographique de Emile Perrot' (prepared by G. Dilleman).

15. On Chevallier, see C. Bonneuil, *Mettre en ordre et discipliner les tropiques: les sciences du vegetal dans l'empire français, 1870–1940* (PhD thesis, Université Paris 7, 1997).

16. A. Chevalier and E. Perrot, *Les kolatiers et lanoix de kola*. Collection *Les végétaux utilres de L'AOF*, vol. 3 (Paris: Chalamel, 1911). On this dimension of Perrot's work, see N. Inckes-Schultze, *La noix de kola comme végétal utile de L'AOF* (Master thesis in the history of science, University Paris 7, 1996).

17. E. Perrot, 'La pharmacognosie', *Bulletin des sciences pharmaceutiques*, 16 (1909), pp. 125–9.

18. A. Goris and E. Perrot, 'Sur la composition chimique des noix de kola', *Bulletin de la Société de Pharmacie*, 14 (1907), pp. 576–653; A. Goris, 'Sur un nouveau principe de la Kola fraîche', *Compte-Rendus de l'Académie des Sciences*, 144 (1907), pp. 1162–4, on p. 1162 (trans. J-PG).

19. J. Chevalier and A. Goris, 'Action pharmacodynamique de la kolatine', *CRAS*, 165 (1907), pp. 354–5, on p. 354 (trans. J-PG).

20. Midy's kola packaging thus claimed: 'contenant intégralement la caféine, la theobromine, le tannin et le ROUGE DE KOLA principe le plus actif de la noix de Kola se transformant en caféine naissante sous l'influence du suc gastrique'.

21. A. Goris and L. Arnould, 'Conservation et stérilisation des noix de kola fraîches', *Bulletin de la Société de Pharmacie*, 14 (1907), pp. 15–161.

22. A. Goris and E. Perrot, 'La stérilisation des plantes médicinales dans ses rapports avec leur activité thérapeutique', *Bulletin des sciences pharmacologiques*, 16 (1909), pp. 380–430 (trans. J-PG).

23. Ibid., pp. 381–90 (trans. J-PG).

24. Brevet, 11 September 1910, INPI 403 312: 'Procédé de stérilisation par tous dispositifs appliqués en vue de la conservation de tous organismes provenant de la flore et de la faune'.

25. On Dausse and the making of *intraits*, see J.-P. Gaudillière in *Making Drugs*.

26. P. Joanin, 'Preface', in A. Joanin (ed.), *Les remèdes galéniques* (Paris: Impr.-édition des Laboratoires Dausse, 1921), (trans. J-PG).

27. On this, see Inckes-Schultze, *Noix de kola*.

28. A. Chevalier and E. Perrot, 'Les Kolatiers et les noix de Kola', *Bulletins des Sciences Pharmaceutiques*, 18 (1911), pp. 1–13, on pp. 10–11 (trans. J-PG).

29. C. Debue-Barazer, *Des simples aux plantes médicinales. Emile Perrot, un pharmagnoste colonial* (DEA d'Histoire Moderne et Contemporaine: Université Paris IV Sorbonne, 2002).

30. Archives Nationales, series F12, box 7710.

31. E. Perrot, 'Dix années d'efforts pour la production des plantes médicinales et aromatiques', *Notice N°32* (Paris: Office Nationale des Matières Premières Végétales pour la Droguerie, la Pharmacie, la Distillerie et la Parfurmerie, 1929).

32. E. Perrot and V. Gatin, 'L'hydrastis canadensis', *Notice n°2* (Office National des Matières Premières Végétales, 1920), p. 18 (trans. J-PG).

33. E. Perrot, *Sur les productions végétales de l'Afrique Occidentale Francaise* (Paris: Office National des Matières Premières Végétales, 1929), p. 99 (trans. J-PG).

34. Ibid., p. 100 (trans. J-PG).

35. Ibid., p. 126.

36. Ibid., p. 125 (trans. J-PG).

37. Ibid., p. 245.

38. Ibid., p. 252 (trans. J-PG).

39. Another interesting example of this pharmaceuticalization is the case of Chaulmoogra's oils, a remedy of Indian origin that Perrot advocated as being active against leprosies and tuberculosis. Perrot successfully made this a topic of inquiry both within his Paris laboratory and in the West African forest, but he failed to transform it into a biological that had been elaborated in the French colonies. See E. Perrot, 'Le chaulmoogra et autres graines utilisables contre la lèpre', *Bulletin des Sciences Pharmacologiques*, 33 (1926), pp. 353–69, on p. 353.

40. Jacob, *Spécialités*.

3 Haller, 'Standardizing the Experimental System: The Development of Corticosteroids and their Impact on Cooperation, Property Rights and Industrial Procedures'

1. E. H. Starling, 'The Croonian Lectures on the Chemical Correlation of the Functions of the Body', *Lancet*, 166:4278 (1905), pp. 339–41, on p. 339.

2. J.-P. Gaudillière, 'Hormones, régimes d'innovation et stratégies d'entreprise: les exemples de Schering et Bayer', *Entreprises et histoire*, 36:2 (2004), pp. 84–102, on pp. 84–6.

3. E. H. Starling, 'The Chemical Control of the Body', *Journal of the American Medical Association*, 50:11 (1908), pp. 835–40, on p. 840.

4. J. A. Secord, 'Knowledge in Transit', *Isis*, 95:4 (2004), pp. 654–72, on p. 667.

5. B. Latour and S. Woolgar, *Laboratory Life: The Social Construction of Scientific Facts* (Beverly Hills: Sage, 1979); H.-J. Rheinberger, *An Epistemology of the Concrete: Twentieth-Century Histories of Life* (Durham, NC: Duke University Press, 2010).

6. C. Bonah, J.-P. Gaudillière, C. Gradmann and V. Hess, 'Standard Drugs and Drugs Standards: A Comparative Historical Study of Pharmaceuticals in the 20th Century', in C. Bonah, C. Masutti, A. Rasmussen and J. Simon (eds), *Harmonizing Drugs: Standards in 20th-Century Pharmaceutical History* (Paris: Editions Glyphe, 2009), pp. 17–27, on p. 20.

7. Secord, 'Knowledge in Transit', p. 670.

8. T. Addison, *On the Constitutional and Local Effects of Disease of the Supra-Renal Capsules* (London: Samuel Highley, 1855).

9. S. Vincent, 'The Present Position of Organotherapy', *Lancet*, 201:1 (1923), pp. 130–2, on p. 130.

10. On the evolving relationship between endocrinology and the meat industry, see N. Pfeffer, 'How Abattoir "Biotrash" Connected the Social Worlds of the University Laboratory and the Disassembly Line', in D. Cantor, C. Bonah and M. Dörries (eds), *Meat, Medicine and Human Health in the Twentieth Century* (London: Pickering & Chatto, 2010), ch. 3.

11. E. C. Kendall, et al., 'Isolation in Crystalline Form of the Hormone Essential to Life From the Suprarenal Cortex; Its Chemical Nature and Physiologic Properties', *Mayo Clinic Proceedings*, 9:17 (1934), pp. 245–50, on p. 246.

12. Haco to Organon, 27 October 1936, Staatsarchiv Basel-Stadt (hereafter StaBS), Korrespondenz betr. Aromaforschung, Vitamine, Nebenniere, 1932–7, PA979a, K 11–1 2.

13. J. W. R. Everse and P. de Fremery, 'On a Method of Measuring Fatigue in Rats and its Application for Testing the Suprarenal Cortical Hormone (Cortin)', *Acta Brevia Neerlandica de Physiologia, Pharmacologia, Microbiologia*, 2 (1932), p. 152.

14. 'Mein Vorschlag, sich den neuen Test von Verzar zu Nutze zu machen, sollte natürlich kein Misstrauensvotum für die bisherigen Methoden sein ... Es scheint allerdings, dass alle Testmethoden bisher besonders gut an dem Ort ausgeführt werden, wo sie erfunden wurden. Ich traue dem Hundetest daher vorläufig nur dann, wenn er wirklich von Dr. Pfiffner ausgeführt wurde, ebenso wie der Everse-de Fremery-Test offenbar nur bei Ihnen richtig durchgeführt wird. Wenn wir Pech haben, so kann es mit dem neuen Test nach Verzar ähnlich herauskommen.' Reichstein to Organon, 3 February 1936, StaBS, Korrespondenz betr. Leberextrakte, 1934–7, PA979a, K 11–2 1 (trans. LH).

15. D. Gugerli, P. Kupper and D. Speich, *Die Zukunftsmaschine. Konjunkturen der ETH Zürich 1855–2005* (Zurich: Chronos, 2005), p. 200.

16. HACO A.G./Prof. Dr. T. Reichstein, Interne Notizen, Novartis Company Archive/ Ciba Archive (hereafter CIBA Archiv), C_RE/V, Recht, Verträge Nr. 386 a/b/c.

17. J.-P. Gaudillière, 'Cartellisation et propriété intellectuelle: l'accord de 1939–1942 sur la Cortin', *Entreprises et histoire*, 36:2 (2004), pp. 150–3; J. Tanner, 'The Swiss Pharmaceutical Industry: The Impact of Industrial Property Rights and Trust in the Laboratory, 1907–1939', in A. S. Travis (ed.), *Determinants in the Evolution of the European Chemical Industry, 1900–1939* (Dordrecht, Boston, MA, and London: Kluwer Academic Publishers, 1998), pp. 257–71.

18. 'Dagegen erscheint es uns ebenso selbstverständlich, dass ein Verfahren, das zu einem cortinartig wirkenden Produkt führt, ausschliesslich der Organon gehört, auch wenn dieses Produkt andere therapeutische interessante Anwendungen finden kann.' HACO A.G./Prof. Dr. T. Reichstein, 7 April 1938, CIBA Archiv, Korrespondenz. Haco to Ciba, C_RE/V, Recht, Verträge Nr. 386 a/b/c (trans. LH).

19. 'Konkret gestellt lautet die uns interessierende Frage: Was geschieht mit solchen Verfahren, welche nicht unter Absatz 2 von Art. IIa fallen, also weder auf unsere Anregung noch mit unserer Unterstützung ausgearbeitet sind, und welche, was ja sehr wohl möglich ist, gleichzeitig zu Cortin, Progesteron und auch Testosteron führen.' Ciba to Haco, 13 April 1938, ibid. (trans. LH).

20. Ciba to Haco, 28 April 1938, ibid.

21. M. Steiger and T. Reichstein, 'Partial Synthesis of a Crystallized Compound with the Biological Activity of the Adrenal-Cortical Hormone', *Nature*, 139:3526 (1937), pp. 925–6, on p. 926.

22. 'Zunächst wird durch eine ziemlich brutale Oxydation die ganze Seitenkette des Cholesterons aboxydiert. Dies ist eine sehr schlecht verlaufende Reaktion, wobei aus einem kg Cholesteron etwa 10 g der nötigen 3-Oxy-äthiocholensäure entsteht.' Referat Reichsteins an der Ärztetagung in Oss, Holland, 13 June 1939, StaBS, Korrespondenz betr. Nebennieren, 1939, PA 979a K 11–2 3 (trans. LH).

23. Protocol from 26 October 1938, CIBA Archiv, Verkauf, Pharmaz. Verkaufscomité, Vf 1.

24. G. Bowker, 'Der Aufschwung der Industrieforschung', in M. Serres (ed.), *Elemente einer Geschichte der Wissenschaften* (Frankfurt/Main: Suhrkamp, 1994), pp. 829–67; D.

Edgerton, '"The Linear Model" Did not Exist: Reflections on the History and Historiography of Science and Research in Industry in the Twentieth Century', in K. Grandin, N. Wormbs and S. Widmalm (eds), *The Science–Industry Nexus: History, Policy, Implications* (Sagamore Beach: Science History Publications, 2004), pp. 31–58.

25. 'Es scheint mir, dass Sie die Schwierigkeiten der ganzen Doca-Fabrikation stark unterschätzen. Auch wenn vorläufig nur beabsichtigt ist, die letzte Fabrikationsstufe in den U.S.A. durchzuführen, so benötigt die praktische Durchführung doch erhebliche Vorbereitungen und vor allem auch die Kontrolle durch einen Fachmann, der nicht nur allgemein gute chemische Kenntnisse besitzt, sondern die in Frage kommenden Reaktionen aus eigener Erfahrung sehr genau kennt', Reichstein to Organon, 20 June 1939, StaBS, Korrespondenz betr. Nebennieren, 1939, PA 979a K 11–2 3 (trans. LH).

26. V. Quirke, 'Standardising Pharmaceutical R&D in the Second Half of the Twentieth Century: ICI's Novadex Development Programme in Historical and Comparative Perspective', in Bonah, Masutti, Rasmussen and Simon (eds), *Harmonizing Drugs*, pp. 148–9.

4 Bächi, 'Cultures of Subjectivity: Coca as a Biologic and the Co-construction of Deviant Subjects and Drug Efficacy, 1880–1900'

1. Special thanks for discussions, comments, hints and critiques go to Bettina Wahrig, Alexander von Schwerin, Heiko Stoff, Christoph Friedrich and the organizers of the Braunschweig workshop on biologics 'Drugs, Living Things and the Problems of Standardization' in 2010.

2. R. Voss, *Drugs Looking for Diseases: Innovative Drug Research and the Development of the Beta Blockers and the Calcium Antagonists* (Dordrecht und Boston, MA: Kluwer, 1991).

3. B. Wahrig, '"Fabelhafte Dinge": Arzneimittelnarrative zu Coca und Cocain im 19. Jahrhundert', *Berichte zur Wissenschaftsgeschichte*, 32:4 (2009), pp. 345–64.

4. Compare J. M. Hoberman, *Mortal Engines: The Science of Performance and the Dehumanization of Sport* (New York: Blackburn Press, 1992), esp. ch. 4; S. B. Karch, *A Brief History of Cocaine* (Boca Raton: CRC Press, 1998); W. Schivelbusch, *Das Paradies, der Geschmack und die Vernunft. Eine Geschichte der Genussmittel* (Frankfurt/Main: Fischer, 1995). Regarding the history of enhancement, see S. M. Rothman and D. J. Rothman, *The Pursuit of Perfection: The Promise and Perils of Medical Enhancement* (New York: Pantheon Books, 2003).

5. See http://herbmuseum.ca/content/parke-davis-co-cocaine-injection-kit [accessed 10 July 2013].

6. For cocaine's role in Freud's (scientific) biography, see H. Markel, *An Anatomy of Addiction: Sigmund Freud, William Halsted and the Miracle Drug Cocaine* (New York: Pantheon Books, 2011).

7. See Wahrig, 'Fabelhafte Dinge'.

8. S. Freud, 'Über Coca', in S. Freud, *Schriften über Kokain*, ed. A. Hirschmüller (1884; Frankfurt/Main: Fischer, 1996), pp. 41–83, on pp. 74–5.

9. Ibid., p. 50.

10. T. Aschenbrand, 'Die physiologische Wirkung und Bedeutung des Cocain. muriat. auf den menschlichen Organismus. Klinische Beobachtungen während der Herbst-

waffenübungen des Jahres 1883 beim H. Bayer. A.-C. 4. Div. 9. Reg. 2. Bat'., *Deutsche medizinische Wochenschrift*, 50 (1883), pp. 730–2 and Wahrig, 'Fabelhafte Dinge', ch. 6.

11. S. Freud, 'Beitrag zur Kenntnis der Cocawirkung', in Freud, *Schriften*, pp. 87–98, on p. 88.

12. C. Windgätter, '"... with mathematic precision": On the Historiography of the Dynamometer', in *The Virtual Laboratory. Essays and Resources on the Experimentation of Life* (2005), at http://vlp.mpiwg-berlin.mpg.de/essays/data/enc42 [accessed 21 October 2010], p. 2. Freud's own discription of a dynamometer is as follows: 'Ein Dynamometer ist bekanntlich eine federnde Metallspange, deren Zusammendrückung einen Zeiger längs eines Gradbogens verschiebt, an welchen die für den Betrag der Zusammendrückung erforderliche Kraft in Pfunden oder Kilo ablesbar ist.' [A dynamometer is, of course, a metal spring that, when compressed, moves a pointer along an arc, enabling one to measure the force in pounds or kilos required to compress the spring.] (trans. BB). S. Freud, 'Über die Allgemeinwirkung des Cocains', in *Schriften über Kokain*, p. 103.

13. A. Hirschmüller, 'E. Merck und das Kokain. Zu Sigmund Freuds Kokainstudien und ihren Beziehungen zu der Darmstädter Firma', *Gesnerus*, 52 (1995), pp. 116–32; A. Hirschmüller, 'Dynamometrie. Zur Messung der Körperkraft des Menschen im 19. Jahrhundert', *Internationale Zeitschrift für Geschichte und Ethik der Naturwissenschaften, Technik und Medizin*, 5 (1997), pp. 104–18.

14. Windgätter, '... with mathematic precision' and C. Windgätter, 'KraftRäume. Aufstieg und Fall der Dynamometrie', in T. Brandstetter and C. Windgätter (eds), *Zeichen der Kraft. Wissensformationen 1800–1900* (Berlin: Kadmos, 2008), pp. 108–37. See also M. Hughes, 'The Dynamometer and the Diemenese', in H. E. Le Grand (ed.), *Experimental Inquiries: Historical, Philosophical and Social Studies of Experimentation in Science* (Dordrecht, Boston, MA, and London: Kluwer, 1990). Nevertheless, the historiography of diagnostic instruments is extensive. For an overview see J. Büttner (ed.), *History of Clinical Chemistry* (Berlin and New York: Walter de Gruyter, 1983); J. Büttner, 'Messende Instrumente im medizinischen Laboratorium des 19. Jahrhunderts und ihre Bedeutung für die ärztliche Erkenntnis', in C. Meinel (ed.), *Instrument – Experiment. Historische Studien* (Berlin, Diepholz: Verlag für Geschichte der Naturwissenschaften und der Technik, 2000), pp. 109–17; M. Dommann, *Durchsicht, Einsicht, Vorsicht. Eine Geschichte der Röntgenstrahlen, 1896–1963* (Zürich: Chronos, 2002); C. Habrich, F. Marguth and J. H. Wolf (eds), *Medizinische Diagnostik in Geschichte und Gegenwart. Festschrift für Heinz Goerke zum sechzigsten Geburtstag* (Munich: Werner Fritsch, 1978); Hoffmann-La Roche, *Sinne, Sensoren und Systeme. Eine Reise durch die Geschichte der Labordiagnostik* (Basel: Editiones Roche, F. Hoffmann-La Roche Ltd. Science, 2003); M. Nicholson, 'The Art of Diagnosis: Medicine and the Five Senses', in W. Bynum and R. Porter (eds), *Companion Encyclopedia of the History of Medicine* (London and New York: Routledge 1993), pp. 801–25; M. Stolberg, *Die Harnschau. Eine Kultur- und Alltagsgeschichte* (Cologne, Weimar and Vienna: Böhlau, 2009).

15. T. Waitz, *Anthropologie der Naturvölker* (Leipzig: Friedrich Fleischer, 1859).

16. Compare J.-H. Fujimura, 'Crafting Science: Standardized Packages, Boundary Objects, and "Translation"', in A. Pickering (ed.), *Science as Practice and Culture* (Chicago, IL: University of Chicago Press, 1992), pp. 168–211; S. L. Star and J. R. Griesemer, 'Institutional Ecology, "Translations" and Boundary Objects: Amateurs and Professionals in Berkeley's Museum of Vertebrate Zoology', *Social Studies of Science*, 19 (1989), pp. 387–420; I. Löwy, 'Unscharfe Begriffe und föderative Experimentalstrategien. Die immunologische Konstruktion des Selbst', in H.-J. Rheinberger and M. Hagner (eds),

Die Experimentalisierung des Lebens. Experimentalsysteme in den biologischen Wissenschaften 1850/1950 (Berlin: Akademie Verlag, 1993), pp. 188–206.

17. A. Rabinbach, *The Human Motor: Energy, Fatigue, and the Origins of Modernity* (Berkeley and Los Angeles, CA: Basic Books, 1990), p. 286. See also A. Rabinbach, 'Ermüdung, Energie und der menschliche Motor', in P. Sarasin and J. Tanner (eds), *Physiologie und industrielle Gesellschaft. Studien zur Verwissenschaftlichung des Körpers im 19. und 20. Jahrhundert* (Frankfurt/Main: Suhrkamp, 1998), pp. 286–321; F. Vatin, *Le travail. Economie et physique 1780–1830* (Paris: Presses Universitaires de France, 1993). For an overview of the impacts of Rabinbach's work and other contributions, see M. R. Levin (ed.), *Cultures of Control* (Amsterdam: Harwood Academic Publishers, 2000).

18. Freud, 'Über die Allgemeinwirkung des Cocains', p. 103.

19. L. Daston and P. Galison, *Objektivität* (Frankfurt/Main: Suhrkamp, 2007), pp. 121–200.

20. Freud, 'Über Coca', p. 68.

21. Windgätter, '... with mathematic precision', pp. 2, 6.

22. Freud, 'Beitrag zur Kenntnis der Cocawirkung', pp. 92–4, 97–8.

23. For the meaning of numerical notation, see esp. Windgätter, '... with mathematic precision', pp. 6–7, 11.

24. On the normal and the pathological, see G. Canguilhem, *Le normal et le pathologique*, 2nd edn (Paris: Presses Universitaires de France, 1988). For a discussion of the normal and the pathological in Freud's work, see J. Link, *Versuch über den Normalismus. Wie Normalität produziert wird*, 2nd edn (Opladen: Westdeutscher Verlag, 1999), pp. 281–3.

25. Freud, 'Beitrag zur Kenntnis der Cocawirkung', p. 91 (trans. BB).

26. Ibid., p. 6.

27. Freud, 'Beitrag zur Kenntnis der Cocawirkung', pp. 96–7.

28. P. Felsch, 'Nach oben. Zur Topologie von Arbeit und Ermüdung im 19. Jahrhundert', in Brandstetter and Windgätter (eds), *Zeichen der Kraft*, pp. 141–69. Regarding the anthropology of work, see U. Bröckling and E. Horn (eds), *Anthropologie der Arbeit* (Tübingen: Gunter Narr Verlag, 2002).

29. N. N., 'Mit oder ohne Cocain?', *Pharmaceutische Zeitung*, 31 (1886), pp. 443–4 (trans. BB).

30. Cited in Windgätter, '... with mathematic precision', p. 9.

31. Ibid., p. 11.

32. D. Gugerli, 'Soziotechnische Evidenzen. Der "pictorial turn" als Chance für die Geschichtswissenschaft', *Traverse*, 3 (1999), pp. 131–59.

33. 'Die mit dem Ergographen angestellten Messungen haben auf die schönste Weise die Thatsachen bekräftigt, welche schon Empirik und die Beobachtung mit gewöhnlichen Mitteln lehrten.' See U. Mosso, 'Ueber die physiologische Wirkung des Cocains. Eine experimentelle Kritik der Arbeiten über den Mechanismus seiner Wirkungsweise', *Archiv für die gesammte Physiologie des Menschen und der Tiere*, 47 (1890), pp. 553–601, on p. 580 (trans. BB).

34. By the 1880s the scientific community had already become acquainted with the method of 'curves', thanks to the electrocardiogram. See C. Borck, 'Das Gehirn im Zeitbild. Populäre Neurophysiologie in der Weimarer Republik', in D. Gugerli and B. Orland (eds): *Ganz normale Bilder. Historische Beiträge zur visuellen Herstellung von Selbstverständlichkeit* (Zurich: Chronos, 2002), pp. 195–225 and S. de Chadarevian, 'Die 'Methode der Kurven' in der Physiologie zwischen 1850 und 1900', in Rheinberger and Hagner (eds), *Experimentalisierung des Lebens*, pp. 28–49. Later on, the graphical method became inter alia important in 'scientific management' as a means of determining the

'one best way'. See esp. P. Sarasin, 'Die Rationalisierung des Körpers. Über "Scientific Management" und "biologische Rationalisierung"', in M. Jeismann (ed.), *Obsessionen. Beherrschende Gedanken im wissenschaftlichen Zeitalter* (Frankfurt/Main: Suhrkamp, 1995), pp. 78–115, H. Mehrtens, 'Schmidts Schaufel (9,5 kg). Frederick W. Taylors Techniken des "Scientific Management"', in W. Sohn and H. Mehrtens (eds), *Normalität und Abweichung. Studien zur Theorie und Geschichte der Normalisierungsgesellschaft* (Opladen: Westdeutscher Verlag, 1999), pp. 85–106 and Windgätter, '... with mathematic precision', pp. 8–11.

35. Mosso, 'Ueber die physiologische Wirkung des Cocains', pp. 588, 592.
36. Ibid., p. 581.
37. See Windgätter, '... with mathematic precision', p. 7.

5 Stoff, 'Vital Regulators of Efficiency: The German Concept of *Wirkstoffe*, 1900–1950'

1. For a history of the concept of '*Wirkstoffe*', see H. Stoff, *Wirkstoffe. Eine Wissenschaftsgeschichte der Hormone, Vitamine und Enzyme, 1920–1970* (Stuttgart: Franz Steiner Verlag, 2012).
2. P. Huijnen, *De belofte van vitamins. Voedingsonderzoek tussen universiteit, industrie en overhead, 1918–1945* (Hilversum: Uitgeverij Verloren, 2011); C. Ratmoko, *Damit die Chemie stimmt. Die Anfänge der industriellen Herstellung von weiblichen und männlichen Sexualhormonen 1914–1938* (Zürich: Chronos, 2010); B. Bächi, *Vitamin C für alle! Pharmazeutische Produktion, Vermarktung und Gesundheitspolitik (1933–1953)* (Zürich: Chronos, 2009); R. Smith, 'The Emergence of Vitamins as Bio-Political Objects during World War I', *Studies in History and Philosophy of Biological and Biomedical Sciences. Part C*, 40:3 (2009), pp. 179–89; H. Kamminga, 'Vitamins and the Dynamics of Molecularization: Biochemistry, Policy and Industry in Britain, 1914–1939', in S. Chadarevian and H. Kamminga (eds), *Molecularizing Biology and Medicine: New Practices and Alliances 1910s–1970s* (Amsterdam: Taylor & Francis, 1998), pp. 83–105. R. D. Apple, *Vitamania: Vitamins in American Culture* (New Brunswick, NJ: Rutgers University Press, 1996).
3. For the concept of problematization, see M. Foucault, 'The Concern for Truth: Interview by François Ewald', in S. Lotringer (ed.), *Foucault Live: Collected Interviews, 1961–1984* (New York: Semiotext(e), 1996), pp. 455–73, on pp. 456–7. See also U. Klöppel, 'Foucaults Konzept der Problematisierungsweise und die Analyse diskursiver Transformationen', in A. Landwehr (ed.), *Diskursiver Wandel* (Wiesbaden: VS, 2010), pp. 255–63.
4. For citation of Culler, see J. Culler, *On Deconstruction. Theory and Criticism after Structuralism* (London, New York: Routledge, 1983), p. 86.
5. B. Latour, 'Networks, Societies, Spheres: Reflections of an Actor-Network Theorist', *International Journal of Communication*, 5 (2011), pp. 796–810, on p. 799.
6. A. Kühn, 'Hormonale Wirkungen in der Insektenentwicklung', *Forschungen und Fortschritte*, 13 (1937), pp. 49–50, on p. 49.
7. The literature on the life-reform movement is vast. For an overview, see F. Fritzen, *Gesünder leben. Die Lebensreformbewegung im 20. Jahrhundert* (Stuttgart: Steiner Verlag, 2006) and D. Kerbs and J. Reulecke (eds), *Handbuch der deutschen Reformbewegungen, 1880–1933* (Wuppertal: Hammer, 1998).

8.   T. Armstrong, *Modernism, Technology, and the Body: A Cultural Study* (Cambridge: Cambridge University Press, 1998).

9.   W. Roux, 'Ankündigung', *Archiv für Entwicklungsmechanik der Organismen*, 44 (1918), pp. 1–4, on pp. 1–3.

10. B. Bühler, *Lebende Körper. Biologisches und anthropologisches Wissen bei Rilke, Döblin und Jünger* (Würzburg: Königshausen & Neumann, 2004), pp. 47–59; R. Mocek, *Die werdende Form. Eine Geschichte der kausalen Morphologie* (Marburg: Basilisken Presse, 1998).

11. Roux, 'Ankündigung', pp. 1–2.

12. C.-E. Brown-Séquard, 'The Effects Produced on Man by Subcutaneous Injections of a Liquid Obtained from the Testicles of Animals', *Lancet*, 67 (1889), pp. 105–7.

13. G. R. Murray, 'Note on the Treatment of Myxoedema by Hypodermic Injections of an Extract of the Thyroid Gland of a Sheep', *British Medical Journal*, 2 (1891), pp. 796–7; C. Sengoopta, *The Most Secret Quintessence of Life. Sex, Glands, and Hormones, 1850–1950* (Chicago, IL, and London: University of Chicago Press, 2006), p. 37. For a history of organotherapy, see V. C. Medvei, *The History of Clinical Endocrinology. A Comprehensive Account of Endocrinology from Earliest Times to the Present Day* (Casterton Hall: Taylor & Francis, 1993), pp. 159–94; H. H. Simmer, 'Organotherapie mit Ovarialpräparaten in der Mitte der neunziger Jahre des 19. Jahrhunderts – Medizinische und pharmazeutische Probleme', in E. Hickel and G. Schröder (eds), *Neue Beiträge zur Arzneimittelgeschichte – Festschrift für Wolfgang Schneider zum 70. Geburtstag* (Stuttgart: WVG, 1991), pp. 229–65; M. Borell, 'Organotherapy, British Physiology and the Discovery of Internal Secretions', *Journal of the History of Biology*, 9 (1976), pp. 235–68.

14. H. Stoff, 'Degenerierte Nervenkörper und regenerierte Hormonkörper. Eine kurze Geschichte der Verbesserung des Menschen zu Beginn des 20. Jahrhunderts', *Historische Anthropologie*, 11:2 (2003), pp. 224–39.

15. C. Roberts, *Messengers of Sex: Hormones, Biomedicine and Feminism* (Cambridge: Cambridge University Press, 2007); A. Fausto-Sterling, *Sexing the Body: Gender Politics and the Construction of Sexuality* (New York: Basic Books, 2000), pp. 155–69; H. Stoff, 'Vermännlichung und Verweiblichung. Wissenschaftliche und utopische Experimente im frühen 20. Jahrhundert', in U. Pasero and F. Braun (eds), *Wahrnehmung und Herstellung von Geschlecht* (Opladen, Wiesbaden: Westdeutscher Verlag, 1999), pp. 47–62; C. Sengoopta, 'Glandular Politics: Experimental Biology, Clinical Medicine, and Homosexual Emancipation in Fin-de-Siècle Central Europe', *Isis*, 89 (1998), pp. 445–73. For rejuvenation, see Sengoopta, *Most Secret Quintessence*, pp. 69–115 and H. Stoff, *Ewige Jugend. Konzepte der Verjüngung vom späten 19. Jahrhundert bis ins Dritte Reich* (Köln, Weimar: Böhlau, 2004).

16. Steinach to Benjamin, 12 May 1926, New York Academy of Medicine, Steinach Papers; Stoff, *Ewige Jugend*, pp. 242–3.

17. W. Sneader, *Drug Discovery: A History* (Chichester: Wiley, 2005), pp. 151–3.

18. For monographs on the history of vitamins, see Huijnen, *De belofte van vitamins*; Bächi, *Vitamin C für alle!*; K. J. Carpenter, *Beriberi, White Rice, and Vitamin B: A Disease, a Cause, and a Cure* (Berkeley, CA: University of California Press, 2000); P. Werner (ed.), *Vitamine als Mythos. Dokumente zur Geschichte der Vitaminforschung* (Berlin: Akademie Verlag, 1998); Apple, *Vitamania*; K. J. Carpenter, *The History of Scurvy and Vitamin C* (Cambridge: Cambridge University Press, 1988). For monographs on the history of hormones, see L. Haller, *Cortison: Geschichte eines Hormons, 1900–1955* (Zürich: Chronos, 2012); Ratmoko, *Damit die Chemie stimmt*; Sengoopta, *The Most Secret Quintessence*; N.

Oudshoorn, *Beyond the Natural Body: An Archeology of Sex Hormones* (London, New York: Routledge, 1994).

19. Carpenter, *Beriberi, White Rice, and Vitamin B*, pp. 31–8.
20. U. Thoms, '"Vitaminfragen – kein Vitaminrummel?" Die deutsche Vitaminforschung in der ersten Hälfte des 20. Jahrhunderts und ihr Verhältnis zur Öffentlichkeit', in S. Nikolow and A. Schirrmacher (eds), *Wissenschaft und Öffentlichkeit als Ressource füreinander. Studien zur Wissenschaftsgeschichte im 20. Jahrhundert* (Frankfurt/Main: Campus, 2007), pp. 75–96, on p. 75.
21. Ibid., p. 77 and Medvei, *History of Clinical Endocrinology*, p. 189.
22. Fausto-Sterling, *Sexing the Body*; Armstrong, *Modernism*.
23. J.-P. Gaudillière, 'Introduction: Drug Trajectories', *Studies in History and Philosophy of Biological and Biomedical Sciences*, 36:4 (2005), pp. 603–11, on p. 603.
24. W. Straub, 'Vitamine, Hormone und Volksgesundheit', *Deutsche Forschung. Aus der Arbeit der Notgemeinschaft der Deutschen Wissenschaft*, 16 (1931), pp. 40–50, on, p. 40.
25. L. L. Okintschitz, 'Ueber die gegenseitigen Beziehungen einiger Drüsen mit innerer Sekretion', *Archiv für Gynäkologie*, 102 (1914), pp. 333–410, on p. 341; Sengoopta, *The Most Secret Quintessence*, p. 37.
26. C. Sengoopta, 'The Modern Ovary: Constructions, Meanings, Uses', *History of Science*, 38 (2000), pp. 425–88.
27. U. Meyer, '"Etwa ein Molekül wie das Morphin". Die Geschichte der Östrogene', *Pharmazie unserer Zeit*, 33 (2004), pp. 352–6, on p. 353.
28. B. Zondek, 'Das Ovarialhormon', *Forschungen und Fortschritte*, 3 (1927), pp. 13–14, on p. 13 and B. Zondek, 'Experimentelle Untersuchungen über den Wert der Organotherapie', *Archiv für Gynäkologie*, 117 (1922), pp. 19–26, on pp. 20, 23, 25.
29. E. Laqueur, 'Bewertung der Ovarialtherapie. Grundlagen', *Deutsche Medizinische Wochenschrift*, 58 (1932), pp. 959–64, on pp. 960–1.
30. A. Bencke, 'Der heutige Stand der Vitaminforschung', *Umschau*, 25 (1921), pp. 282–3, on p. 282.
31. C. Bonah, J.-P. Gaudillière, C. Gradmann and V. Hess, 'Standard Drugs and Drug Standards: A Comparative Historical Study of Pharmaceuticals in the 20th Century', in C. Bonah, C. Masutti, A. Rasmussen and J. Simon (eds), *Harmonizing Drugs: Standards in 20th-Century Pharmaceutical History* (Paris: Editions Glyphe, 2009), pp. 17–27.
32. I. Herzog, 'Die neuen Arzneimittel im Wechsel der letzten 40 Jahre', *Archiv der Pharmazie und Berichte der Deutschen Pharmazeutischen Gesellschaft*, 41 (1931), pp. 183–201, on pp. 195–6.
33. C. Auffray, 'The Difference between Inventions and Discoveries', in I. Wilczek (ed.), *Biomedical Research and Patenting: Ethical, Social, and Legal Aspects* (Baarn: European Platform for Patients' Organization, Science, and Industry, 1996), pp. 67–72.
34. F. Laquer, 'Chemie der Vitamine und Hormone. Nach dem gegenwärtigen Stand der Forschung', *Klinische Wochenschrift*, 9 (1930), pp. 97–102, on p. 97; R. Bud, *The Uses of Life: A History of Biotechnology* (Cambridge: Cambridge University Press, 1994), p. 45.
35. C. Oppenheimer, 'Chemie der Hormone und Vitamine. Ein Überblick über die neuesten Entdeckungen', *Deutsche Medizinische Wochenschrift*, 58 (1932), pp. 17–19, on p. 17.
36. D. J. Finney, 'The Principles of Biological Assay', *Supplement to the Journal of the Royal Statistical Society*, 9:1 (1947), pp. 46–91, on pp. 46–7.
37. C. Oppenheimer, 'Neue Gebiete und neue Forschungen der Hormonlehre', *Deutsche Medizinische Wochenschrift*, 58 (1932), pp. 1691–3, on p. 1692.

38. On holism, see D. Cantor (ed.), *Reinventing Hippocrates* (Aldershot: Ashgate, 2002); A. Harrington, *Reenchanted Science: Holism in German Culture from Wilhelm II to Hitler* (Princeton, NJ: Princeton University Press, 1999), and C. Lawrence and G. Weisz (ed.), *Greater than the Parts: Holism in Biomedicine, 1920–1950* (New York: Oxford University Press, 1998).

39. J. Kühnau, 'Die Wirkungsweise der Vitamine im Organismus', *Umschau*, 38 (1934), pp. 750–1, on p. 750; Straub, 'Vitamine, Hormone und Volksgesundheit', p. 40; M. Dohrn, 'Über Hormon', *Archiv der Pharmazie und Berichte der Deutschen Pharmazeutischen Gesellschaft*, 39 (1929), pp. 60–76, on p. 62 and H. E. Voss, 'Das Fluidum der Geschlechtlichkeit', *Umschau*, 31 (1927), pp. 1029–33, on p. 1030.

40. H. Stoff, '"Dann schon lieber Lebertran". Staatliche Rachitisprophylaxe und das wohl entwickelte Kind', in N. Eschenbruch, V. Balz, U. Klöppel and M. Hulverscheidt (eds), *Arzneimittel des 20. Jahrhunderts. Historische Skizzen von Lebertran bis Contergan* (Bielefeld: transcript Verlag, 2009), pp. 53–76.

41. Stoff, *Wirkstoffe*, pp. 59–60.

42. Ibid., pp. 123–38.

43. A. Butenandt, 'Entwicklungslinien in der künstlichen Darstellung natürlicher Steroidhormone', *Naturwissenschaften*, 30 (1942), pp. 4–17, on p. 6; J.-P. Gaudillière, 'Professional or Industrial Order? Patents, Biological Drugs, and Pharmaceutical Capitalism in Early Twentieth Century Germany', *History and Technology*, 24 (2008), pp. 107–33, on p. 119; J.-P. Gaudillière, 'Hormones at Risk: Cancer and the Medical Uses of Industrially-Produced Sex Steroids in Germany, 1930–1960', in T. Schlich and U. Tröhler (eds), *The Risks of Medical Innovation: Risk Perception and Assessment in Historical Context* (London/New York: Routledge, 2006), pp. 148–69, on pp. 150–1.

44. E. A. Schäfer, 'Address in Physiology: On Internal Secretions', *Lancet*, 73 (1895), pp. 321–4, on p. 324 and H.-J. Rheinberger, *An Epistemology of the Concrete: Twentieth-Century Histories of Life* (Durham, NC: Duke University Press, 2010), p. 46.

45. B. Steininger, 'Katalysator – Annäherung an einen Schlüsselbegriff des 20. Jahrhunderts', in E. Müller and F. Schmieder (eds), *Begriffsgeschichte der Naturwissenschaften. Zur historischen und kulturellen Dimension naturwissenschaftlicher Konzepte* (Berlin and New York: De Gruyter, 2008), pp. 53–71; I. Stengers, 'The Challenge of Complexity: Unfolding the Ethics of Science. In Memomoriam Ilya Prigogine', *E:CO*, 6 (2004), pp. 92–9, on p. 97.

46. C. Brandt, *Metapher und Experiment. Von der Virusforschung zum genetischen Code* (Göttingen: Wallstein, 2004), pp. 72–4.

47. R. E. Kohler, 'The Enzyme Theory and the Origin of Biochemistry', *Isis*, 64 (1973), pp. 181–96, on p. 189. For a history of enzymes, see J. S. Fruton, *Proteins, Enzymes, Genes: The Interplay of Chemistry and Biology* (New Haven, CT, and London: Yale University Press, 1999); A. Kornberg, *For the Love of Enzymes: The Odyssey of a Biochemist* (Cambridge: Cambridge University Press, 1989) and R. E. Kohler, *From Medical Chemistry to Biochemistry* (Cambridge: Cambridge University Press, 1982).

48. F. Cramer, 'Biochemical Correctness: Emil Fischer's Lock and Key Hypothesis, a Hundred Years After – An Essay', *Pharmaceutica Acta Helvetiae*, 69 (1995), pp. 193–203, on p. 195.

49. A. Mittasch, 'Über Katalyse und Katalysatoren in Chemie und Biologie', *Naturwissenschaften*, 24 (1936), pp. 770–7, 785–90, on pp. 773–4.

50. L. E. Kay, *Who Wrote the Book of Life? A History of the Genetic Code* (Stanford: Stanford University Press, 2000), pp. 38–72.

51. Oppenheimer, 'Chemie der Hormone und Vitamine', p. 19.

52. Mittasch, 'Über Katalyse und Katalysatoren', pp. 785–6.

53. J. Link, '"Normativ" oder "normal". Diskursgeschichtliches zur Sonderstellung der Industrienorm im Normalismus, mit einem Blick auf Walter Cannon', in W. Sohn and H. Mehrtens (eds), *Normalität und Abweichung. Studien zur Theorie und Geschichte der Normalisierungsgesellschaft* (Opladen: Westdeutscher Verlag, 1999), pp. 30–44.

54. G. Canguilhem, 'La formation du concept de régulation biologique', in G. Canguilhem, *Idéologie et rationalité dans l'histoire des sciences de la vie, Nouvelles études d'histoire et de philosophie des sciences* (Paris: Vrin, 1977), pp. 79–100, on p. 82.

55. Dohrn, 'Über Hormon', p. 60–1.

56. Druckrey to Butenandt, 21 September 1938, MPG-Archiv, III. Abt., Rep. 84/2, Nr. 1359.

57. H. Stieve, 'Abhängigkeit der Keimdrüsen vom Zustand des Gesamtkörpers und von der Umgebung', *Forschungen und Fortschritte*, 3 (1927), pp. 228–9 and V. Roelcke, '"Gesund ist der moderne Culturmensch keineswegs ...": Natur, Kultur und die Entstehung der Kategorie "Zivilisationskrankheit" im psychiatrischen Diskurs des 19. Jahrhunderts', in A. Barsch and P. M. Hejl (eds), *Menschenbilder. Zur Pluralisierung der Vorstellungen von der menschlichen Natur (1850–1914)* (Frankfurt/Main: Suhrkamp, 2000), pp. 215–36.

58. M. Kaasch, 'Sensation, Irrtum, Betrug? – Emil Abderhalden und die Geschichte der Abwehrfermente', *Acta historica Leopoldina*, 36 (2000), pp. 145–210.

59. R. Ammon and W. Dirscherl, *Fermente, Hormone und Vitamine und die Beziehungen dieser Stoffe zueinander* (Stuttgart: Thieme, 1938).

60. 'Rummel' can be accurately translated as 'hype'.

61. Bächi, *Vitamin C für alle!*

62. Clauberg to Himmler, 30 May 1942, Bundesarchiv Berlin, NS 19/1583.

63. Stoff, *Wirkstoffe*, pp. 240–5.

64. Bächi, *Vitamin C für alle!*

65. Stoff, *Wirkstoffe*, pp. 273–4.

66. R. B. Goldschmidt, *Theoretical Genetics*. 2nd edn (London: Cambridge University Press, 1958), p. 248; B. Gausemeier, *Natürliche Ordnungen und politische Allianzen: biologische und chemische Forschung an Kaiser-Wilhelm-Instituten 1933–1945* (Göttingen: Wallstein, 2005), pp. 94–122.

67. A. Butenandt, 'Neue Probleme der biologischen Chemie', *Angewandte Chemie*, 51 (1938), pp. 617–22, on p. 617.

68. H. J. Jusatz, 'Experimentelle Untersuchungen über den Synergismus der Vitamine', *Zeitschrift für die gesamte experimentelle Medizin*, 87 (1933), pp. 529–44, on p. 529.

69. W. Kollath, 'Natürliche Nahrung, wissenschaftliche Ernährungslehre und ihre Synthese', *Ernährung*, 7 (1942), pp. 7–14, on pp. 7, 10–14.

70. Ibid.; Kollath to Notgemeinschaft, 8 August 1934, Bundesarchiv Koblenz, R 73/12308.

71. W. Kollath, 'Neue Befunde und neue Begriffe in der Ernährungslehre', *Forschungen und Fortschritte*, 18 (1942), pp. 181–3 and W. Kollath, *Die Ordnung unserer Nahrung. Grundlagen einer dauerhaften Ernährungslehre* (Stuttgart: Hippokrates, 1942). See also U. Spiekermann, 'Der Naturwissenschaftler als Kulturwissenschaftler. Das Beispiel Werner Kollaths', in G. Neumann, A. Wierlacher and R. Wild (eds), *Essen und Lebensqualität: Natur- und kulturwissenschaftliche Perspektiven* (Frankfurt/Main: Campus, 2001), pp. 247–74.

72. G. A. Wagner, 'Bewertung der Ovarialtherapie. II. Vom Standpunkt des Gynäkologen', *Deutsche Medizinische Wochenschrift*, 58 (1932), pp. 964–68, on p. 976.

73. H. Schroeder, 'Kritische Bewertung der Vitamintherapie (Allgemeine Vitaminwirkung)', *Deutsche Medizinische Wochenschrift*, 68 (1942), pp. 833–5.

74. W. Stepp and H. Schroeder, 'C-Vitamin und klinische Erfahrung', *Deutsche Medizinische Wochenschrift*, 67 (1941), pp. 179, 208; A. Kuhn and H. Gerhard, 'Zur Kenntnis der Wirkung des natürlichen C-Vitamins', *Hippokrates* (1941), p. 1284.

75. W. Alter, 'Zur Bewertung der synthetischen Vitamine und Hormone', *Zeitschrift für Vitaminforschung*, 12 (1942), pp. 297–9; W. Alter, 'Vitamine und Vitaminoide', *Münchener Medizinische Wochenschrift*, 36 (1941), p. 779. See also Bächi, *Vitamin C für alle!*, pp. 102–25, 172–87.

76. Die Schriftleitung der Chemiker-Zeitung 1941.

77. Scheunert to Abderhalden, 24 September 1942, Akademiearchiv, Berlin, Historische Abteilung, Institut für Ernährung, Nr. 52 and Abderhalden to Scheunert, 4 August 1942, ibid., Nr. 54.

78. E. Abderhalden, 'Natürliche und künstliche Vitamine', *Chemiker-Zeitung*, 65 (1941), pp. 443–4, on p. 443.

79. K. Maier, 'Natürliche oder synthetische Vitamine?', *Chemiker-Zeitung*, 65 (1941), pp. 444–5.

80. W. Stepp and H. Schroeder, 'Gibt es Vitaminoide?', *Münchener Medizinische Wochenschrift*, 36 (1941), p. 1186.

81. Abderhalden, 'Natürliche und künstliche Vitamine', pp. 443–4.

82. Stoff, *Wirkstoffe*, pp. 261–4.

83. Ibid., pp. 280–322.

84. B. Wahrig, H. Stoff, A. von Schwerin and V. Balz, 'Precarious Matters: An Introduction', in V. Balz, A. von Schwerin, H. Stoff and B. Wahrig (eds), *Precarious Matters/Prekäre Stoffe: The History of Dangerous and Endangered Substances in the 19th and 20th Centuries*, Preprint series 356 (Berlin: Max Planck Institute for the History of Science, 2008), pp. 5–14 and Gaudillière, 'Hormones at Risk'.

85. A. Butenandt, 'Neuere Beiträge der biologischen Chemie zum Krebsproblem', *Angewandte Chemie*, 53 (1940), pp. 345–52, on p. 345 and Gaudillière, 'Hormones at Risk'.

86. H.-A. Schweigart, *Biologie der Vitalstoffe. 1. Band* (Dachau: Zauner, 1964), pp. 15, 17; Stoff, *Wirkstoffe*, pp. 286–7 and J. M. Melzer, *Vollwerternährung. Diätetik, Naturheilkunde, Nationalsozialismus, sozialer Anspruch* (Stuttgart: Steiner, 2003), p. 311.

6 Bergmann, 'The Detachability of Reproductive Cells: On Body Politics in Sperm and Egg Donation'

1. This essay is based on my PhD research on the practice of gamete donation in different European countries. The research was financed by a scholarship of the German Research Foundation (DFG) in the Research Training Group 'Gender as a Category of Knowledge' at the Humboldt University in Berlin and a fellowship at the Max Planck Institute for the History of Science. I am very grateful to Emily Ngubia Kuria, Carola Pohlen, Heiko Stoff and an anonymous reviewer for proofreading and commenting on versions of this essay and for their helpful comments and critique.

2. L. F. Hogle, *Recovering the Nation's Body: Cultural Memory, Medicine, and the Politics of Redemption* (New Brunswick, NJ: Rutgers University Press, 1999), p. 159.

3. A. C. Kramer and E. R. Goldmark, 'Postmortem Sperm Extraction', in J. P. Mulhall (ed.), *Fertility Preservation in Male Cancer Patients* (Cambridge and New York: Cambridge University Press, 2013), pp. 322–8.

4. G. Gallup, Jr, R. Burch and S. Platek, 'Does Semen Have Antidepressant Properties?', *Archives of Sexual Behavior*, 31:3 (2002), pp. 289–93.

5. K. S. Rajan, *Biocapital: The Constitution of Postgenomic Life* (Durham, NC: Duke University Press, 2006), p. 42.

6. Compare F. Vienne, 'Vom Samentier zur Samenzelle: Die Neudeutung der Zeugung im 19. Jahrhundert', *Berichte zur Wissenschaftsgeschichte*, 32:3 (2009), pp. 215–29.

7. Compare A. Clarke, *Disciplining Reproduction: Modernity, American Life Sciences, And 'The Problems of Sex'* (Berkeley, CA: University of California Press, 1998). See also C. Schreiber, *Natürlich künstliche Befruchtung? Eine Geschichte der In-Vitro-Fertilisation von 1878 bis 1950* (Göttingen: Vandenhoeck & Ruprecht, 2007).

8. For other perspectives, see C. Fortier, 'Blood, Sperm and the Embryo in Sunni Islam and in Mauritania: Milk Kinship, Descent and Medically Assisted Procreation', *Body & Society*, 13:3 (2007), pp. 15–36; M. C. Inhorn, 'Masturbation, Semen Collection and Men's IVF Experiences: Anxieties in the Muslim World', *Body & Society*, 13:3 (2007), pp. 37–53; S. M. Kahn, *Reproducing Jews: A Cultural Account of Assisted Reproduction in Israel* (Durham, NC: Duke University Press, 2000) and M. Strathern, *Reproducing the Future: Essays on Anthropology, Kinship and the New Reproductive Technologies* (New York: Routledge, 1992).

9. K. Nayernia, J. H. Lee, N. Drusenheimer, J. Nolte, G. Wulf, R. Dressel, G. Jörg and W. Engel, 'Derivation of Male Germ Cells from Bone Marrow Stem Cells', *Laboratory Investigation*, 86 (2006), pp. 654–63.

10. B. Latour, *We Have Never Been Modern* (Cambridge, MA: Harvard University Press, 1993), p. 21.

11. P. Lutjen, A. Trounson, J. Leeton, J. Findlay, C. Wood and P. Renou, 'The Establishment and Maintenance of Pregnancy Using *In Vitro* Fertilization and Embryo Donation in a Patient with Primary Ovarian Failure', *Nature*, 307 (1984), pp. 174–5.

12. M. Strathern, *After Nature: English Kinship in the Late Twentieth Century* (Cambridge: Cambridge University Press, 1992), p. 52.

13. Vienne, *Samentier*, pp. 216–7.

14. Ibid., pp. 220–4.

15. E. Martin, 'The Egg and the Sperm: How Science Has Constructed a Romance Based on Stereotypical Male–Female Roles', *Signs*, 16:3 (1991), pp. 485–501.

16. C. Haber, 'Anti-Aging Medicine: The History Life Extension and History: The Continual Search for the Fountain of Youth', *Journals of Gerontology Series A: Biological Sciences and Medical Sciences*, 59:6 (2004), pp. B515–22; see also H. Stoff, *Wirkstoffe. Eine Wissenschaftsgeschichte der Hormone, Vitamine und Enzyme, 1920–1970* (Stuttgart: Franz Steiner Verlag 2012), p. 36.

17. H. Landecker, *Culturing Life: How Cells Became Technologies* (Cambridge, MA and London: Harvard University Press, 2007), p. 226.

18. Ibid., p. 153.

19. S. Franklin and M. Lock, 'Animation and Cessation: The Remaking of Life and Death', in S. Franklin and M. Lock (eds), *Remaking Life & Death: Toward an Anthropology of the Biosciences* (Santa Fe, NM: School of American Research Press, 2001), pp. 3–22.

20. B. Bock von Wülfingen, *Genetisierung der Zeugung. Eine Diskurs- und Metaphernanalyse reproduktionsgenetischer Zukünfte* (Bielefeld: transcript, 2007), p. 325.

21. L. Mamo, *Queering Reproduction: Achieving Pregnancy in the Age of Technoscience* (Durham, NC: Duke University Press, 2007), p. 47. See also T. W. Laqueur, '"From Generation to Generation". Imaging Connectedness in the Age of Reproductive Tech-

nologies', in P. E. Brodwin (ed.), *Biotechnology and Culture: Bodies, Anxieties, Ethics* (Bloomington, IN: Indiana University Press, 2000), pp. 75–98, on p. 79.

22. C. M. Thompson, *Making Parents: The Ontological Choreography of Reproductive Technologies* (Cambridge, MA: The MIT Press, 2005), pp. 179–204; Mamo, *Queering Reproduction*, pp. 157–89; S. Hess, 'Flexible reproduktive Biografisierung: Zum Kinder-Machen im Zeitalter biopolitischer Möglichkeiten – von Zeugungsstreiks und Spielermentalitäten', *Berliner Blätter. Ethnographische und ethnologische Beiträge*, 42 (2007), pp. 109–23.

23. Commission Directive 2006/86/EC of 24 October 2006 implementing Directive 2004/23/EC of the European Parliament and of the Council as regards traceability requirements, notification of serious adverse reactions and events and certain technical requirements for the coding, processing, preservation, storage and distribution of human tissues and cells, at http://eur-lex.europa.eu/LexUriServ/LexUriServ.do?uri=O J:L:2006:294:0032:0050:en:pdf [accessed 22 May 2012].

24. These observations are based on my fieldwork notes taken during participant observation in an IVF clinic in Barcelona (2006, 2011), Prague (2007) and two sperm banks in Denmark (2007).

25. All names of research participants are pseudonyms.

26. Compare D. Kulick and M. Willson (eds), *Taboo: Sex, Identity, and Erotic Subjectivity in Anthropological Fieldwork* (London and New York: Routledge, 1995).

27. K. Wylie and A. A. Pacey, 'Using Erotica in Government-Funded Health Service Clinics', *Journal of Sexual Medicine*, 8:5 (2011), pp. 1261–5.

28. L. Williams, *Hard Core: Power, Pleasure, and the 'Frenzy of the Visible'* (Berkeley, CA: University of California Press, 1999).

29. P. B. Marshburn, M. Alanis, M. L. Matthews, R. Usadi, M. H. Papadakis, S. Kullstam and B. S. Hurst, 'A Short Period of Ejaculatory Abstinence before Intrauterine Insemination is Associated with Higher Pregnancy Rates', *Fertility and Sterility*, 93:1 (2010), pp. 286–8.

30. M. López-Teijón, F. García, O. Serra, M. Moragas, A. Rabanal, R. Olivares and J. G. Álvarez, 'Semen Quality in a Population of Volunteers from the Province of Barcelona', *Reproductive BioMedicine Online*, 15:4 (2007), pp. 434–44.

31. H. Pearson, 'Health Effects of Egg Donation May Take Decades to Emerge', *Nature*, 442:7103 (2006), pp. 607–8.

32. R. Almeling, 'Selling Genes, Selling Gender: Egg Agencies, Sperm Banks, and the Medical Market in Genetic Material', *American Sociological Review*, 72:3 (2007), pp. 319–40.

33. Martin, 'The Egg and the Sperm'.

34. Landecker, *Culturing Life*, p. 4.

35. Ibid., p. 67.

36. D. Mortimer and S. T. Mortimer, *Quality and Risk Management in the IVF Laboratory* (Cambridge: Cambridge University Press, 2008), pp. 94–100.

37. Results in egg freezing over the last years challenges these reservations, see M. C. Magli, M. Lappi, A. P. Ferraretti, A. Capoti, A. Ruberti and L. Gianaroli, 'Impact of Oocyte Cryopreservation on Embryo Development', *Fertility and Sterility*, 93:2 (2010), pp. 510–6. While during my fieldwork in Barcelona in autumn 2006 egg freezing was not practised, at my follow-up visit to the same clinic in 2011 the clinic had installed its own programme of oocyte vitrification.

38. G. C. Bowker and S. L. Star, *Sorting Things Out: Classifications and its Consequences* (Cambridge, MA: The MIT Press, 1999), pp. 15, 286.

39. WHO, *WHO Laboratory Manual for the Examination and Processing of Human Semen*, 5th edn (2010), at http://whqlibdoc.who.int/publications/2010/9789241547789_eng.pdf [accessed 28 February 2013], p. 226.
40. F. Vienne, 'Der Mann als medizinisches Wissensobjekt: Ein blinder Fleck in der Wissenschaftsgeschichte', *NTM Zeitschrift für Geschichte der Wissenschaften, Technik und Medizin*, 14 (2006), pp. 222–30, on p. 226.
41. A. F. Heinitz and R. Roscher, 'The Making of German Sperm: Überlegungen zum Zusammenhang von Spermakonservierung, Männlichkeiten und Nationalsozialismus', *Berliner Blätter. Ethnographische und ethnologische Beiträge*, 51 (2010), pp. 29–67, on p. 53.
42. B. Bartoov, A. Berkovitz, F. Eltes, A. Kogosovsky, A. Yagoda, H. Lederman, S. Artzi, M. Gross and Y. Barak, 'Pregnancy Rates are Higher with Intracytoplasmic Morphologically Selected Sperm Injection than with Conventional Intracytoplasmic Injection', *Fertility and Sterility*, 80:6 (2003), pp. 1413–19.
43. S. X. Y. Wang, 'The Past, Present, and Future of Embryo Selection in *In Vitro* Fertilization', *Yale Journal of Biology and Medicine*, 84:4 (2011), pp. 487–90.
44. M. Greuner, S. Winkler, B. Maxraths, M. Montag and H. Schmiady, 'Charakterisierung des morphologischen Entwicklungspotenzials von der Oozyte bis zum Embryo', *Journal of Reproductive Medicine and Endocrinology*, 9:1 (2012), pp. 13–9.
45. WHO, *Laboratory Manual*, p. 44.
46. B. C. Heng, 'Regulatory Safeguards Needed for the Travelling Foreign Egg Donor', *Human Reproduction*, 22:8 (2007), pp. 2350–2.
47. S. McKinnon, 'The Economies in Kinship and the Paternity of Culture: Origin Stories in Kinship Theory', in S. Franklin and S. McKinnon (eds), *Relative Values: Reconfiguring Kinship Studies* (Durham, NC: Duke University Press, 2001), pp. 277–301, on pp. 288–9.
48. S. Bergmann, 'Resemblance That Matters: On Transnational Anonymized Egg Donation in Two European IVF Clinics', in M. Knecht, M. Klotz and S. Beck (eds), *Reproductive Technologies as Global Form: Ethnographies of Knowledge, Practices, and Transnational Encounters* (Frankfurt/Main: Campus, 2012), pp. 331–55.
49. Interview with Jesper Lindberg, 12 April 2007.
50. Interview with Bjarke Mortensen, 11 April 2007.
51. Ibid.
52. Ibid.
53. D. M. Tober, 'Semen as Gift, Semen as Goods: Reproductive Workers and the Market in Altruism', *Body & Society*, 7:2–3 (2001), pp. 137–60, on p. 137.
54. Hogle, *Recovering the Nation's Body*, p. 146.
55. K. Haggerty and R. V. Ericson, 'The Surveillant Assemblage', *British Journal of Sociology*, 51:51 (2000), pp. 605–22.
56. Interview with Bjarke Mortensen, 11 April 2007.
57. Mamo, *Queering Reproduction*, p. 222.
58. While according to US regulations donation can be anonymous or open, most European countries favour only one possibility: in the UK and Sweden regulation opts for disclosure and only open donor systems, in Spain and the Czech Republic only anonymous donation is permitted (see ESHRE website for detailed information for every country, at www.eshre.eu/ESHRE/English/Guidelines-Legal/Legal-documentation/page.aspx/145 [accessed 22 May 2012]).

59. S. W. Adrian, 'Sperm Stories: Policies and Practices of Sperm Banking in Denmark and Sweden', *European Journal of Women's Studies*, 17:4 (2010), pp. 393–411, on p. 401. However, these marketing strategies are changing. Other research on Danish sperm banks shows how these Viking images are becoming much more multicultural, especially for the increasing number of US customers. Compare C. Krøløkke, 'Click a Donor: Viking Masculinity on the Line', *Journal of Consumer Culture*, 9:1 (2009), pp. 7–30.

60. In most European countries law or medical directives regulate egg donation, therefore in most cases only reimbursement is allowed. Nevertheless, forms of reimbursements differ significantly (e.g. in the UK the maximum compensation rate for one cycle is £250; in most Spanish private clinics egg donors receive €900).

61. A. B. Weiner, *Inalienable Possessions: The Paradox of Keeping-while-Giving* (Berkeley, CA: University of California Press, 1992).

62. See K. Marx, *Das Kapital, Marx-Engels-Werke*, ed. H. Scheibler, vol. 23 (Berlin: Dietz, 1986), pp. 54–5.

63. J. A. Grifo and N. Noyes, 'Delivery Rate Using Cryopreserved Oocytes is Comparable to Conventional in Vitro Fertilization Using Fresh Oocytes: Potential Fertility Preservation for Female Cancer Patients', *Fertility and Sterility*, 93:2 (2010), pp. 391–6.

64. Californian sperm banks also promote deposits for groups with high risk-levels (like soldiers) to achieve future reproductive goals.

65. D. Dowling-Lacey, et al, 'Live Birth from a Frozen-Thawed Pronuclear Stage Embryo Almost 20 Years after its Cryopreservation', *Fertility and Sterility*, 95:3 (2011), pp. 1120–1.

66. M. Nahman, 'Reverse Traffic: Intersecting Inequalities in Human Egg Donation', *Reproductive BioMedicine Online*, 23:5 (2011), pp. 626–33.

67. Compare K. R. Daniels, R. Curson and G. M. Lewis, 'Semen Donor Recruitment: A Study of Donors in Two Clinics', *Human Reproduction*, 11:4 (1996), pp. 746–51; C. Murray and S. Golombok, 'Oocyte and Semen Donation: A Survey of UK Licensed Centres', *Human Reproduction*, 15:10 (2000), pp. 2133–9.

68. M. Konrad, 'Ova Donation and Symbols of Substance: Some Variations on the Theme of Sex, Gender and the Partible Body', *Journal of the Royal Anthropological Institute*, 4:1 (1998), pp. 643–67, on p. 655.

69. P. Rivière, 'Unscrambling Parenthood: The Warnock Report', *Anthropology Today*, 4 (1985), pp. 2–7.

70. Strathern, *After Nature*, p. 40.

71. Gesetz zum Schutz von Embryonen (Embryonenschutzgesetz). 13 December 1990, at www.gesetze-im-internet.de/eschg/index.html [accessed 22 May 2012].

72. A. Hieb, *Die gespaltene Mutterschaft im Spiegel des deutschen Verfassungsrechts. Die verfassungsrechtliche Zulässigkeit reproduktionsmedizinischer Verfahren zur Überwindung weiblicher Unfruchtbarkeit. Ein Beitrag zum Recht auf Fortpflanzung* (Berlin: Logos, 2005).

73. Landecker, *Culturing Life*, p. 227.

74. Konrad, 'Ova Donation and Symbols of Substance'; Martin, 'The Egg and the Sperm'.

75. M. Konrad, *Nameless Relations: Anonimity, Melanesia and Reproductive Gift Exchange between British Ova Donors and Recipients* (New York and Oxford: Berghahn Books, 2005), p. 130.

76. M. Lock, 'The Alienation of Body Tissue and the Biopolitics of Immortalized Cell Lines', in N. Scheper-Hughes and L. Wacquant (eds), *Commodifying Bodies* (London: Sage, 2003), pp. 63–92, on p. 71.

77. However, in the realm of substituting human tissue and substance, questions of kinship, ownership rights and patents are contiguous: The case of *John Moore* v. *The State of California* about the proprietorship of his cell line illustrates forms of personalization of bodily detached material. C. Hayden, 'Taking as Giving: Bioscience, Exchange, and the Politics of Benefit-Sharing', *Social Studies of Science*, 37:5 (2007), pp. 729–58.

78. E. Porqueres i Gené and J. Wilgaux, 'Incest, Embodiment, Genes and Kinship', in J. Edwards and C. Salazar (eds), *European Kinship in an Age of Biotechnology* (New York and Oxford: Berghahn, 2009), pp. 112–27.

79. Gallup, Burch and Platek, 'Antidepressant Properties'.

80. S. Franklin, *Embodied Progress: A Cultural Account of Assisted Conception* (London, New York: Routledge, 1997), p. 103.

81. I. Kopytoff, 'The Cultural Biography of Things: Commoditization as Process', in A. Appadurai (ed.), *The Social Life of Things: Commodities in Cultural Perspective* (Cambridge: Cambridge University Press, 1986), pp. 64–91, on p. 86.

7 Chauveau, 'Human Tissues and Organs: Standardization and "Commodification" of the Human Body'

1. S. Chauveau, 'From Human Blood to Blood Products. Blood Collection and Blood Derived Products in France after 1950: A Third Way of Standardising Therapeutic Agents?', in C. Bonah, C. Masutti, A. Rasmussen and J. Simon (eds), *Harmonizing Drugs: Standards in 20th-Century Pharmaceutical History* (Paris: Editions Glyphe, 2009), pp. 181–201.

2. S. J. Youngner, M. W. Anderson and R. Schapiro (eds), *Transplanting Human Tissue: Ethics, Policy and Practice* (Oxford: Oxford University Press, 2004); Y. Eglert (ed.), *Organ and Tissue Transplantation in the European Union: Management of Difficulties and Health Risks Linked to Donors* (Dordrecht: Martinus Nijhoff Publishers, 1995).

3. C. Gradmann, 'Commentary and Concluding Remarks at the Braunschweig Conference', 27 March 2010. For a definition of 'trust', see K. Zachmann and P. Østby, 'Food, Technology, and Trust: An Introduction', *History and Technology*, 27 (2011), pp. 1–10.

4. C. Waldby and R. Mitchell, *Tissue Economies: Blood Organs and Cell Lines in Late Capitalism* (Durham, NC: Duke University Press, 2006).

5. N. Scheper-Hughes and L. Wacquant (eds), *Commodifying Bodies* (London: Sage Publications, 2002).

6. A. Wahlberg and S. Bauer, 'Introduction: Categories of Life', in S. Bauer and A. Wahlberg (eds), *Contested Categories: Life Sciences in Society* (London: Ashgate, 2009), pp. 7–8.

7. P. Steiner, *La transplantation d'organes. Un commerce nouveau entre les humains* (Paris: Gallimard, 2010).

8. R. G. Simmons, S. Klein Marine and R. L. Simmons (eds), *Gift of Life: The Effect of Organ Transplantation on Individual, Family and Social Dynamics* (Chichester: John Wiley & Sons, 1977).

9. M. J. Radin, *Contested Commodities: The Trouble with Trade in Sex, Children, Body Parts and Other Things* (Cambridge, MA: Harvard University Press, 2001).

10. L. A. Sharp, *Strange Harvest: Organ Transplants, Denatured Bodies and the Transformed Self* (Berkeley, CA: University of California Press, 2006), p. 15.

11. R. Fox and J. P. Swazey, *Spare Parts: Organ Replacement in American Society* (New York: Oxford University Press, 1992).

12. P. Mollaret and M. Goulon, 'Le coma dépassé. Mémoire préliminaire', *Revue neurologique*, 101:1 (1959), pp. 3–15.
13. Circulaire n° 67 du 24 avril 1968 relative aux autopsies et aux prélèvements, dite 'circulaire Jeanneney', *Bulletin Officiel du Ministère de la Santé*, 24 April 1968.
14. R. D. Truog and F. G. Miller, 'The Dead Donor Rule and Organ Transplantation', *New England Journal of Medicine*, 359:7 (2008), pp. 674–5; F. G. Miller and R. D. Truog, *Death, Dying, and Organ Transplantation: Reconstructing Medical Ethics at the End of Life* (Oxford: Oxford University Press, 2011).
15. M. Morioka, 'Bioethics and Japanese Culture: Brain Death, Patients' Rights and Cultural Factors', *Eubios Journal of Asian and International Bioethics*, 5 (1997), pp. 87–90.
16. M. Lock, *Twice Dead: Organ Transplants and the Reinvention of Death* (Berkeley, CA: University of California Press, 2002), p. 8.
17. Steiner, *La transplantation d'organes*, pp. 37–49; P. Steiner, 'Mort encéphalique et don d'organes: la "productivisation" de la mort', *Quaderni*, 62 (2006), pp. 69–80.
18. Chauveau, 'From Human Blood to Blood Products'.
19. Comité de transparence, Organes et Tissus, Rapport d'activité, février 1993, Archives de l'Assistance Publique-Hôpitaux de Paris (hereafter Archives de l'AP-HP), 620 W-3-1.
20. IGAS, *Rapport d'étape sur les banques de tissus d'origine humaine* (Paris, 1993).
21. Création d'une commission de la transplantation, arrêté du 23 mars 1989 et lettre d'information de Jean Choussat, Rapport de la Direction des Affaires Médicales, mars 1989, Archives de l'AP-HP, 620 W-2-4-A. Du.
22. Compte rendu de la réunion du groupe de travail 'tissus', 8 avril 1992, Archives de l'AP-HP, 620 W-2-4-A.
23. Compte-rendu de la séance du Comité d'Ethique des Hôpitaux de Paris, 16 septembre 1991, Archives de l'AP-HP, 620 W-2-4-A.
24. L. F. Hogle, 'Standardization across Non-Standard Domains: The Case of Organ Procurement', *Science, Technology and Human Values*, 20:4 (1995), pp. 482–500.
25. K. Wailoo, J. Livingston and P. Guarnaccia (eds), *A Death Retold: Jesica Santillan, The Bungled Transplant and Paradoxes of Medical Citizenship* (Chapel Hill, NC: The University of North Carolina Press, 2006).
26. I. Braun and B. Joerges, 'How to Recombine Large Systems: The Case of European Organ Transplantation', in J. Summerton (ed.), *Changing Large Technical Systems* (Boulder, CO: Westview Press, 1994), pp. 25–52; N. Machado, *Using the Bodies of the Dead: Legal, Ethical and Organisational Dimensions of Organ Transplantation* (Aldershot: Ashgate, 1998).
27. K. Healy, *Last Best Gifts: Altruism and the Market for Human Blood and Organs* (Chicago, IL: University of Chicago Press, 2006), pp. 47–9.
28. S. Chauveau, 'Le monde associatif face à l'hôpital: France-Transplant', *Entreprises et Histoire*, 56 (2009), pp. 145–8. The law on associations promulgated in 1901 represents a legal milestone of the French Republic: it provides a legal framework primarily for religious activities, but also for a variety of non-profit associations such as trade unions, sports clubs, alumni organizations, charities, as well as health-related associations, such as patients' rights groups or blood and organ donation and collection agencies (these agencies were disbanded in 1992–3).
29. C. Boileau, *Dans le dédale du don d'organes. Le cheminement de l'ethnologue* (Paris: Editions des Archives Contemporaines, 2002); F. Paterson, 'Solliciter l'inconcevable ou le consentement des morts. Prélèvement d'organes, formes de circulation des greffons et normes de compétence', *Sciences sociales et santé*, 15:1 (1997), pp. 35–74.
30. Ibid., p. 47.

31. Boileau, *Dans le dédale*; Healy, *Last Best Gifts*, pp. 23–42; Fox and Swazey, *Spare Parts*.

32. Healy, *Last Best Gifts*, p. 15; M. Sque and S. A. Payne, 'Gift Exchange Theory: A Critique in Relation to Organ Transplantation', *Journal of Advanced Nursing*, 19 (1994), pp. 45–51.

33. Direction des Affaires Médicales, Dossiers relatifs aux activités de greffes, rapports de l'Inspection Générale des Affaires Sociales, Comité de transparence et Commission de la transplantation, dates extrêmes, 1970–1993, Archives de l'Assistance Publique Hôpitaux de Paris.

34. IGAS, *Rapport sur les transplantations d'organes en France* (Paris: 1992).

35. Simmons, Klein Marine and Simmons (eds), *Gift of Life*.

36. S. Chauveau, 'L'épreuve du vivant: santé publique et marché en France depuis les années 1970', *Le Mouvement Social*, 229 (2009), pp. 79–101.

37. A. Tesnière, *Les yeux de Christophe. L'affaire d'Amiens* (Paris: Editions du Rocher, 1993); S. Chauveau, *L'affaire du sang contaminé (1983–2003)* (Paris: Les Belles Lettres, 2011); Paterson, 'Solliciter l'inconcevable', pp. 47–9.

38. Wahlberg and Bauer, 'Introduction: Categories of Life', p. 4.

39. Sharp, *Strange Harvest*, p. 14.

40. P. Pharo, 'Introduction: justice et respect', *Sciences sociales et santé*, 15:1 (1997), pp. 9–19.

41. Compte-rendu de la réunion avec les coordonnateurs des centres de prélèvement, 7 October 1992, Archives de l'AP-HP, 620 W-3.

42. For more information, see: http://optn.transplant.hrsa.gov/optn/ [accessed 30 May 2012].

43. M.-J. Festle, 'Enemies or Allies? The Organ Transplant Medical Community, the Federal Government and the Public in the United States, 1967–2000', *Journal of the History of Medicine and Allied Sciences*, 65:1 (2010), pp. 48–80.

44. Al Gore's testimony, quoted in Festle, 'Enemies of Allies?', p. 59.

45. IGAS, *Rapport sur la transplantation rénale à l'hôpital Necker*, January 1991, Archives de l'AP-HP, 620 W-1-5-B.

46. E. Hirsch and M. Guerrier, 'Transplantation: la répartition des organes', in E. Hirsch (ed.), *Ethique, médecine et société. Comprendre, réfléchir, décider* (Paris: Vuibert, 2007), pp. 768–76.

47. For an overview of public debates, see www.etatsgenerauxdelabioethique.fr/ [accessed 28 October 2012].

48. Festle, 'Enemies or Allies?'

49. R. Rhodes, 'Justice in Organ Allocation', in Wailoo, Livingston and Guarnaccia (eds), *A Death Retold*, pp. 158–79; J. A. Gross, 'Playing with Matches without Getting Burned: Public Confidence in Organ Allocation', ibid., pp. 180–204.

50. M. J. Cherry, *Kidney for Sale by Owner: Human, Organs, Transplantation and the Market* (Washington, DC: Georgetown University Press, 2005).

51. Hogle, 'Standardization'.

52. Healy, *Last Best Gifts*.

53. D. Thouvenin, 'L'obtention des organes: le don comme finalité et le prélèvement comme modalité', in B. Feuillet-Le Mintier (ed.), *Les lois 'bioéthique' à l'épreuve des faits: réalités et perspectives* (Paris: PUF, 1999), pp. 77–131.

54. C. Waldby, 'Stem Cells, Tissue Cultures and the Production of Biovalue', *Health: An Interdisciplinary Journal for the Social Study of Health, Illness and Medicine*, 6:3 (2002), pp. 305–23, on p. 309.

55. D. Fassin, 'Les économies morales revisitées', *Annales HSS*, 64:6 (2009), pp. 1237–66.

56. N. Rose, *The Politics of Life Itself: Biomedicine, Power and Subjectivity in the Twenty-First Century* (Princeton, NJ: Princeton University Press, 2007).

8 Huijnen, 'The Science of Measuring Vitamins: Quality Control and Competition in the Dutch Vitamin Industry before the Second World War'

1. H. G. K. Westenbrink, 'Bij het vijfentwintigjarig doctoraat van prof. B.C.P. Jansen 1912 – 10 juli – 1937', *Chemisch Weekblad*, 34 (1937), pp. 471–7, on p. 471 (trans. PH).

2. H. Kamminga, 'Vitamins and the Dynamics of Molecularization: Biochemistry, Policy and Industry in Britain, 1914–1939', in S. de Chadarevian and H. Kamminga (eds), *Molecularizing Biology and Medicine: New Practices and Alliances 1910s–1970s* (Amsterdam: Harwood Academic Publishers, 1998), pp. 78–98.

3. S. M. Horrocks, 'The Business of Vitamins: Nutrition Science and the Food Industry in Inter-War Britain', in H. Kamminga and A. Cunningham (eds), *The Science and Culture of Nutrition, 1840–1940* (Amsterdam and Atlanta, GA: Rodopi Bv Divisions, 1995), pp. 235–58; S. M. Horrocks, 'Nutrition Science and the Food and Pharmaceutical Industries in Inter-War Britain', in D. Smith (ed.), *Nutrition in Britain: Science, Scientists and Politics in the Twentieth Century* (London and New York: Routledge, 1997), pp. 53–74.

4. R. D. Apple, *Vitamania. Vitamins in American Culture* (New Brunswick, NJ: Rutgers University Press, 1996); B. Bächi, *Vitamin C für alle! Pharmazeutische Produktion, Vermarktung und Gesundheitspolitik (1933–1953)* (Zürich: Chronos Verlag, 2009); P. Werner (ed.), *Vitamine als Mythos. Dokumente zur Geschichte der Vitaminforschung* (Berlin: Akademie Verlag, 1998); H. Stoff, '"Dann schon lieber Lebertran". Staatliche Rachitisprophylaxe und das wohl entwickelte Kind', in N. Eschenbruch, V. Balz, U. Klöppel and M. Hulverscheidt (eds), *Arzneimittel des 20. Jahrhunderts. Historische Skizzen von Lebertran bis Contergan* (Bielefeld: transcript Verlag, 2009), pp. 53–76; H. Stoff, *Wirkstoffe. Eine Wissenschaftsgeschichte der Hormone, Vitamine und Enzyme, 1920–1970* (Stuttgart: Franz Steiner Verlag, 2012). See also Kamminga and Cunningham (eds), *Science and Culture of Nutrition*; Smith (ed.), *Nutrition in Britain*; A. Fenton (ed.), *Order and Disorder: The Health Implications of Eating and Drinking in the Nineteenth and Twentieth Centuries* (Edinburgh: Tuckwell Press, 2000).

5. Bächi, for example, writes that 'scientific knowledge could be generated' only after vitamin C had been purified. Only then, he argues, was it 'possible to determine the exact quantities to be used in experiments'. Bächi, *Vitamin C für alle* (trans. PH).

6. J.-P. Gaudillière, 'Introduction: Drug Trajectories', *Studies in History and Philosophy of Biological and Biomedical Sciences*, 36:4 (2005), pp. 603–11, on p. 606.

7. K. J. Carpenter, *Beriberi, White Rice, and Vitamin B: A Disease, a Cause, and a Cure* (Berkeley, CA: University of California Press, 2000), pp. 98–100.

8. E. V. McCollum, *The Newer Knowledge of Nutrition: The Use of Food for the Preservation of Vitality and Health* (New York: The MacMillan Company, 1918).

9. Carpenter, *Beriberi, White Rice, and Vitamin B*, pp. 105–9.

10. See, for example, the highly readable account on the early discoveries of vitamins by K. J. Carpenter, 'The Nobel Prize and the Discovery of Vitamins', at http://nobelprize.org/ nobel_prizes/medicine/articles/carpenter [accessed 28 March 2011].

11. Ibid.; G. Wolf, 'The Discovery of Vitamin D: The Contribution of Adolf Windaus', *Journal of Nutrition*, 134 (2004), pp. 1299–302.
12. R. Bud, 'Upheaval in the Moral Economy of Science? Patenting, Teamwork, and the World War II Experience of Penicillin', *History and Technology*, 24 (2008), pp. 173–90, on pp. 176–8. See also R. D. Apple, 'Patenting University Research: Harry Steenbock and the Wisconsin Alumni Research Foundation', *Isis*, 80 (1989), pp. 374–94.
13. M. Tausk, *Organon. De geschiedenis van een bijzondere Nederlandse onderneming* (Nijmegen: Dekker & Van de Vegt, 1978), p. 9.
14. N. Oudshoorn, 'United We Stand: The Pharmaceutical Industry, Laboratory, and Clinic in the Development of Sex Hormones into Scientific Drugs, 1920–1940', *Science, Technology, & Human Values*, 18 (1993), pp. 5–24.
15. Tausk, *Organon*, pp. 17–33.
16. Ibid., p. 46.
17. B. C. P. Jansen, 'Over de voorziening der bevolking met antirhachitis-vitamine', *Nederlandsch Tijdschrift voor Geneeskunde*, 79 (1935), pp. 1674–6, on p. 1675; E. Gorter and J. J. Soer, 'Rhachitis-behandeling met ultra-violetlicht', *Nederlandsch Tijdschrift voor Geneeskunde*, 74 (1930), pp. 4310–15, on p. 4315; O. A. Driessen, E. Gorter, J. Haverschmidt and J. J. Soer, 'Rhachitisbehandeling met D-vitamine, I', *Nederlandsch Tijdschrift voor Geneeskunde*, 74 (1930), pp. 4205–18.
18. Stoff, 'Dann schon lieber Lebertran', p. 67.
19. See, for example, L. K. Wolff to Organon, 30 December 1929, Organon Company Archives [hereafter: OCA], correspondence with the Hygienics Laboratory Utrecht, HA 25–6. This practice would remain of great significance for Organon. This becomes clear when looking at the soaring Davitamon sales during the first few months of the German occupation of the Netherlands in the summer of 1940. Organon saw no other option to meet the sudden increase in demand than to break with its authorization rule. Tausk, as scientific head of Organon, described this course of action as 'highly unpleasant' and 'an intentional transgressing of my competences'. H. W. Julius, Wolff's successor, understood Organon's position. Nonetheless, he reserved the right to withdraw the batches from the market if the tests he was still planning to conduct called for it. See the correspondence between H. W. Julius and Organon, 7 and 12 August and 9 September 1940, OCA, HA 35–2.
20. See, for example, Organon to Wolff, 22 April 1930, OCA, HA 26–2 and E. C. van Leersum, 'Over het aantoonen van vitamines, in het bijzonder de vitamines A en D', *Nederlandsch Tijdschrift voor Geneeskunde*, 73 (1929), pp. 3997–4009.
21. R. M. Sprenger, *'Ten behoeve van de gezondheid van mens, dier en plant'. De geschiedenis van Duphar 1930–1980* (Weesp: Solvay Duphar B.V., 1992), p. 8.
22. Ibid. p. 10; Driessen, et al., 'Rhachitisbehandeling met D-vitamine', p. 4205.
23. Sprenger, *'Ten behoeve'*, p. 10. For the connection between Gorter and Philips-Van Houten, see Wolff to Organon, 12 February 1931, OCA, HA 26–5.
24. Driessen, et al., 'Rhachitisbehandeling met D-vitamine', p. 4205.
25. Ibid., p. 4207.
26. M. Tausk, 'Rhachitisbehandeling met D-vitamine', *Nederlandsch Tijdschrift voor Geneeskunde*, 74 (1930), pp. 5643–4.
27. E. Gorter, 'Rhachitisbestrijding', *Nederlandsch Tijdschrift voor Geneeskunde*, 74 (1939), p. 4953.
28. Tausk, 'Rhachitisbehandeling met D-vitamine', p. 5643.

29. J. W. R. Everse and J. van Niekerk, 'Het standaardiseren van vitamine-D-praeparaten', *Nederlandsch Tijdschrift voor Geneeskunde*, 75 (1931), pp. 1101–7.
30. Ibid., p. 1101.
31. Tausk, 'Rhachitisbehandeling met D-vitamine', p. 5644.
32. League of Nations Health Organization, *Vitamin Standards: Report of the Permanent Commission on Biological Standardisation* (London: George Allen & Unwin Ltd., 1931); see also, for example, 'Vitamin Standards and Units: Recommendations of the London Conference', *British Medical Journal*, 7 November (1931), pp. 862–3.
33. Wolff to J. W. R. Everse and J. van Niekerk, 19 March 1931, OCA, HA 26–5.
34. See, from many examples, K. Grandin, N. Wormbs and S. Widmalm (eds), *The Science-Industry Nexus: History, Policy, Implications* (Sagamore Beach: Science History Publications, 2002) and J. P. Gaudillière and I. Löwy (eds), *The Invisible Industrialist: Manufacturers and the Production of Scientific Knowledge* (Basingstoke: Palgrave MacMillan, 1998).
35. Oudshoorn, 'United We Stand'.
36. Ibid., p. 21.
37. Ibid., p. 20.
38. Ibid., p. 21.
39. Organon to Wolff, 29 January 1937, OCA, HA 31–4.
40. Wolff to Organon, 31 January 1937, OCA, HA 31–4.
41. Ibid.
42. Merck to Wolff, 25 February 1937, OCA, HA 31–4.
43. Apple, *Vitamania*, p. 44; P. Huijnen, *De belofte van vitamins. Voedingsonderzoek tussen universiteit, industrie en overhead, 1918–1945* (Hilversum: Uitgeverij Verloren, 2011), p. 55; P. Huijnen, 'Het wondermiddel van professor Buytendijk. Het vitaminepreparaat Eviunis en de risico's van wetenschappelijke voorspraak', *Studium*, 3 (2010), pp. 155–69.
44. Horrocks, 'The Business of Vitamins', pp. 235–6.
45. E. Gorter, *Engelsche ziekte* (Rotterdam: Nijgh & Van Ditmar, 1932), p. 35.
46. Apple, *Vitamania*, p. 13.
47. Julius to Organon, 21 May 1940, OCA, HA 35–1.

9 Thoms, 'The German Pharmaceutical Industry and the Standardization of Insulin before the Second World War'

1. See, for example, M. Bliss, *The Discovery of Insulin* (Chicago, IL: Chicago University Press, 2007); for the German context, see P. Dilg, 'Zur Frühgeschichte der industriellen Insulin-Herstellung in Deutschland', *Pharmazie in unserer Zeit*, 30 (2001), pp. 10–15 and K. Federlin, *75 Jahre Insulin Hoechst. Vom Naturstoff zum Designerprotein* (Frankfurt/Main: Hoechst, 1999).
2. C. Sinding, 'Making the Unit of Insulin: Standards, Clinical Work, and Industry, 1920–1925', *Bulletin of the History of Medicine*, 76 (2002), pp. 231–70.
3. N. N., 'Das neue Heilmittel Insulin', *Rhein-Ruhr-Zeitung*, Duisburg, no. 67, 13 February 1924, Bayer Archive, Leverkusen (hereafter BAL), Einzelne Produkte: Insulin, Nr. 166/08 (trans. UT).
4. C. Lewin, 'Diabetesbehandlung mit Insulin. Kongress für innere Medizin', *Berliner Tageblatt*, no. 197, 25 April 1924, BAL, Einzelne Produkte: Insulin, Nr. 116/08 (trans. UT).

5. See, for example, Werner Grohnert to Prof. Bartung, 9 May 1923, Archive of the University of Toronto (hereafter AUT), A1982–0001/005/10. I owe special thanks to Tricia Close-Koenig for organizing copies of these sources for me.
6. See the collection at BAL, Einzelne Produkte: Insulin, Nr. 166/08.
7. Chris Feudtner has nicely described how this system was developed at the clinic of the diabetes specialist, Elliot Joslin. C. Feudtner, *Bittersweet: Diabetes, Insulin and the Transformation of Illness* (Chapel Hill, NC: The University of North Carolina Press, 2003).
8. D. P. Carpenter, *Regulation and Power: Organizational Image and Pharmaceutical Regulation at the FDA* (Princeton, NJ: Princeton University Press, 2010).
9. Federlin, *75 Jahre Insulin Hoechst*, p. 19.
10. M. Bliss, *The Discovery of Insulin* (Chicago, IL: Chicago University Press, 1984).
11. F. G. Banting, C. H. Best, J. P. Collip, W. B. Campbell and A. A. Fletcher, 'Pancreatic Extracts in the Treatment of Diabetes Mellitus. Preliminary Report', *Journal of the Canadian Medical Association Journal*, 2 (1922), pp. 141–6; Bliss, *Discovery of Insulin*.
12. Over time the influence of industry increased, as more industrial representatives and a patent lawyer became involved.
13. Sinding, 'Making the Unit', p. 240. For Lilly's history, see J. P. Swann, 'Insulin: A Case Study in the Emergence of Collaborative Pharmacomedical Research', *Pharmacy in History*, 28 (1986), pp. 2–13, 65–74; J. H. Madison, 'Manufacturing Pharmaceuticals: Eli Lilly and Company, 1876–1948', *Business and Economic History, Second Series*, 18 (1989), pp. 72–8; J. H. Madison, *Eli Lilly: A Life 1885–1977* (Indianapolis, IN: Indiana Historical Society, 1989).
14. Sinding, 'Making the Unit', p. 240.
15. Ibid., p. 243.
16. H. M. Marks, 'Trust and Mistrust in the Marketplace. Statistics and Clinical Research, 1945–1960', *History of Science*, 38 (2000), pp. 343–55.
17. The standard unit used by the Danish researcher Krogh, for example, relied on mice. Compare Sinding, 'Making the Unit', p. 247.
18. See the different regimes in D. Oyen, E. A. Chantelau and M. Berger, *Zur Geschichte der Diabetesdiät* (Berlin and Heidelberg: Springer, 1985).
19. Sinding, 'Making the Unit', p. 253.
20. Ibid., pp. 254–5.
21. Ibid., p. 265.
22. It was only at this point that Banting's and Best's paper was published, because they had not delivered their data before.
23. W. Griesbach, 'Mitteilungen der englischen Literatur über Insulin', *Klinische Wochenschrift*, 2 (1923), p. 147; W. Griesbach, 'Weitere Mitteilungen der englischen und amerikanischen Literatur über Insulin', ibid., p. 619.
24. Fuld to University of Toronto, 28 November 1922, AUT, A1982–0001–5/11.
25. N. N., '"Insulin"-Fabrikation durch das "Connaught"-Laboratory in Toronto', *Chemische Industrie*, 46 (1923), p. 188.
26. Letter no. 301, Verkaufskontor München to Farbenfabriken, 27 April 1923 and newspaper clippings in BAL, Einzelne Produkte A-Z: Insulin, 166/08.
27. Ibid.
28. See, for example, the report on Umber's presentation to the Berlin Medical Society on 17 August 1923, *Deutsche Medizinische Wochenschrift*, 49 (1923), p. 1972.
29. For the role of this argument in the context of the development of standardized trial procedures see Marks, 'Trust and Mistrust'.

30. See T. Close-Koenig and U. Thoms, 'A Balancing Act: Antidiabetic Products and Diabetic Markets in Germany and France', in J.-P. Gaudillière and U. Thoms, *The Birth of Scientific Marketing* (forthcoming).

31. A. Daemmrich, *Pharmacopolitics: Drug Regulation in the United States and Germany* (Chapel Hill. NC: The University of North Carolina Press, 2004), p. 109.

32. Fuld to Macleod, 28 November 1922, AUT, A1982–0001/005/011.

33. Fuld to Minkowski, 2 February 1923, ibid.

34. MacLeod to Minkowski respectively Fuld, 6 April 1923, ibid.

35. Insulin Committee to Fuld, 18 April 1923, ibid.; Minkowski to MacLeod, 28 April 1923, ibid.

36. Fuld to MacLeod, 5 May 1923, ibid.

37. Helbig, 23 March 1923, BAL, Einzelne Produkte: Insulin, Nr. 166/08.

38. Verkaufskontor München to Farbenfabriken Bayer, 4 April 1923, ibid.

39. Duisberg to Minkowski, 20 July 1923, ibid.

40. Sinding, 'Making the Unit', p. 253.

41. Minkowski to von Noorden, 19 April 1923, BAL, Einzelne Produkte: Insulin, Nr. 166/08.

42. Minkowski to Bayer, 5 July 1923, ibid. (trans. UT).

43. Hoffmann and Thümler to Sales Office Munich, 13 September 1923, ibid.

44. Letter no. 846, Dr Linder, scientific office Berlin, to Elberfeld, 10 September 1923, ibid.

45. Letter no. 21 to Farbwerke, vorm. Meister Lucius & Brüning, Wissenschaftliche Abteilung, 31 January 1923, ibid. (trans. UT).

46. M. Rosenberg, 'Ueber den heutigen Stand der Insulinforschung', *Münchener Medizinische Wochenschrift*, 70 (1923), pp. 1290–4, on p. 1290.

47. Fuld to MacLeod, 2 February 1923, AUT, A1982–0001/005–11.

48. Report, 31 January 1923, BAL, Einzelne Produkte: Insulin, BA 166/08 and Organon to Bayer, 2 October 1923, ibid., Nr. 166/08. The negotiations between Organon and Bayer about the delivery of dried pancreas illustrate Bayer's problems in producing enough insulin to satisfy demand. Bayer ended up purchasing dried insulin from Organon and putting its own label on it just in order to be in the market. Organon to Bayer, 3 October 1923, ibid.

49. Merck bought dried extract from Schering, but found that this extract varied widely in quality and was delivered only irregularly. W. Ried, *Zur Insulingeschichte in Deutschland: naturwissenschaftlich-pharmazeutische sowie sozialmedizinische und diätetische Aspekte seit der Isolierung des Insulins im Jahre 1921 bis zur Währungsreform 1948* (Dissertation, University of Frankfurt, 1986), pp. 46–9.

50. Thus Bayer's representative in Leipzig claimed, after a local practitioner had asked him to provide insulin for his hospital: 'Concerning the permanent willingness of Hoffmann's clinic, I strongly recommend giving the gentlemen a free sample. Manus manum lavat'. Extract from the report No. 56 from Dr Thünen about his visits to doctors in Düsseldorf, 21 September 1923, BAL, Einzelne Produkte: Insulin, Nr. 166/08.

51. Bayer's Office in Berlin played a central role in the communication because most of the members of the Insulin Committee lived and worked there. Lomnitz and Thümler to Dr Strickrodt, Breslau, 11 October 1923, ibid.

52. 'On the occasion of our discussion of today with Geheimrat Minkowski, Minkowski presented us with a letter, which he sent to you yesterday and in which he approves the official permission to launch Insulin'. Sales Office Leipzig to Pharmaceutical-Scientific Office Leverkusen, 12 October 1923, ibid. (trans. UT).

53. Letter no. 2955, Zwergel, Scientific Office Berlin, to Scientific Department Leverkusen, 2 November 1928, ibid. (trans. UT).
54. This was a result of inflation, because Bayer had to pay for the pancreatic glands in foreign currency. Minkowski to Farbenfabriken vorm. Friedr. Bayer & Co, Leverkusen, 25 July 1923, ibid.; Lomnitz and Müller to Verkaufskontor Leipzig, 13 August 1923, ibid.
55. 'Die Angriffe gegen das Deutsche Insulin-Komitee', *Klinische Wochenschrift*, 8 (1929), pp. 1983–4 and O. Minkowski, 'In Sachen des Insulin', *Münchener Medizinische Wochenschrift*, 76 (1929), p. 1702. The discussion came up because leftist journals published critical articles on the high price of insulin, due to the exclusion of the firm that produced the cheaper 'Seaxulin'.
56. Dorfmüller and Henneberg to Prof. Gutzeit, Breslau, and to Prof. Grafe, Würzburg, 11 September 1942, Landesarchiv Berlin, (hereafter LAB), A Rep 229, Nr. 263.
57. This is surprising, as there were also academic researchers who were occupied with more technical questions, for example Hans Staub, who published numerous articles on the problems of standardization. Ried, *Insulingeschichte*, appendix, pp. 398–403.
58. On the different national models of drug regulation and therapeutic cultures, see Daemmrich *Pharmacopolitics*, p. 109.
59. The president of the Imperial Health Office had commissioned a report on insulin for the office's publications by August 1923, i.e. shortly after the end of the conference. Note by Rost, 28 August 1923, Bundesarchiv, Berlin (hereafter BA Berlin), R 86/1648–1, fol. 8. It then took until October before Rost wrote the requested article, which was approved by the president on 17 October 1923 and published in the office's journal under the title 'Miscellaneous'. 'Vermischtes. Das neue Heilmittel Insulin auf der Internationalen Standardisierungs-Konferenz und dem Internationalen Physiologen-Kongress in Edinburgh 1923', *Veröffentlichungen des Reichsgesundheitsamtes*, 47 (1923), pp. 742–3.
60. BA Berlin, R 86/1648–1, fol. 13.
61. *Deutsche Medizinische Wochenschrift*, 49 (1923), p. 1972; H. Strauss, 'Ueber Insulinbehandlung bei Diabetes mellitus', *Deutsche Medizinische Wochenschrift*, 49 (1923), pp. 971–2. The insulin file contains a publication in the social-democratic journal, *Vorwärts*. 'Neuestes von dem neuen Mittel gegen Zuckerkrankheit', *Vorwärts*, no. 416, 6 September 1923. In October 1923 the journal published a second article. It rated insulin's efficacy as high as that of the diphtheria serum, but warned against the obstacles of treatment and insisted that only an experienced doctor use it. 'Prof. von Noorden über Insulin', *Vorwärts*, no. 525, 9 November 1923. Both articles are clippings in BA Berlin, R86/1648–1, fol. 9.
62. Note by Rost from 7 July 1923, BA Berlin, R86/1648–1, fol. 5.
63. See, for example, the report on Umber's presentation in the Berlin Medical Society on 18 July 1923. 'Berlin, Medizinische Gesellschaft, 18 July 1923', *Deutsche Medizinische Wochenschrift*, 49 (1923), p. 1972; Strauss, 'Ueber Insulinbehandlung bei Diabetes mellitus'.
64. Note from 16 July 1923, BA Berlin, R86/1648–1, fol. 5 and Report from the sitting of the Berlin Medical Association, 19 July 1923, *Deutsche Medizinische Wochenschrift*, 49 (1923), p. 1972.
65. Letter from 10 July 1923, BA Berlin, R86/1648–1, fol. 5.
66. On these, see C. Gradmann and J. Simon (eds), *Evaluating and Standardizing Therapeutic Agents, 1890–1950* (New York: Palgrave Macmillan, 2010).
67. Minkowski to Imperial Health Office, 22 April 1924, BA Berlin, R 86/1648–1, fol. 53 and minutes from the meeting of the Insulin Committee, 22 April 1924, ibid., fols 54–5.
68. Fuld to Hutchison, 10 October 1924, AUT, A1982–0001/005/011.

69. Fuld to Huchison, 14 October 1924, ibid.; Mestern to Fuld, 24 November 1924, ibid.
70. Fuld to Hutchison, 7 January 1925, ibid.
71. Report of the discussion held 23 November 1925 in the Imperial ('National') Health Office (*Reichsgesundheitsamt*) on the testing of insulin preparations, AUT, A1982-0001/005/011. The citations are not taken from the German original in this file, but from the English translation made by the committee.
72. Ibid.
73. Ibid., p. 3 of the minutes.
74. Fuld to unnamed [Hutchison], 7 December 1925, ibid.
75. Note by G. A. from 10 July 1923, BA Berlin, R86/1648-1, fol. 5.
76. See the report on Umber's lecture on his trials with insulin, *Klinische Wochenschrift*, 2 (1923), pp. 1522–4 and C. von Noorden and S. Isaac, 'Allgemeine Bemerkungen über 50 mit Insulin behandelte Diabetesfälle', *Klinische Wochenschrift*, 2 (1923), pp. 1968–70; H. Staub, 'Insulin', *Klinische Wochenschrift*, 2 (1923), pp. 2082–139; Strauss, 'Ueber Insulinbehandlung bei Diabetes mellitus'; W. Ercklentz, 'Über die Behandlung des Diabetes mit Insulin', *Deutsche Medizinische Wochenschrift*, 49 (1923), pp. 1073–4; O. Minkowski, 'Zur Insulinbehandlung des Diabetes', *Deutsche Medizinische Wochenschrift*, 49 (1923), pp. 1107–8; E. Grafe, 'Über die praktische und theoretische Bedeutung des Insulins', *Deutsche Medizinische Wochenschrift*, 49 (1923), pp. 1141–3, 1177–9. A comprehensive bibliography of the insulin literature up to the year 1960 can be found in J. Schuhmacher, *Index zum Diabetes mellitus* (Munich and Berlin: Urban & Schwarzenberg, 1961).
77. Mann and Lomnitz to sales office Berlin, Nr. 657, 7 August 1923, BAL, Einzelne Produkte: Insulin, Nr. 166/08.
78. Bonhoeffer and Hörlein to Willstätter, 1 August 1923, ibid.
79. Lomnitz and Thümen to sales offices at Berlin, Munich, Leipzig, 5 October 1923, ibid. and subsequent letter, 4 October 1923, ibid.
80. Sales Office Munich no. 595 to scientific department, 5 October 1923, ibid.
81. Minkowski from 17 November 1923, ibid.
82. Federlin, *75 Jahre Insulin Höchst*, p. 32.
83. F. Umber, 'Werden und Wirken des Deutschen Insulinkomitees', *Deutsche Medizinische Wochenschrift*, 58 (1932), pp. 1150–60.
84. The patent question is somewhat unclear. Although the German documents clearly speak of a free right to use the patent, Sinding points to the enormous income the patent produced for its owner, the University of Toronto.
85. Umber, 'Werden und Wirken', p. 1158.
86. From the rich literature, see only H. S. Chawla, 'Patenting of Biological Material and Biotechnology', *Journal of Intellectual property Rights*, 10 (2005), pp. 44–51 and 'Biotechnology in European Patents – Threat or Promise?', at www.eop.org/news-issues/issues/biotechnology.html [accessed 30 January 2012].
87. A. Grevenstuk and E. Laquer, 'Insulin – Seine Darstellung, physiologische und pharmakologische Darstellung mit besonderer Berücksichtigung seiner Wertbestimmung (Eichung)', in L. Asher and K. Spiro (eds), *Ergebnisse der Physiologie*, vol. 23, II. Abteilung (Munich: Bergmann, 1925).
88. K. Wentzel, 'Ist der Name "Insulin" ein schutzfähiges Warenzeichen', *Pharmazeutische Zeitung*, 71 (1926), p. 1299.
89. H. Schadewaldt, 'Die Geschichte des Diabetes mellitus', in D. von Engelhardt (ed.), *Diabetes in Medizin- und Kulturgeschichte* (Berlin: Springer Verlag, 1989), pp. 47–110, on p. 87; Ried, *Insulingeschichte*, p. 417; P. Drügemöller and L. Norpoth, 'Wege und Irrwege

der deutschen Insulin-Forschung', *Deutsche Medizinische Wochenschrift*, 78 (1953), pp. 919–22.

90. Ried, *Insulingeschichte*, p. 41–3.

91. See, for example, Dilg, 'Frühgeschichte', p. 13.

92. Letter no. 825, Lindner to Bayer, Scientific Department, 30 August 1923, BAL, Einzelne Produkte: Insulin, 166/08. For the prices of English and American insulin, see C. von Noorden, 'Ist Insulin bereits in Deutschland erhältlich?', *Klinische Wochenschrift*, 2 (1923), p. 1483.

93. Letter no. 21 to Farbwerke Meister, Lucius & Brüning, 20 November 1923, BAL, Einzelne Produkte: Insulin, Nr. 166/08.

94. Dr. Lindner to Leverkusen, 10 October 1923, ibid.

95. District President Düsseldorf to Imperial Health Office, 11 March 1924, BA Berlin, R86/1648–1, fol. 20.

96. The Prussian Minister of Welfare to Imperial Health Office, 5 April 1924, BA Berlin, R86/1649, fol. 22.

97. Von Noorden to Minkowsiki, 29 April 1923, AUT, A1982–0001/005–11.

98. Evidence of this can be seen to this day in discussions about generic drugs and their comparison with the originally patented brand products and the life-cycle theories of goods, which are especially prominent in the pharmaceutical industry.

99. Rosenberg, 'Stand der Insulinforschung', p. 1292, fn. 1.

100. G. Klemperer, 'Ist deutsches Insulin vollwertig?', *Therapie der Gegenwart*, 66 (1925), pp. 41–3.

101. But as Krehl put it in a personal conversation with Bayer's sales representative, animal trials would help 'to unravel this trick'. Sales office Munich to Scientific Department Bayer Leverkusen, 12 December 1923, BAL, Einzelne Produkte: Insulin, Nr. 166/08.

102. Ried, *Insulingeschichte*, p. 400. This contrasts with the findings of Christiane Sinding, who acted as if the standard of the Canadian Insulin Committee was maintained. Sinding, 'Making the Unit'.

103. Letter to Minkowski, 11 November 1928, AUT, A1982–0001/005–11.

104. Ried, *Insulingeschichte*, p. 399.

105. Sinding, 'Making the Unit', p. 247; Ried, *Insulingeschichte*, p. 400.

106. For a description of the many problems associated with the rabbits and the measures taken to deal with them, see 'Vorschrift für die Eichung von Insulin-Präparaten [1946]', Schering Archives, Bayer AG, S1–412.

107. H. Dale, 'League of Nations: Second International Conference on the Biological Standardization of Certain Remedies (31 August to 3 September 1925)', *Publications of the League of Nations*, C 532. M. 1983. 1925, III, C.H. 350.

108. Ried, *Insulingeschichte*, p. 403.

109. Sinding, 'Making the Unit', p. 266.

110. Letter, Umber to Degewop, October 1940, LAB, A Rep. 229, Nr. 263.

111. Umber, 'Werden und Wirken'.

112. For his biography, see H-G. Dercken, *Zur Entwicklung der I. Medizinischen Klinik im Krankenhaus Westend in der Ära Professor Friedrich Umber* (Dissertation, FU Berlin, 1992). This publication does not mention Umber's role in the national socialist health system.

113. This attitude follows clearly from the first letter Fuld wrote to the University of Toronto. Fuld to University of Toronto, 28 November 1922, AUT, A1982–0001/005–11. Moreover, he hosted visitors of the international Peace Congress from Britain in Octo-

ber 1924. Fuld to Hutchison, 14 October 1924, ibid. In 1940, Minkowski's Jewish wife, Marie, emigrated to Argentina with some support from the University of Toronto. AUT, A1982–0001/012/04.

114. H. Jenss, *Hermann Strauss. Internist und Wissenschaftler in der Charité und im jüdischen Krankenhaus Berlin* (Berlin: Hentrich & Hentrich, 2010).

115. Oyen, Chantelau and Berger, *Geschichte der Diabetesdiät*.

116. U. Knödler, 'Das Insulinproblem. Eine Studie zum Zusammenbruch der Arzneimittelversorgung der Zivilbevölkerung im Zweiten Weltkrieg', in C. Pross and G. Aly (eds), *Der Wert des Menschen. Medizin in Deutschland 1918–1945* (Berlin: Hentrich, 1989), pp. 250–60.

117. I cannot discuss the related problems here for reasons of space, but I am currently writing a book on the development of the nutritional sciences, which will deal with this problem in great detail. For the problem of insulin rationalization in Germany during the Second World War, see Knödler, 'Insulinproblem'.

118. J. Tanner, 'Standards and Modernity', in C. Bonah, C. Masutti, A. Rasmussen and J. Simon (eds), *Harmonizing Drugs: Standards in 20th-Century Pharmaceutical History* (Paris: Editions Glyphe, 2010), pp. 45–60.

119. Letter, concerning Arbeitsgebiet Insulin, Adlershof, 29 April 1938, LAB, A Rep. 229/124.

120. Insulin [product specification, dated August 1924], Schering Archive, Bayer AG, S1–407; insulin [product specification], 11 March 1946, ibid., S1–412.

121. Bericht der Insulin-Abteilung über Monat Januar 1942, 18 February 1942, LAB, A Rep. 229, Nr. 161.

122. E. Putter, 'Die Standardisierung des Insulins', *Medizinische Mitteilungen*, 2 (1929), pp. 109–11; E. Putter, 'Über Insulin', *Medizinische Mitteilungen*, 4 (1932), pp. 160–5.

10 Angerer, '"There is a Frog in South America / Whose Venom is a Cure": Poison Alkaloids and Drug Discovery'

1. This essay is derived from ongoing research for my PhD thesis on the investigation and the uses of biological materials in pharmaceutical companies and other institutions. I wish to thank the *Andrea von Braun Stiftung* for providing funding for my dissertation project and the European Science Foundation (ESF) for awarding me a research travel grant to visit Cermes3 (Villejuif). I would also like to thank many members of the ESF Network DRUGS for their helpful suggestions and comments, especially Jean-Paul Gaudillière and Alexander von Schwerin. I would like to thank the *Sociedad Peruana de Derecho Ambiental* (Peruvian Society of Environmental Law) for funding the consultancy project 'Analysis of the Real and Potential Value of Genetic Resources in Latin America and the Caribbean' that supported the research for this essay. This chapter is based on an earlier paper focusing on the case of epibatidine and the regulation of biodiversity, see K. Angerer, 'Frog Tales – on Poison Dart Frogs, Epibatidine, and the Sharing of Biodiversity', *Innovation: The European Journal of Social Science Research*, 24:3 (2011), pp. 353–69.

2. D. Bradley, 'Frog Venom Cocktail Yields A One-Handed Painkiller', *Science*, 261:5125 (1993), p. 1117.

3. Almost all earlier sources follow Daly and refer to another poison frog species endemic to Ecuador, *Epipedobates tricolor*, as the source of epibatidine; however, ever since a

recent taxonomic revision it has been assumed – based on the collection sites – that Daly actually collected frogs belonging to *E. anthonyi*. C. R. Darst, P. A. Menéndez-Guerrero, L. A. Coloma and D. C. Cannatella, 'Evolution of Dietary Specialization and Chemical Defense in Poison Frogs (Dendrobatidae): a Comparative Analysis', *American Naturalist*, 165:1 (2005), pp. 56–69, on p. 59; T. Grant, et al., 'Phylogenetic Systematics of Dart-Poison Frogs and their Relatives (Amphibia: Athesphatanura: Dendrobatidae)', *Bulletin of the American Museum of Natural History*, 299 (2006), pp. 1–262.

4. D. J. Newman and G. M. Cragg, 'Natural Products As Sources of New Drugs over the 30 Years from 1981 to 2010', *Journal of Natural Products*, 75:3 (2012), pp. 311–35, on p. 316.

5. R. W. Fitch and C. A. Bewley, 'John W. Daly (1933–2008)', *Journal of Natural Products*, 73:3 (2010), pp. 299–300, on p. 299; A. M. Gillis, 'Serendipity and Sweat in Science. "Frog Man" Daly Follows Curiosity To Ends of the Earth', *NIH Record*, 44:18 (2002), at http://nihrecord.od.nih.gov/newsletters/09_03_2002/story01.htm [accessed 15 March 2013].

6. J. W. Daly, B. Witkop, P. Bommer and K. Biemann, 'Batrachotoxin. The Active Principle of the Colombian Arrow Poison Frog, Phyllobates Bicolor', *Journal of the American Chemical Society*, 87:1 (1965), pp. 124–6; T. Tokuyama and J. Daly, 'Structure of Batrachotoxin, a Steroidal Alkaloid from the Colombian Arrow Poison Frog, Phyllobates Aurotaenia, and Partial Synthesis of Batrachotoxin and its Analogs and Homologs', *Journal of the American Chemical Society*, 91:14 (1969), pp. 3931–8.

7. Gillis, 'Serendipity and Sweat in Science'.

8. Ibid.

9. J. W. Daly, et al., 'Alkaloids from Frog Skin: The Discovery of Epibatidine and the Potential for Developing Novel Non-opioid Analgesics', *Natural Product Reports*, 17:2 (2000), pp. 131–5, on p. 131.

10. M. Williams, H. M. Garraffo and T. F. Spande, 'Epibatidine: From Frog Alkaloid to Analgesic Clinical Candidates. A Testimonial to "True Grit"!', *HETEROCYCLES*, 79:1 (2009), pp. 207–17, on p. 213.

11. Gillis, 'Serendipity and Sweat in Science'. An early publication evidencing their interdisciplinary approach is C. W. Myers and J. W. Daly, 'Preliminary Evaluation of Skin Toxins and Vocalizations in Taxonomic and Evolutionary Studies of Poison-dart Frogs (Dendrobatidae)', *Bulletin of the American Museum of Natural History*, 157:3 (1976), pp. 173–262.

12. Fitch and Bewley, 'John W. Daly', p. 299.

13. Gillis, 'Serendipity and Sweat in Science'.

14. Ibid.

15. Williams, Garraffo and Spande, 'Epibatidine', p. 214.

16. For the citation, see ibid., p. 215.

17. Daly, et al., 'Alkaloids from Frog Skin', p. 132; H. M. Garraffo and T. F. Spande, 'Discovery of Batrachotoxin: The Launch of the Frog Alkaloid Program at NIH', *HETEROCYCLES*, 79:1 (2009), pp. 195–205, on p. 196; Williams, Garraffo and. Spande, 'Epibatidine', p. 208.

18. B. Parry, 'The Fate of the Collections: Social Justice and the Annexation of Plant Genetic Resources', in C. Zerner (ed.), *People, Plants, and Justice: The Politics of Nature Conservation* (New York & Chichester: Columbia University Press, 2000), pp. 374–402, on p. 375.

19. Gillis, 'Serendipity and Sweat in Science'.

20. Williams, Garraffo and Spande, 'Epibatidine', p. 213.
21. Garraffo and Spande, 'Discovery of Batrachotoxin', p. 195.
22. Ibid., p. 198.
23. Ibid., p. 196.
24. Williams, Garraffo and Spande, 'Epibatidine', p. 214.
25. Ibid., quoted on p. 207.
26. Ibid.
27. Daly, et al., 'Alkaloids from Frog Skin', p. 132.
28. Williams, Garraffo and Spande, 'Epibatidine', p. 208.
29. Ibid., p. 209.
30. Daly and his colleagues experienced this first-hand when they reported the isolation, structure and pharmacology of epiquinamide, another novel alkaloid from *E. tricolor*. Its bioactivity later turned out to be due to contamination from co-occurring epibatidine in the isolated sample. R. W. Fitch, et al., 'Epiquinamide: A Poison That Wasn't from a Frog That Was', *Journal of Natural Products*, 72:2 (2009), pp. 243–7.
31. Williams, Garraffo and Spande, 'Epibatidine', p. 210.
32. R. W. Fitch, et al., 'Bioassay-Guided Isolation of Epiquinamide, a Novel Quinolizidine Alkaloid and Nicotinic Agonist from an Ecuadoran Poison Frog, Epipedobates Tricolor', *Journal of Natural Products*, 66:10 (2003), pp. 1345–50, on p. 1349.
33. J. W. Daly, 'Thirty Years of Discovering Arthropod Alkaloids in Amphibian Skin', *Journal of Natural Products*, 61:1 (1998), pp. 162–72, on p. 169; 'Checklist of CITES species', at www.cites.org/eng/resources/pub/checklist11/History_of_CITES_listings.pdf [accessed 8 March 2013].
34. 'What is CITES?', at http://www.cites.org/eng/disc/what.php [accessed 22 March 2013].
35. Ibid.
36. See 'How CITES works', at http://www.cites.org/eng/disc/how.php [accessed 22 March 2013].
37. Daly, 'Thirty Years', p. 169. Actually, a query in the CITES Trade Database shows that there was a sharp rise in the number of export permits granted for live specimens of *E. tricolor* from Ecuador between 1994 and 1997, possibly due to increased interest following the publication of the molecular structure of epibatidine in 1992; while only 41 specimens were exported between 1987 and 1993, more than 4,000 were exported between 1994 and 1997. Query at http://www.cites.org/eng/resources/trade.shtml [accessed 8 March 2013].
38. J. W. Daly, 'Amphibian Skin: A Remarkable Source of Biologically Active Arthropod Alkaloids', *Journal of Medicinal Chemistry*, 46:4 (2003), pp. 445–52, on p. 449.
39. Williams, Garraffo and Spande, 'Epibatidine', pp. 209–10, 215.
40. This new detection technology was called 'inverse detection' and focused on detecting the nuclear spin of 1H-atoms instead of 13C-atoms. It became widely used in the early 1990s and, according to a natural product researcher interviewed during my PhD fieldwork, radically improved the conditions for structure determination via NMR.
41. Williams, Garraffo and Spande, 'Epibatidine', p. 210; T. F. Spande, et al., 'Epibatidine: A Novel (Chloropyridyl)azabicycloheptane with Potent Analgesic Activity from an Ecuadoran Poison Frog', *Journal of the American Chemical Society*, 114:9 (1992), pp. 3475–8.
42. Garraffo and Spande, 'Discovery of Batrachotoxin', p. 203.
43. Daly, 'Thirty Years', p. 168.
44. Garraffo and Spande, 'Discovery of Batrachotoxin', p. 195.

45. Williams, Garraffo and Spande, 'Epibatidine', p. 209.
46. See the introduction to this volume, on pp. 28–9.
47. Williams, Garraffo and Spande, 'Epibatidine', p. 210.
48. Ibid., p. 214.
49. B. Parry, 'Bodily Transactions: Regulating a New Space of Flows in "Bio-information"', in K. Verdery and C. Humphrey (eds), *Property in Question: Value Transformation in the Global Economy* (Oxford and New York: Berg, 2004), pp. 29–48, on p. 43.
50. J.-P. Gaudillière, 'Introduction: Drug Trajectories', *Studies in History and Philosophy of Biological and Biomedical Sciences*, 36:4 (2005), pp. 603–11.
51. M. Dukat and R. Glennon, 'Epibatidine: Impact on Nicotinic Receptor Research', *Cellular and Molecular Neurobiology*, 23:3 (2003), pp. 365–78, on p. 365. Furthermore, on 3 March 1992, a patent on 'Epibatidine and derivatives, compositions and methods of treating pain' was filed by Daly and his colleagues. J. W. Daly, T. F. Spande and H. M. Garraffo, 'United States Patent: 5314899 – Epibatidine and Derivatives, Compositions and Methods of Treating Pain'.
52. Bradley, 'Frog Venom Cocktail', p. 1117.
53. Ibid.
54. B. Badio and J. W. Daly, 'Epibatidine, a Potent Analgetic and Nicotinic Agonist', *Molecular Pharmacology*, 45:4 (1994), pp. 563–9.
55. For example, a paper submitted in July of 1994 and published in 1995 mentions in its methods section that epibatidine had been purchased. See A. W. Bannon, K. L. Gunther and M. W. Decker, 'Is Epibatidine Really Analgesic? Dissociation of the Activity, Temperature, and Analgesic Effects of (±)-epibatidine', *Pharmacology Biochemistry and Behavior*, 51:4 (1995), pp. 693–8, on p. 694.
56. A. W. Bannon, et al., 'Broad-Spectrum, Non-opioid Analgesic Activity by Selective Modulation of Neuronal Nicotinic Acetylcholine Receptors', *Science*, 279:5347 (1998), pp. 77–81, on p. 77.
57. S. P. Arneric, M. Holladay and M. Williams, 'Neuronal Nicotinic Receptors: A Perspective on Two Decades of Drug Discovery Research', *Biochemical Pharmacology*, 74:8 (2007), pp. 1092–101, on p. 1094.
58. AP, 'Painkiller Based Onfrog Poison', *Augusta Chronicle*, 2 January 1998, at http://chronicle.augusta.com/stories/1998/01/02/tec_219951.shtml [accessed 12 March 2013].
59. Arneric, Holladay and Williams, 'Neuronal Nicotinic Receptors', p. 1097.
60. Ibid. Daly was generally known for his generous and informal sharing of knowledge, a fact that is highlighted in the acknowledgments of many articles on epibatidine. In Daly's obituary, a former colleague is even quoted as saying: 'You could milk the guy (for information) and he would love to be milked'. Fitch and Bewley, 'John W. Daly', p. 300.
61. Dukat and Glennon, 'Epibatidine', p. 365.
62. Williams, Garraffo and Spande, 'Epibatidine', p. 211.
63. Arneric, Holladay and Williams, 'Neuronal Nicotinic Receptors', p. 1097. The article in *Science* mentioned in the quotation is Bannon, et al., 'Broad-Spectrum'.
64. Daly, et al., 'Alkaloids from Frog Skin', p. 134.
65. Paul Simon, 'Señorita with a Necklace of Tears', © 2000 Words and Music by Paul Simon, see http://www.paulsimon.com/us/music/youre-one/se%C3%B1orita-necklace-tears [accessed 7 March 2013].

66. J. P. Sullivan, et al., '(+/-)-Epibatidine Elicits a Diversity of in Vitro and in Vivo Effects Mediated by Nicotinic Acetylcholine Receptors', *Journal of Pharmacology and Experimental Therapeutics*, 271:2 (1994), pp. 624–31.

67. Arneric, Holladay and Williams, 'Neuronal Nicotinic Receptors', p. 1097.

68. Dukat and Glennon, 'Epibatidine', p. 375.

69. For a review of the role of natural products as an inspiration in the so-called diversity-oriented synthesis of compound libraries, see C. Cordier, et al., 'Natural Products as an Inspiration in the Diversity-Oriented Synthesis of Bioactive Compound Libraries', *Natural Product Reports*, 25:4 (2008), pp. 719–37. Diversity-oriented synthesis is not exactly the same as the synthesis of structurally optimized derivatives of a known natural compound, but this article is a good example of the many ways that a compound can serve as an inspiration in the design of libraries of derivatives.

70. See 'History of the Convention', at http://www.cbd.int/history/ and 'List of Parties', at http://www.cbd.int/convention/parties/list/default.shtml [accessed 23 March 2013].

71. K. McAfee, 'Selling Nature to Save It? Biodiversity and Green Developmentalism', *Environment and Planning D: Society and Space*, 17:2 (1999), pp. 133–54, on p. 140; C. Hamilton, 'Biodiversity, Biopiracy and Benefits: What Allegations of Biopiracy tell us about Intellectual Property', *Developing World Bioethics*, 6:3 (2006), pp. 158–73, on p. 161.

72. D. L. Kleinman and J. R. Kloppenburg, 'Seeds of Controversy: National Property Versus Common Heritage', in J. R. Kloppenburg (ed.), *Seeds and Sovereignty: The Use and Control of Plant Genetic Resources* (Durham, NC, and London: Duke University Press, 1988), pp. 173–203, on p. 194; for the historical background of the CBD, see also J. R. Kloppenburg, *First the Seed: The Political Economy of Plant Biotechnology, 1492–2000*, 2nd edn (Madison, WI: University of Wisconsin Press, 2004) and M. Flitner, *Sammler, Räuber und Gelehrte: Die Politischen Interessen an Pflanzengenetischen Ressourcen 1895–1995* (Frankfurt/Main: Campus, 1995).

73. C. Hayden, *When Nature Goes Public: The Making and Unmaking of Bio-Prospecting in Mexico* (Princeton, NJ: Princeton University Press, 2003), p. 64.

74. Ibid.

75. McAfee, 'Selling Nature to Save It?', p. 133. According to McAfee, '[b]y the logic of this paradigm, nature is constructed as a world currency and ecosystems are recoded as warehouses of genetic resources for biotechnology industries'. Ibid.

76. Hayden, *When Nature Goes Public*, p. 65.

77. McAfee, 'Selling Nature to Save It?', p. 133.

78. Daly, et al., 'Alkaloids from Frog Skin', p. 132.

79. H. Werning, 'Streit um Froschgene', *Reptilia*, 15 (1999), pp. 11–13, at https://blogs.taz.de/reptilienfonds/2010/09/30/wem_gehoeren_die_gene_der_froesche/ [accessed 6 March 2013].

80. Bradley, 'Frog Venom Cocktail', p. 1117.

81. See Angerer, 'Frog Tales', pp. 360–1.

82. Almost half of the article published on this expedition consists of an ethnographic description of the practices of dart poisoning, blowgun fabrication and dart fabrication. Given that one specimen of *P. terribilis* contains enough poison to kill a dozen people, the researchers readily admitted to paying close attention to the way locals treated the frogs: '[W]e heeded the advice of our Indian friends and handled [the frog] with appropriate caution, especially after accidentally killing a few of their domestic animals that got into our contaminated garbage'. C. W. Myers, J. W. Daly and B. Malkin, 'A Dan-

gerously Toxic New Frog (Phyllobates) used by Emberá Indians of Western Colombia, with Discussion of Blowgun Fabrication and Dart Poisoning', *Bulletin of the American Museum of Natural History*, 161:2 (1978), pp. 307–66, on p. 312.

83. This remains true even after the adoption of the 'Protocol on Access to Genetic Resources and the Fair and Equitable Sharing of Benefits Arising from their Utilization' at the tenth conference of the parties to the CBD at Nagoya (Japan) in 2010. On the pitfalls of access and benefit sharing, see for example J. H. Vogel, et al., 'The Economics of Information, Studiously Ignored in the Nagoya Protocol on Access to Genetic Resources and Benefit Sharing', *LEAD. Law, Environment & Development Journal*, 7:1 (2011), pp. 52–65.

84. M. Ribadeneira Sarmiento, 'La Biopiratería, El Desafío De Construir Un Camino Entre Una Acusación Política y Una Categoría Legal', in M. V. Lottici (ed.), *Conservación De La Biodiversidad y Política Ambiental. Sexta Convocatoria, Premio De Monografía Adriana Schiffrin 2007, Trabajos Premiados* (Buenos Aires: Fundación Ambiente y Recursos Naturales, 2008), pp. 87–117, on p. 104.

85. J. Martinez-Alier, *The Environmentalism of the Poor: A Study of Ecological Conflicts and Valuation* (Cheltenham and Northampton: Edward Elgar Publishing, 2002), p. 134.

86. L. Á. Saavedra, 'Invasion of the Frog-Snatchers', *New Internationalist*, 311 (April 1999), at http://newint.org/columns/currents/1999/04/01/ecuador/ [accessed 13 March 2013].

87. No further source is given for this claim, however it is difficult to believe that Daly and his colleagues had to smuggle frogs out of Ecuador, given the high numbers of specimens they routinely collected over many years in several countries. Furthermore, the original Spanish print version of the bulletin of the Ecuadorian NGO *Acción Ecológica* doesn't make this claim. But the English translation available on the website of the NGO contains this direct accusation (and constitutes its putative source), as do other later Spanish and English versions of the same bulletin. See Acción Ecológica, 'Epipedobates Triqué? Tan Pequeño y Tan Grande', *Alerta Verde. Boletín De Acción Ecológica*, 58 (1999), at http://www.accionecologica.org/alerta-verde-el-boletin-de-ae/1238-58-epipedobates-tricolor-nombre-largo-para-algo-tan-pequeno [accessed 13 March 2013].

88. Hayden, *When Nature Goes Public*, p. 65.

89. B. Parry, *Trading the Genome: Investigating the Commodification of Bio-information* (New York and Chichester: Columbia University Press, 2004), p. 105.

90. Daly, et al., 'Alkaloids from Frog Skin', p. 132.

91. Fitch and Bewley, 'John W. Daly', p. 300.

92. R. A. Saporito, et al., 'A Review of Chemical Ecology in Poison Frogs', *Chemoecology*, 22:3 (2012), pp. 159–68, on p. 161; Daly, 'Amphibian Skin', p. 449. On the key role of biodiversity below the species level in the case of epibatidine, see also Angerer, 'Frog Tales', pp. 358–60.

93. Nagoya Protocol on Access to Genetic Resources and the Fair and Equitable Sharing of Benefits Arising from Their Utilization to the Convention on Biological Diversity, Art. 2 (e), at http://www.cbd.int/abs/text/default.shtml [accessed 13 March 2003].

94. Vogel, et al., 'The Economics of Information', pp. 54–5.

95. See J.-P. Gaudillière's contribution to this volume on p. 62.

96. See for example C. Z. Zhu, et al., 'Potentiation of Analgesic Efficacy but not Side Effects: Co-administration of an A4β2 Neuronal Nicotinic Acetylcholine Receptor Agonist and Its Positive Allosteric Modulator in Experimental Models of Pain in Rats', *Biochemical Pharmacology*, 82:8 (2011), pp. 967–76.

97. Arneric, Holladay and Williams, 'Neuronal Nicotinic Receptors', p. 1094; Data-monitor, 12 February 2009, 'NeuroSearch: ABT-894 remains viable option for ADHD following neuropathic pain failure', at www.datamonitor.com/store/News/neurosearch_abt_894_remains_viable_option_for_adhd_following_neuropathic_pain_failure?productid=2D5D97F8-CBDA-4B2D-A291-253ADB570F10 [accessed 14 March 2013].
98. See for example Saporito, et al., 'Review of Chemical Ecology'; Darst, et al., 'Evolution of Dietary Specialization'.
99. J. Miller, 'The Discovery of Medicines from Plants: A Current Biological Perspective', *Economic Botany*, 65:4 (2011), pp. 396–407, on pp. 396–7.
100. G. F. Pauli, et al., 'Analysis and Purification of Bioactive Natural Products: The AnaPurNa Study', *Journal of Natural Products*, 75:6 (2012), pp. 1243–55, on p. 1244.
101. W. R. Strohl, 'The Role of Natural Products in a Modern Drug Discovery Program', *Drug Discovery Today*, 5:2 (2000), pp. 39–41, on p. 40.
102. A. L. Harvey, 'Strategies for Discovering Drugs from Previously Unexplored Natural Products', *Drug Discovery Today*, 5:7 (2000), pp. 294–300, on p. 298.
103. Strohl, 'Role of Natural Products', p. 40.

Gradmann, 'Commentary: Biologics, Medicine and the Therapeutic Revolution: Towards Understanding the History of Twentieth-Century Medicine'

1. I wish to thank Jean-Paul Gaudillière (Paris) for a critical reading and valuable suggestions for improvement.
2. On the contemporary history of medicine and science, see R. E. Doel and T. Söderqvist, *The Historiography of Contemporary Science, Technology and Medicine. Writing recent Science* (London and New York: Routledge, 2006); compare R. Cooter and J. Pickstone (eds), *Medicine in the Twentieth Century* (Amsterdam: Harwood Academic Publishers, 2000).
3. F. Huisman and J. H. Warner (eds), *Locating Medical History. The Stories and Their Meanings* (Baltimore, MD, and London: The Johns Hopkins University Press, 2004).
4. C. Bonah, J.-P. Gaudillière, C. Gradmann and V. Hess, 'Standard Drugs and Drug Standards: A Comparative Historical Study of Pharmaceuticals in the 20th Century', in C. Bonah, C. Masutti, A. Rasmussen and J. Simon (eds), *Harmonizing Drugs: Standards in 20th-Century Pharmaceutical History* (Paris: Editions Glyphe, 2009), pp. 17–27; compare M. J. Vogel and C. E. Rosenberg (eds), *The Therapeutic Revolution: Essays in the Social History of American Medicine* (Philadelphia, PA: University of Pennsylvania Press, 1979). Vogel and Rosenberg used the term in reference to nineteenth-century medicine. A good introduction to twentieth-century pharmaceuticals can be found in N. Eschenbruch, V. Balz, U. Klöppel and M. Hulverscheidt (eds), *Arzneimittel des 20. Jahrhunderts. Historische Skizzen von Lebertran bis Contergan* (Bielefeld: transcript Verlag, 2009). A recent paper discussing the history of late twentieth-century medicine from a comparative vantage point is V. Quirke and J.-P. Gaudillière, 'The Era of Biomedicine: Science, Medicine, and Public Health in Britain and France after the Second World War', *Medical History*, 52 (2008), pp. 441–52.
5. H. M. Marks, *The Progress of Experiment: Science and Therapeutic Reform in the United States, 1900–1990* (Cambridge: Cambridge University Press, 1997); S. Timmermanns

and M. Berg, *The Gold Standard: The Challenge of Evidence-Based Medicine and the Standardization in Health Care* (Philadelphia, PA: Temple University Press, 2003).

6. C. Connolly, J. Golden and B. Schneider, 'A Startling New Chemotherapeutic Agent: Pediatric Infectious Disease and the Introduction of Sulfonamides at Baltimore's Sydenham Hospital', *Bulletin of the History of Medicine*, 86 (2012), pp. 66–93.

7. The notorious question of whether there was a bacteriological revolution in medicine is intimately connected to this. Michael Worboys has reminded everyone that the promises of the bacteriological laboratory remained precisely that for a long time. M. Worboys, 'Was there a Bacteriological Revolution in Late Nineteenth-Century Medicine?', *Studies in History and Philosophy of Biologic and Biomedical Sciences*, 38 (2007), pp. 20–42.

8. I have argued this point with regard to models of infectious causation in which, beyond a certain bustle of technological invention, the basic assumptions about man, microbe and disease remained almost constant from 1880 to 2000. C. Gradmann, 'Alles eine Frage der Methode. Zur Historizität der Kochschen Postulate 1840–2000', *Medizinhistorisches Journal*, 43 (2008), pp. 121–48. Thomas Schlich's work on organ transplantation could be read in a similar fashion. T. Schlich, *The Origins of Organ Transplantation: Surgery and Laboratory Science, 1880–1930* (Rochester, NY: University of Rochester Press, 2010).

9. J. den Hollander, 'Contemporary History and the Art of Self-Distancing', *History and Theory*, 50 (2011), pp. 51–67.

10. L. Schiebinger, *Plants and Empire: Colonial Bioprospecting in the Atlantic World* (Cambridge, MA: Harvard University Press, 2004).

11. C. Gradmann and J. Simon (eds), *Evaluating and Standardizing Therapeutic Agents, 1890–1950* (Basingstoke: Palgrave Macmillan, 2010).

12. D. Cantor, C. Bonah and M. Dörries (eds), *Meat, Medicine, and Human Health in the Twentieth Century* (London: Pickering & Chatto, 2010); R. Bud, *The Uses of Life: A History of Biotechnology* (Cambridge: Cambridge University Press, 1993).

13. D. Greenwood, *Antimicrobial Drugs: Chronicle of a Twentieth Century Triumph* (Oxford: Oxford University Press, 2008).

14. R. E. Kohler, *Lords of the Fly: Drosophila Genetics and the Experimental Life* (Chicago, IL: University of Chicago Press, 1994); K. Rader, *Making Mice: Standardizing Animals for American Biomedical Research, 1900–1955* (Princeton, NJ: Princeton University Press, 2004).

15. P. Sizaret, 'Evolution of Activities in International Biological Standardisation since the Early Days of the Health Organisation of the League of Nations', *Bulletin of the World Health Organization*, 66 (1988), pp. 1–6.

16. J.-P. Gaudilliere, 'New Wine in Old Bottles? The Biotechnology Problem in the History of Molecular Biology', *Studies in History and Philosophy of Biological and Biomedical Sciences*, 40 (2009), pp. 20–8; P. Rabinow, *Making PCR: A Story of Biotechnology* (Chicago, IL: University of Chicago Press, 1996).

17. A. M. Brandt and M. Gardner, 'The Golden Age of Medicine?', in R. Cooter and J. Pickstone (eds), *Companion to Medicine in the Twentieth Century* (London and New York: Routledge, 2000), pp. 21–37.

18. J. Greene, *Prescribing by Numbers: Drugs and the Definition of Disease* (Baltimore, MD: The Johns Hopkins University Press, 2007).

19. C. Gradmann, 'Locating Therapeutic Vaccines in Nineteenth-Century History', *Science in Context*, 21 (2008), pp. 145–60.

INDEX

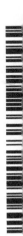